Y0-CCN-563

COLOR ATLAS AND SYNOPSIS OF WOMEN'S CARDIOVASCULAR HEALTH

NOTICE

COLOR ATLAS AND SYNOPSIS OF WOMEN'S CARDIOVASCULAR HEALTH

EDITOR

Martha Gulati, MD, MS, FACC, FAHA

Associate Professor of Medicine, Division of Cardiology

Associate Professor of Clinical Public Health, Division of Epidemiology

Sarah Ross Soter Chair in Women's Cardiovascular Health

Section Director for Preventive Cardiology and Women's Cardiovascular Health

The Ohio State University

Columbus, Ohio

SERIES EDITOR

William T. Abraham, MD, FACP, FACC, FAHA, FESC

Professor of Medicine, Physiology, and Cell Biology

Chair of Excellence in Cardiovascular Medicine

Director, Division of Cardiovascular Medicine

Deputy Director, Davis Heart and Lung Research Institute

The Ohio State University

Columbus, Ohio

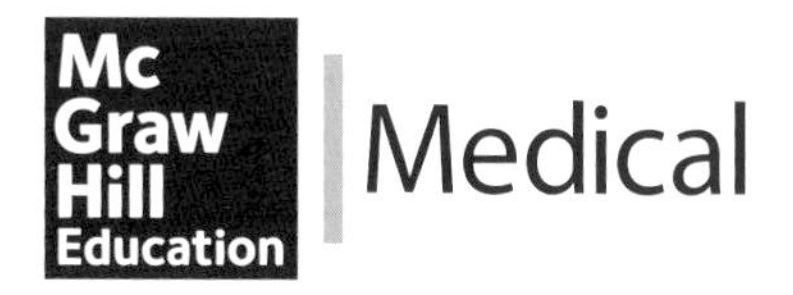

New York Chicago San Francisco Athens London Madrid Mexico City
Milan New Delhi Singapore Sydney Toronto

Color Atlas and Synopsis of Women's Cardiovascular Health

1 2 3 4 5 6 7 8 9 0 CTP/CTP 18 17 16 15 14

ISBN 978-0-07-178620-1
MHID 0-07-178620-1

This book was set in Perpetua by Cenveo® Publisher Services.
The editors were Christine Diedrich and Robert Pancotti.
The production supervisor was Richard Ruzycka.
Project management was provided by Harry Popli, Cenveo Publisher Services.
The cover designer was Thomas De Pierro.
China Translation & Printing Services Ltd. was the printer and binder.

Library of Congress Cataloging-in-Publication Data

Color atlas and synopsis of women's cardiovascular health/[edited by] Martha Gulati.—First edition.
p. ; cm.
Includes bibliographical references and index.
ISBN-13: 978-0-07-178620-1 (hardcover)
ISBN-10: 0-07-178620-1 (hardcover)
I. Gulati, Martha, 1969- editor of compilation.
[DNLM: 1. Cardiovascular Diseases—Atlases. 2. Women's Health—Atlases. WG 17]
RC669.9
616.10022'3—dc23

2014000499

DEDICATION

I dedicate this book to the men who have always supported my every step: my dad (Deep Gulati), my brother (Justin Gulati), and my love and my best friend Gareth Gwyn.

I also dedicate this book to all the women whom my coauthors and I have had the honor of taking care of as patients. It is all of you who inspire us to understand your hearts.

CONTENTS

Lana Alghothani, MD
Resident in Internal Medicine
The Ohio State University
Columbus, Ohio

Grace Ayafor, MD
Department of Medicine (Cardiology)
The Ohio State University
Columbus, Ohio

Khadijah Breathett, MD
Department of Medicine (Cardiology)
The Ohio State University
Columbus, Ohio

Juan Crestanello, MD
Assistant Professor of Surgery
Division of Cardiothoracic Surgery
The Ohio State University
Columbus, Ohio

Jennifer Dickerson, MD
Assistant Professor of Internal Medicine
Department of Cardiovascular Disease
The Ohio State University
Columbus, Ohio

JoAnne Foody, MD, FACC, FAHA
Cardiovascular Division
Brigham and Women's Hospital
Boston, Massachusetts

Veronica Franco, MD, MSPH
Assistant Professor of Clinical Cardiology
Section of Pulmonary Hypertension
Section Head, Pulmonary Hypertension Research Studies
Davis Heart and Lung Research Institute
The Ohio State University
Columbus, Ohio

Martha Gulati, MD, MS, FACC, FAHA
Associate Professor of Medicine, Division of Cardiology
Associate Professor of Clinical Public Health, Division of Epidemiology
Sarah Ross Soter Chair in Women's Cardiovascular Health
Section Director for Preventive Cardiology and Women's Cardiovascular Health
The Ohio State University
Columbus, Ohio

Ayesha Hasan, MD, FACC
Associate Professor of Clinical Internal Medicine
Medical Director, Cardiac Transplant Program
Director, Heart Failure Fellowship Program
The Ohio State University
Columbus, Ohio

Nkechinyere Ijioma, MBBS
Department of Medicine (Cardiology)
The Ohio State University
Columbus, Ohio

Priya Kohli, MD, MPH
Brigham and Women's Cardiovascular Associates
Memorial Hospital of Rhode Island
Pawtucket, Rhode Island

Kameswari Maganti, MD
Associate Professor of Medicine
Director of Cardiac Rehabilitation
Northwestern University Feinberg School of Medicine
Chicago, Illinois

Gina G. Mentzer, MD
Medical Director of Heart Failure Program
Attending Cardiologist
Heart Failure, Transplant, and Mechanical Circulatory Support Specialist
Nebraska Heart Institute
Lincoln, Nebraska

Adam Pleister, MD
Department of Medicine (Cardiology)
The Ohio State University
Columbus, Ohio

Sharon L. Roble, MD
Assistant Professor of Internal Medicine
Division of Cardiovascular Medicine
The Ohio State University
Columbus, Ohio

Molly Sachdev, MD, MPH
Division of Cardiovascular Medicine
The Ohio State University
Columbus, Ohio

Christina Salazar, MD
Attending Cardiologist
Lawrence Memorial Hospital
Lawrence, Kansas

Kavita Sharma, MD
Assistant Professor of Clinical Cardiology
Department of Medicine (Cardiology)
The Ohio State University
Columbus, Ohio

Jean Starr, MD, FACS, RPVI
Division of Vascular Diseases and Surgery
The Ohio State University
Columbus, Ohio

Rita Szymanski, RN, BSN
Division of Cardiology
Northwestern University Feinberg School of Medicine
Chicago, Illinois

Jennifer M. Worth, MD
Lancaster General Health
Lancaster, Pennsylvania

PREFACE

Cardiovascular disease remains the number one killer of women in the United States, but great strides have been made in terms of our knowledge and treatment of cardiovascular disease in women. In just the past two decades, there has been a heightened awareness of cardiovascular disease in women, in what previously had been thought of as a man's disease. As a result, in the past decade we have seen a continuous decline in mortality from cardiovascular disease in women, and most recently, it has demonstrated a more prominent decline in cardiovascular mortality for women than men. Nonetheless, more women than men die from cardiovascular disease in the United States and there are more deaths from cardiovascular causes in women than from all cancers combined. We are just at the earliest stages of understanding the cardiovascular disease process in women. Nonetheless, recent research has demonstrated important sex differences in the pathophysiology and clinical presentation of cardiovascular disease in women.

Many risk factors for cardiovascular disease are similar for men and women, but for many risk factors their impact on cardiovascular disease differs by sex. This is discussed in Chapter 2. There are risk assessment tools that do exist and should be incorporated routinely into clinical practice, assessing both short-term and lifetime risk on a regular basis (Chapter 3).

There remains a difference in how we treat women, even once we have recognized that a woman has cardiovascular disease. This difference ultimately impacts outcome differences between sexes. In addition, the pathophysiology of ischemic heart disease may differ for women, with women often having nonobstructive coronary artery disease even in the setting of a myocardial infarction. In the past, such a pattern of disease was not thought to be clinically significant. However, more recent research has shown that symptomatic women with symptoms and signs of ischemia are at an increased risk of future cardiovascular events, despite this nonobstructive coronary disease pattern. Further work needs to be done to determine optimal treatment for such women, but the definition of patterns of ischemic heart disease is already possible (Chapter 4).

Noninvasive imaging is a useful tool for an accurate diagnosis of cardiovascular disease in women, allowing earlier and more precise disease detection in women. Consideration of the choice of test in women depends on many variables, including consideration regarding the impact of radiation. Gender-related aspects are covered in Chapter 6.

Cardiac surgery also has many sex-specific issues, which are visually demonstrated in Chapter 5. Heart failure, cardiac arrhythmias, and arterial vascular disease are common in women, with some highly sex-specific issues in terms of their diagnosis, prognosis, and treatment (Chapters 8, 9, and 11). Pulmonary hypertension is far more common in women than in men, and in light of this finding, this book includes an entire chapter that addresses the unique cardiac issues concerning women with this disease (Chapter 12). An issue that is obviously unique for women is pregnancy. During pregnancy, cardiac issues can arise in women, even in those without congenital heart disease. The clinical issues that can arise in pregnancy, in women with and without congenital heart disease, are discussed using a case-based manner in Chapter 10.

I would like to thank the authors of each chapter in this book for their excellent work in describing the unique risk factors and cardiovascular issues that are specific to women. In addition, I am grateful to the assistance that I have received from Ms Janice Whitmire, as this project unfolded, and her assistance in the preparation of this book. I would like to thank Sarah Ross Soter and Bill Soter and their family for their unrelenting support and for helping us to make the Ross Heart Hospital and The Ohio State University Wexner Medical Center a leader in women's cardiovascular health. I am very grateful for the opportunity provided by Dr William Abraham for making this series possible and for deciding that no atlas series on cardiovascular disease would be complete without addressing the issues of cardiovascular disease in women. My hope is that this book helps us to better understand the issues relating to women and their ever-precious hearts.

Martha Gulati, MD, MS, FACC, FAHA

INTRODUCTION

Nkechinyere Ijioma, MBBS
Martha Gulati, MD, MS, FACC, FAHA

INTRODUCTION

Cardiovascular disease (CVD) is the leading cause of death in women. For more than 2 decades, more women have died from CVD compared to men.[1] However, for several decades, CVD was regarded as a male disease. Women were underrepresented in cardiovascular clinical trials and comprised <27% of trial participants.[2] Only 33% of clinical trials reported sex-specific outcomes.[2] These low enrolment numbers resulted in most clinical trials being underpowered to evaluate for gender-specific outcomes. This has had significant implications because for carrying out clinical translation of research in a specific population group, that population group should adequately represented in research study. This has not been the case for women in most major cardiovascular trials. Moreover, a growing body of evidence has suggested that there may be differences in the clinical presentation of CVDs in men and women, in addition to sex differences in terms of impact of cardiovascular risk factors, CVD prevention, and even the pathophysiology of CVD.

The first milestone toward reducing the cardiovascular disparities in women, was the 1985 Report of the Public Health Service Task Force on Women's Health Issues.[3] This report highlighted concerns that there was a scarcity of health information available to women, and that women were underrepresented in clinical research. In 1991 the National Institute of Health (NIH), under the direction of Dr Bernadine Healy, established a policy that all NIH-funded trials must include both women and men in studies of conditions that affect both genders. As a result, the majority of studies on women and CVD commenced following this mandate. In 1992, the National Heart, Lung and Blood Institute (NHLBI) conducted a conference on Cardiovascular Health and Disease in Women.[4] This conference identified several knowledge gaps affecting ideal cardiovascular health-care delivery in women. The Heart and Estrogen/Progestin Replacement Study (HERS)[5] and the Women's Health Initiative (WHI)[6] were the next 2 important landmarks in women's health. The WHI was initiated in 1992 and was designed to evaluate the efficacy of hormone replacement therapy for the primary prevention of coronary heart disease (CHD) in postmenopausal women.[7] In 1993, the HERS study began enrolment of postmenopausal women with a uterus and with CHD to study the efficacy and safety of estrogen plus progestin therapy for secondary prevention of CHD in women.[8] Both studies showed that menopausal hormonal therapy did not reduce the risk of CVD in menopausal women. Rather the risk of myocardial infarction and stroke increased in the healthy women in the WHI study who were on hormone replacement therapy compared with placebo. These 2 studies redirected the clinical focus on implementing standard cardiovascular management strategies in women, rather than focusing on hormonal replacement therapy as the solution for CVD in women. The 2001 Institute of Medicine (IOM) report took sex disparity in CVD to the next level by stating that sex differences in disease and medical research should be explored and implemented in the translation of research into clinical practice.[9] The results from the HERS and the WHI studies provided the stimuli for the initiation of the 2004 evidence-based guidelines for CHD prevention in women.[10] In the past decade, more studies have examined the effect of preventive measure in women. The Women's Health Study showed that the use of aspirin in women did not prevent coronary artery disease (CAD),[11] in contrast to what was well established in men.[12] Aspirin appeared to reduce the risk of stroke in women, with more benefit than risks (bleeding) seen in women over the age of 65 years.

The Can Rapid Risk Stratification of Unstable Angina Patients Suppress Adverse Outcomes with Early Implementation of the American College of Cardiology/American Heart Association Guidelines (CRUSADE) study demonstrated that women with non-ST elevation myocardial infarction had worse outcomes compared to male counterparts.[13] Women were less likely to receive guideline-recommended therapies when compared with men, resulting in worse outcomes. The NHLBI Women's Ischemia Syndrome Evaluation (WISE) study was the first study to show the high prevalence of non-obstructive CAD in the setting of cardiac symptoms of ischemia and evidence of myocardial ischemia.[14] The American Heart Association (AHA) released a consensus statement (2005) regarding the criteria for appropriate choice of noninvasive cardiac test for CVD evaluation in women.[15] The AHA also released guidelines for prevention of CVD in women.[16] In 2008, the Get with the Guidelines CAD data showed sex disparities in the treatment of acute myocardial infarction in women.[17] In 2011, The AHA released an updated guideline for CVD in women, in which an effectiveness model for CVD prevention in women was emphasized. History of pregnancy complications (gestational diabetes, preeclampsia, pregnancy-induced hypertension) were also highlighted as important facets of history taking in women, as these may be early indicators of increased cardiovascular risk.[18]

Women are different from men. Acute myocardial infarction or sudden cardiac death is the most common initial presentation of ischemic heart disease (IHD) in women.[19] Women more commonly present with atypical symptoms of IHD such as dyspnea, jaw pain, nausea, and back pain compared to men.[14,20] Atrioventricular nodal reentrant tachycardia is more common in women than men.[21] Women have longer rate-corrected QT intervals (QTc), higher baseline (resting) heart rates,[22] and are more likely to sustain torsades de pointes with long QT syndromes compared to men.[23,24]

Traditional risk factors for CVD remain the same regardless of sex, but the impact of these risk factors do differ by sex. Psychosocial stressors (work, marital stress) have been associated with an increase in CVD in women[25] and stress-induced cardiomyopathy occurs more often in older women compared to men.[26] Female-specific risk factors have also been identified. Preeclampsia and pregnancy-associated hypertension are both associated with a greater risk for the onset of hypertension, diabetes, and ischemic stroke.[27-29] A recent cohort analysis has shown that any form of gestational hypertension is associated with an increased risk for CVD, chronic kidney disease, and hypertension.[30] Also unique to women is the risk factor of gestational diabetes. Gestational diabetes doubles the risk of diabetes 4 months postpartum and remains a lifelong risk factor for diabetes.[31,32] A recent study involving 3416 women showed that preeclampsia and gestational diabetes are associated with an increased risk for future CVD (odds ratio 1.31, 95% confidence interval 1.11-1.53 and odds ratio 1.26, 95% confidence interval 0.95-1.68, respectively).[33] Besides, androgen excess in polycystic ovarian syndrome (PCOS) has been associated with increased atherosclerosis and IHD[34,35] and aging and menopause lead to unfavorable lipid profiles.[36] Premenopausal estrogen deficiency may increase the risk for IHD in young women,[34] and menstrual irregularity is associated with increased adverse cardiovascular events.[37] It is hypothesized that estrogen levels in premenopausal women may explain the reduced incidence of CVD in younger women compared to men of similar age.[38] Despite these potential sex-related CVD risk factors, the guidelines for CVD prevention in women do not include these risk factors, as their impact and predictive value are not well established. Valvular heart disease and congestive heart failure play a greater role as risk factors for atrial fibrillation in women compared to IHD as a risk factor for atrial fibrillation in men.[39-41] In addition, embolic stroke is more often a complication of atrial fibrillation in women compared to men.[42] The lifetime risk for a 40-year-old to develop heart failure without a preceding myocardial infarction is 1 in 6 for women, compared with 1 in 9 in men.[43] Unique risk factors for the development of heart failure in women include cardiac toxicity from chemotherapeutic drugs used for treatment of breast cancer and peripartum cardiomyopathy.

In the pathophysiology of CAD, women have been shown to have less coronary plaque disease compared to men.[44,45] About 10% to 30% of women with chest pain do not have obstructive CAD on coronary angiogram.[46,47] Unlike men and older women who develop the classical plaque rupture with subsequent thrombus formation, young women usually have plaque erosion with subsequent distal embolization of microemboli.[48-50] The term *microvascular angina* describes the occurrence of chest pain suggestive of myocardial ischemia in the setting of nonobstructive CAD.[51,52]

The sex paradox has been used to describe the phenomenon that although women with acute coronary syndrome have less extensive obstructive coronary artery disease compared to their male counterparts; women still have a much higher mortality rate when compared with men.[53,54] Sex difference in mortality after acute coronary syndrome (ACS) occurs specifically in the ST-elevation myocardial infarction female population[17,55,56] and in younger female patients (age <50) with myocardial infarction.[56-61] These subgroups of women have higher mortality post ACS compared to their male counterparts.

An additional growing concern is the fact that women are undertreated once a diagnosis of heart disease is established. Women with stable angina are less likely to be referred for coronary angiography,[62] and women with CVD and/or ACS with non-ST elevation are less likely to receive percutaneous coronary intervention compared to male counterparts.[63-66] In addition, women are less likely to be referred for cardiac rehabilitation or attend or complete a cardiac rehabilitation program.[67] Sex disparities have been demonstrated in the utilization of device therapy (pacemakers and implantable cardioverter defibrillator) in systolic dysfunction heart failure, with fewer women receiving devices compared to their male counterparts.[68-70] Women are less likely to be referred for atrial fibrillation ablation, when compared with men.[71,72]

Developing an optimal treatment or preventive management strategy begins with making the right diagnosis or proper risk stratification. However, studies have shown that the traditional Framingham risk score underestimates the risk of CVD in women. Recently, attempts have been made to identify risk markers and develop alternative risk-scoring models to predict CAD risk in women. High-sensitivity C-reactive protein (hs-CRP) has been noted to add prognostic value to traditional risk factors for detecting cardiovascular events in women.[73,74] The Reynolds risk score, which includes hs-CRP and family history of CAD in the scoring model, may be a better risk predictor of CVD in women compared to the Framingham scoring system.[75]

A barrier to achieving optimum cardiovascular health in women is the underestimation of CVD burden in women and health-care providers.[76] Recent surveys showed that <60% of women knew they had to call 911 for symptoms of a heart attack[77,78] and only 41% knew both the clinical features of a heart attack and need to call 911.[77] More women need to be represented in CVD prevention trials to provide answers to the questions regarding the sex differences in therapy benefit.[79] The first step in addressing the disparity in women outcomes is to eliminate the knowledge gap both among health-care providers and the general public. This has been the thrust of several awareness campaign groups, including the Red Dress Campaign, The Go Red Campaign, Women Heart and the National Coalition for Women With Heart Disease. The goal of this book is to address this knowledge gap and provide to the reader, evidence-based data highlighting the sex-related differences in the pathophysiology, the clinical presentation, and treatment of heart disease in women. In the following chapters, the reader will learn the unique characteristics of heart disease in women, the studies that have been done in women in terms of diagnosing and treating heart disease, and the current treatment and management guidelines. We hope that in the next decade the disparities in cardiovascular care for women will be eliminated.

REFERENCES

1. Roger VL, Go AS, Lloyd-Jones DM, et al. Executive summary: heart disease and stroke statistics—2012 update: a report from the American Heart Association. *Circulation.* Janury 3 2012;125(1):188-197.

2. Johnson SM, Karvonen CA, Phelps CL, et al. Assessment of analysis by gender in the Cochrane reviews as related to treatment of cardiovascular disease. *J Womens Health (Larchmt).* June 2003;12(5):449-457.

3. Women's health: report of the Public Health Service Task Force on Women's Health Issues. *Public Health Rep.* January-February 1985;100(1):73-106.

4. Wenger NK, Speroff L, Packard B. Cardiovascular health and disease in women. *N Engl J Med.* 1993;329(4):247-256.

5. Hulley S, Grady D, Bush T, et al. Randomized trial of estrogen plus progestin for secondary prevention of coronary heart

disease in postmenopausal women. Heart and Estrogen/progestin Replacement Study (HERS) Research Group. *JAMA.* August 19 1998;280(7):605-613.

6. Rossouw JE, Anderson GL, Prentice RL, et al. Risks and benefits of estrogen plus progestin in healthy postmenopausal women: principal results from the Women's Health Initiative randomized controlled trial. *JAMA.* July 17 2002;288(3):321-333.
7. The Women's Health Initiative Study Group. Design of the Women' s Health Initiative clinical trial and observational study. *Control Clin Trials.* February 1998;19(1):61-109.
8. Grady D, Applegate W, Bush T, et al. Heart and Estrogen/progestin Replacement Study (HERS): design, methods, and baseline characteristics. *Control Clin Trials.* August 1998;19(4):314-335.
9. Exploring the biological contributions to human health: does sex matter? *J Womens Health Gend Based Med.* June 2001;10(5):433-439.
10. Mosca L, Appel LJ, Benjamin EJ, et al. Evidence-based guidelines for cardiovascular disease prevention in women. *Circulation.* February 10 2004;109(5):672-693.
11. Ridker PM, Cook NR, Lee IM, et al. A randomized trial of low-dose aspirin in the primary prevention of cardiovascular disease in women. *N Engl J Med.* March 31 2005;352(13):1293-1304.
12. Steering Committee of the Physicians' Health Study Research Group. Final report on the aspirin component of the ongoing Physicians' Health Study. *N Engl J Med.* July 20 1989;321(3):129-135.
13. Blomkalns AL, Chen AY, Hochman JS, et al. Gender disparities in the diagnosis and treatment of non-ST-segment elevation acute coronary syndromes: large-scale observations from the CRUSADE (Can Rapid Risk Stratification of Unstable Angina Patients Suppress Adverse Outcomes With Early Implementation of the American College of Cardiology/American Heart Association Guidelines) National Quality Improvement Initiative. *J Am Coll Cardiol.* March 15 2005;45(6):832-837.
14. Bairey Merz CN, Shaw LJ, Reis SE, et al. Insights from the NHLBI-Sponsored Women's Ischemia Syndrome Evaluation (WISE) Study: Part II: gender differences in presentation, diagnosis, and outcome with regard to gender-based pathophysiology of atherosclerosis and macrovascular and microvascular coronary disease. *J Am Coll Cardiol.* February 7 2006;47(3 suppl):S21-S29.
15. Mieres JH, Shaw LJ, Arai A, et al. Role of noninvasive testing in the clinical evaluation of women with suspected coronary artery disease: consensus statement from the Cardiac Imaging Committee, Council on Clinical Cardiology, and the Cardiovascular Imaging and Intervention Committee, Council on Cardiovascular Radiology and Intervention, American Heart Association. *Circulation.* February 8 2005;111(5):682-696.
16. Mosca L, Banka CL, Benjamin EJ, et al. Evidence-based guidelines for cardiovascular disease prevention in women: 2007 update. *Circulation.* March 20 2007;115(11):1481-1501.
17. Jneid H, Fonarow GC, Cannon CP, et al. Sex differences in medical care and early death after acute myocardial infarction. *Circulation.* December 16 2008;118(25):2803-2810.
18. Mosca L, Benjamin EJ, Berra K, et al. Effectiveness-based guidelines for the prevention of cardiovascular disease in women—2011 update: a guideline from the American Heart Association. *J Am Coll Cardiol.* March 22 2011;57(12):1404-1423.
19. Lerner DJ, Kannel WB. Patterns of coronary heart disease morbidity and mortality in the sexes: a 26-year follow-up of the Framingham population. *Am Heart J.* February 1986;111(2):383-390.
20. DeVon HA, Ryan CJ, Ochs AL, et al. Symptoms across the continuum of acute coronary syndromes: differences between women and men. *Am J Crit Care.* January 2008;17(1):14-24; quiz 25.
21. Rodriguez LM, de Chillou C, Schlapfer J, et al. Age at onset and gender of patients with different types of supraventricular tachycardias. *Am J Cardiol.* November 1 1992;70(13):1213-1215.
22. Rautaharju PM, Zhou SH, Wong S, et al. Sex differences in the evolution of the electrocardiographic QT interval with age. *Can J Cardiol.* September 1992;8(7):690-695.
23. Zareba W, Moss AJ, Locati EH, et al. Modulating effects of age and gender on the clinical course of long QT syndrome by genotype. *J Am Coll Cardiol.* July 2 2003;42(1):103-109.
24. Lehmann MH, Hardy S, Archibald D, et al. Sex difference in risk of torsade de pointes with D,L-sotalol. *Circulation.* November 15 1996;94(10):2535-2541.
25. Orth-Gomer K, Leineweber C. Multiple stressors and coronary disease in women. The Stockholm Female Coronary Risk Study. *Biol Psychol.* April 2005;69(1):57-66.
26. Prasad A, Lerman A, Rihal CS. Apical ballooning syndrome (Tako-Tsubo or stress cardiomyopathy): a mimic of acute myocardial infarction. *Am Heart J.* March 2008;155(3):408-417.
27. Lykke JA, Langhoff-Roos J, Sibai BM, et al. Hypertensive pregnancy disorders and subsequent cardiovascular morbidity and type 2 diabetes mellitus in the mother. *Hypertension.* 2009 June;53(6):944-951.
28. Brown DW, Dueker N, Jamieson DJ, et al. Preeclampsia and the risk of ischemic stroke among young women: results from the Stroke Prevention in Young Women Study. *Stroke.* April 2006;37(4):1055-1059.
29. Bellamy L, Casas JP, Hingorani AD, et al. Pre-eclampsia and risk of cardiovascular disease and cancer in later life: systematic review and meta-analysis. *BMJ.* November 10 2007;335(7627):974.
30. Mannisto T, Mendola P, Vaarasmaki M, et al. Elevated blood pressure in pregnancy and subsequent chronic disease risk. *Circulation.* February 12 2013;127(6):681-690.
31. Ratner RE. Prevention of type 2 diabetes in women with previous gestational diabetes. *Diabetes Care.* July 2007;30(suppl 2):S242-S245.
32. Schaefer-Graf UM, Buchanan TA, Xiang AH, et al. Clinical predictors for a high risk for the development of diabetes mellitus in the early puerperium in women with recent gestational diabetes mellitus. *Am J Obstet Gynecol.* April 2002;186(4):751-756.
33. Fraser A, Nelson SM, Macdonald-Wallis C, et al. Associations of pregnancy complications with calculated cardiovascular disease

risk and cardiovascular risk factors in middle age: the Avon Longitudinal Study of Parents and Children. *Circulation.* March 20 2012;125(11):1367-1380.

34. Bairey Merz CN, Johnson BD, Sharaf BL, et al. Hypoestrogenemia of hypothalamic origin and coronary artery disease in premenopausal women: a report from the NHLBI-sponsored WISE study. *J Am Coll Cardiol.* February 5 2003;41(3):413-419.
35. Shaw LJ, Bairey Merz CN, Azziz R, et al. Postmenopausal women with a history of irregular menses and elevated androgen measurements at high risk for worsening cardiovascular event-free survival: results from the National Institutes of Health—National Heart, Lung, and Blood Institute sponsored Women's Ischemia Syndrome Evaluation. *J Clin Endocrinol Metab.* April 2008;93(4):1276-1284.
36. Knopp RH. Risk factors for coronary artery disease in women. *Am J Cardiol.* June 20 2002;89(12A):28E-34E; discussion 34E-35E.
37. Solomon CG, Hu FB, Dunaif A, et al. Menstrual cycle irregularity and risk for future cardiovascular disease. *J Clin Endocrinol Metab.* May 2002;87(5):2013-2017.
38. Kannel WB, Hjortland MC, McNamara PM, et al. Menopause and risk of cardiovascular disease: the Framingham study. *Ann Intern Med.* October 1976;85(4):447-452.
39. Benjamin EJ, Wolf PA, D'Agostino RB, et al. Impact of atrial fibrillation on the risk of death: the Framingham Heart Study. *Circulation.* Sep 8 1998;98(10):946-952.
40. Kaufman ES, Zimmermann PA, Wang T, et al. Risk of proarrhythmic events in the Atrial Fibrillation Follow-up Investigation of Rhythm Management (AFFIRM) study: a multivariate analysis. *J Am Coll Cardiol.* September 15 2004;44(6):1276-1282.
41. Rienstra M, Van Veldhuisen DJ, Hagens VE, et al. Gender-related differences in rhythm control treatment in persistent atrial fibrillation: data of the Rate Control Versus Electrical Cardioversion (RACE) study. *J Am Coll Cardiol.* October 4 2005;46(7):1298-1306.
42. Dagres N, Nieuwlaat R, Vardas PE, et al. Gender-related differences in presentation, treatment, and outcome of patients with atrial fibrillation in Europe: a report from the Euro Heart Survey on Atrial Fibrillation. *J Am Coll Cardiol.* February 6 2007;49(5):572-577.
43. Hsich EM, Pina IL. Heart failure in women: a need for prospective data. *J Am Coll Cardiol.* August 4 2009;54(6):491-498.
44. Nicholls SJ, Wolski K, Sipahi I, et al. Rate of progression of coronary atherosclerotic plaque in women. *J Am Coll Cardiol.* April 10 2007;49(14):1546-1551.
45. Han SH, Bae JH, Holmes DR, Jr., et al. Sex differences in atheroma burden and endothelial function in patients with early coronary atherosclerosis. *Eur Heart J.* June 2008;29(11):1359-1369.
46. Johnson BD, Shaw LJ, Pepine CJ, et al. Persistent chest pain predicts cardiovascular events in women without obstructive coronary artery disease: results from the NIH-NHLBI-sponsored Women's Ischaemia Syndrome Evaluation (WISE) study. *Eur Heart J.* June 2006;27(12):1408-1415.
47. Bugiardini R, Bairey Merz CN. Angina with "normal" coronary arteries: a changing philosophy. *JAMA.* January 26 2005;293(4):477-484.
48. Kramer MC, Rittersma SZ, de Winter RJ, et al. Relationship of thrombus healing to underlying plaque morphology in sudden coronary death. *J Am Coll Cardiol.* January 12 2010;55(2):122-132.
49. Pepine CJ, Anderson RD, Sharaf BL, et al. Coronary microvascular reactivity to adenosine predicts adverse outcome in women evaluated for suspected ischemia results from the National Heart, Lung and Blood Institute WISE (Women's Ischemia Syndrome Evaluation) study. *J Am Coll Cardiol.* June 22 2010;55(25):2825-2832.
50. Burke AP, Farb A, Malcom GT, et al. Effect of risk factors on the mechanism of acute thrombosis and sudden coronary death in women. *Circulation.* June 2 1998;97(21):2110-2116.
51. Shaw LJ, Bugiardini R, Merz CN. Women and ischemic heart disease: evolving knowledge. *J Am Coll Cardiol.* October 20 2009;54(17):1561-1575.
52. Cannon RO, 3rd. Microvascular angina and the continuing dilemma of chest pain with normal coronary angiograms. *J Am Coll Cardiol.* September 1 2009;54(10):877-885.
53. Gulati M, Cooper-DeHoff RM, McClure C, et al. Adverse cardiovascular outcomes in women with nonobstructive coronary artery disease: a report from the Women's Ischemia Syndrome Evaluation Study and the St James Women Take Heart Project. *Arch Intern Med.* May 11 2009;169(9):843-850.
54. Arant CB, Wessel TR, Ridker PM, et al. Multimarker approach predicts adverse cardiovascular events in women evaluated for suspected ischemia: results from the National Heart, Lung, and Blood Institute-sponsored Women's Ischemia Syndrome Evaluation. *Clin Cardiol.* May 2009;32(5):244-250.
55. Berger JS, Elliott L, Gallup D, et al. Sex differences in mortality following acute coronary syndromes. *JAMA.* August 26 2009;302(8):874-882.
56. Champney KP, Frederick PD, Bueno H, et al. The joint contribution of sex, age and type of myocardial infarction on hospital mortality following acute myocardial infarction. *Heart.* June 2009;95(11):895-899.
57. Vaccarino V, Parsons L, Every NR, et al. Sex-based differences in early mortality after myocardial infarction. National Registry of Myocardial Infarction 2 Participants. *N Engl J Med.* July 22 1999;341(4):217-225.
58. Koek HL, de Bruin A, Gast F, et al. Short- and long-term prognosis after acute myocardial infarction in men versus women. *Am J Cardiol.* October 15 2006;98(8):993-999.
59. Rosengren A, Spetz CL, Koster M, et al. Sex differences in survival after myocardial infarction in Sweden; data from the Swedish National Acute Myocardial Infarction Register. *Eur Heart J.* February 2001;22(4):314-322.
60. Mahon NG, McKenna CJ, Codd MB, et al. Gender differences in the management and outcome of acute myocardial infarction in unselected patients in the thrombolytic era. *Am J Cardiol.* April 15 2000;85(8):921-926.

61. Andrikopoulos GK, Tzeis SE, Pipilis AG, et al. Younger age potentiates post myocardial infarction survival disadvantage of women. *Int J Cardiol.* April 14 2006;108(3):320-325.

62. Daly C, Clemens F, Lopez Sendon JL, et al. Gender differences in the management and clinical outcome of stable angina. *Circulation.* January 31 2006;113(4):490-498.

63. Akhter N, Milford-Beland S, Roe MT, et al. Gender differences among patients with acute coronary syndromes undergoing percutaneous coronary intervention in the American College of Cardiology-National Cardiovascular Data Registry (ACC-NCDR). *Am Heart J.* January 2009;157(1):141-148.

64. Singh M, Rihal CS, Gersh BJ, et al. Mortality differences between men and women after percutaneous coronary interventions. A 25-year, single-center experience. *J Am Coll Cardiol.* June 17 2008;51(24):2313-2320.

65. Peterson ED, Shah BR, Parsons L, et al. Trends in quality of care for patients with acute myocardial infarction in the National Registry of Myocardial Infarction from 1990 to 2006. *Am Heart J.* December 2008;156(6):1045-1055.

66. Poon S, Goodman SG, Yan RT, et al. Bridging the gender gap: insights from a contemporary analysis of sex-related differences in the treatment and outcomes of patients with acute coronary syndromes. *Am Heart J.* January 2012;163(1):66-73.

67. Caulin-Glaser T, Blum M, Schmeizl R, et al. Gender differences in referral to cardiac rehabilitation programs after revascularization. *J Cardiopulm Rehabil.* January-February 2001;21(1):24-30.

68. El-Chami MF, Hanna IR, Bush H, et al. Impact of race and gender on cardiac device implantations. *Heart Rhythm.* November 2007;4(11):1420-1426.

69. Gauri AJ, Davis A, Hong T, Burke MC, Knight BP. Disparities in the use of primary prevention and defibrillator therapy among blacks and women. *Am J Med.* February 2006;119(2): 167.e117-167.e121.

70. Santangeli P, Pelargonio G, Dello Russo A, et al. Gender differences in clinical outcome and primary prevention defibrillator benefit in patients with severe left ventricular dysfunction: a systematic review and meta-analysis. *Heart Rhythm.* July 2010;7(7):876-882.

71. Forleo GB, Tondo C, De Luca L, et al. Gender-related differences in catheter ablation of atrial fibrillation. *Europace.* August 2007;9(8):613-620.

72. Patel D, Mohanty P, Di Biase L, et al. Outcomes and complications of catheter ablation for atrial fibrillation in females. *Heart Rhythm.* 2010;7(2):167-172.

73. Ridker PM, Buring JE, Shih J, et al. Prospective study of C-reactive protein and the risk of future cardiovascular events among apparently healthy women. *Circulation.* August 25 1998;98(8):731-733.

74. Ridker PM, Rifai N, Rose L, et al. Comparison of C-reactive protein and low-density lipoprotein cholesterol levels in the prediction of first cardiovascular events. *N Engl J Med.* November 14 2002;347(20):1557-1565.

75. Ridker PM, Buring JE, Rifai N, et al. Development and validation of improved algorithms for the assessment of global cardiovascular risk in women: the Reynolds Risk Score. *JAMA.* February 14 2007;297(6):611-619.

76. Lindquist R, Boucher JL, Grey EZ, et al. Eliminating untimely deaths of women from heart disease: highlights from the Minnesota Women's Heart Summit. *Am Heart J.* January 2012;163(1):39-48.e31.

77. Giardina EG, Sciacca RR, Foody JM, et al. The DHHS Office on Women's Health Initiative to Improve Women's Heart Health: focus on knowledge and awareness among women with cardiometabolic risk factors. *J Womens Health (Larchmt).* June 2011;20(6):893-900.

78. Mosca L, Mochari-Greenberger H, Dolor RJ, et al. Twelve-year follow-up of American women's awareness of cardiovascular disease risk and barriers to heart health. *Circ Cardiovasc Qual Outcomes.* March 2010;3(2):120-127.

79. Melloni C, Berger JS, Wang TY, et al. Representation of women in randomized clinical trials of cardiovascular disease prevention. *Circ Cardiovasc Qual Outcomes.* March 2010;3(2):135-142.

1 HEART DISEASE IN WOMEN

Kavita Sharma, MD
Martha Gulati, MD, MS, FACC, FAHA

INTRODUCTION

Cardiovascular disease (CVD) is the leading cause of death in the United States (Figure 1-1).[1] The burden of CVD is shared by men and women alike (Figures 1-2 and 1-3), although CVD's impact on women has been traditionally underappreciated. For far too long, women were not represented in major cardiovascular trials (Figure 1-4 and Table 1-1).[2] In addition, both patients and physicians have displayed a lack of awareness regarding CVD's prevalence in women, although this scenario is changing now (Figure 1-5).[3,4] The pathophysiology of CVD has unique characteristics in women. Furthermore, as women are increasingly being included in cardiovascular trials, management strategies specific to women are being defined.[5-9] In this *Atlas and Synopsis of Women's Cardiovascular Health*, we hope to highlight the impact of CVD on women, its unique characteristics in women, and important topics in CVD that have female-specific management strategies.

PREVALENCE OF CARDIOVASCULAR DISEASE

In the United States more women than men die of CVD (Figure 1-6).[1] Moreover, more women have died of CVD than cancer (including breast cancer), chronic lower respiratory disease, Alzheimer disease, and accidents combined (Figure 1-7).[1] From 1998 to 2008, though the overall death rates attributable to CVD declined to 30.6%, these have shown an increasing trend among young women (<55 years).[1,10] Of particular concern is the rise in obese American population, with its subsequent impact on diabetes and development of CVD in future. According to NHANES 2007-2008, 34% of men and women in the United States are obese.[11] However, the impact of obesity on the development of CVD appears to be greater on women than men. Among individuals in the Framingham Heart Study, obesity increased the relative risk of CVD by 64% in women, as opposed to 46% in men.[12]

The average age of first myocardial infarction (MI) is 64.5 years for men and 70.3 years for women.[1] The onset of CVD in women is on average 10 years later than men and incidence serious clinical events such as MI and sudden death usually lag behind by 20 years.[13] The consequences of CVD are worse in women than in men. Women with premature MI (<50), experience a 2-fold increase in mortality after acute MI (Figure 1-8);[14] however among older individuals (>65), women are more likely to die within the first year after MI.[1] In individuals ages 45 to 64 years, women are more likely than men to have heart failure within 5 years of MI.[1]

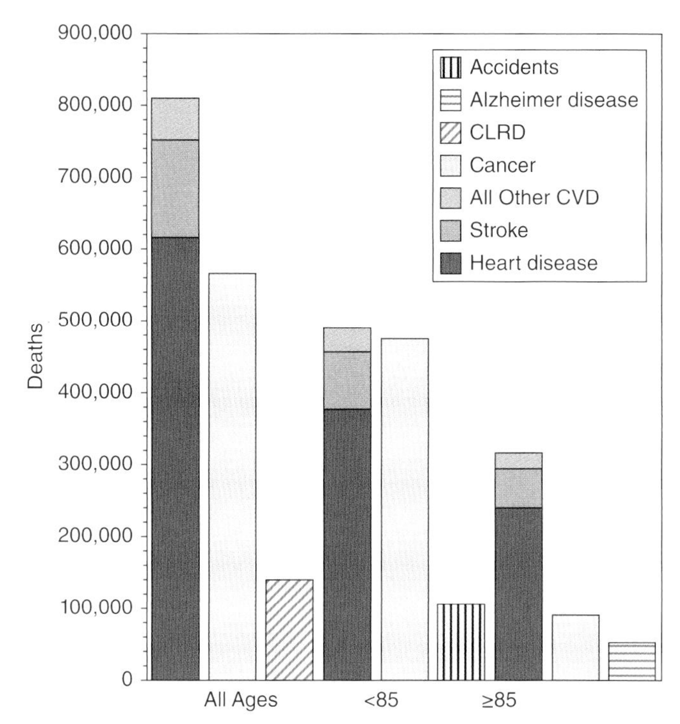

FIGURE 1-1 Cardiovascular disease (CVD) and other major causes of death: total, <85 years of age, and ≥85 years of age. Deaths among both sexes, United States, 2008, CLRD indicates chronic lower respiratory disease. Heart disease include International Classification of Diseases, 10th Revision codes I00-I09, I11, I13, I20-I51; stroke, I60-I69; all other CVD, I10, I12, I15, I70-I99; cancer, C00-C97; CLRD, J40-J47; Alzheimer disease, G30; and accidents, V01-X59, Y85-Y86. Reproduced with permission from Roger VL et al. Heart disease and stroke statistics—2012 update: a report from the American Heart Association. Circulation, 2012. 125(1): p. e2-e220.

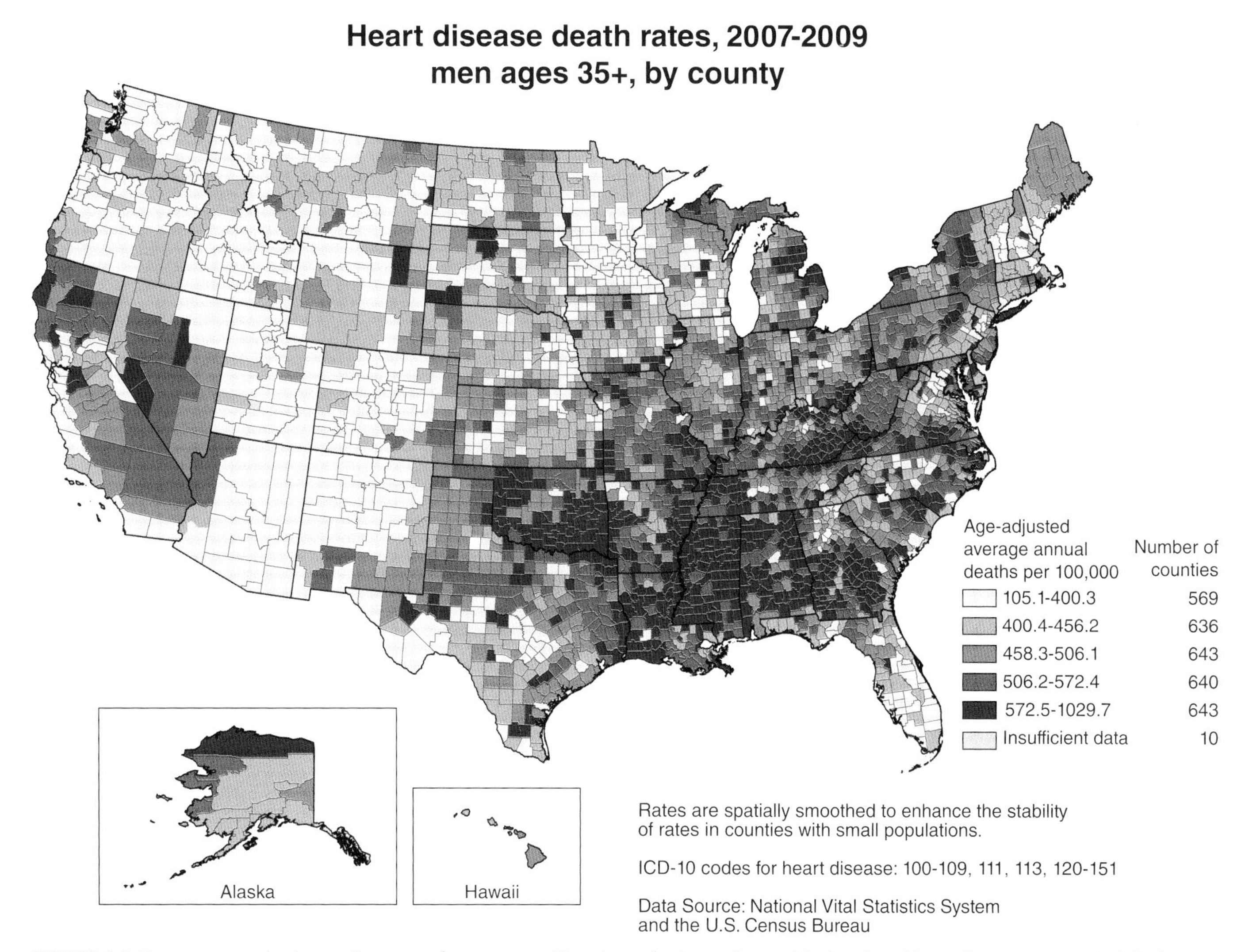

FIGURE 1-2 Demonstrates death rates by county for men ages 35 and over for heart disease. The burden of heart disease is particularly high in the South.
CDC, Behavioral risk factor surveillance system. http://www.cdc.gov/dhdsp/data_statistics/fact_sheets/fs_men_heart.htm. Accessed December 26, 2012.

The burden of CVD is high among women. However, it appears that the pathophysiology of CVD varies between women and men. On cardiovascular computed tomography (CT), women have been shown to have smaller coronary artery diameters.[15] They are less likely to have obstructive coronary artery disease at time of coronary angiography.[16,17] Despite the lack of obstructive disease visualized on cardiac catheterization at time of acute coronary syndrome (ACS), the prognosis of these women is not benign. Over half of symptomatic women without obstructive coronary artery disease continue to have signs and symptoms of ischemia, undergo repeat hospitalization, and coronary angiography.[18,19]

Recently, disorders of the coronary microvasculature and endothelial dysfunction have been implicated in the occurrence of CVD without obstructive coronary artery disease in women. Han et al[20] studied men and women with early coronary artery disease and found that men have higher degrees of atheroma and epicardial endothelial dysfunction, whereas women have more incidence of the microvasculature. Retinal artery narrowing has been shown to be a marker for

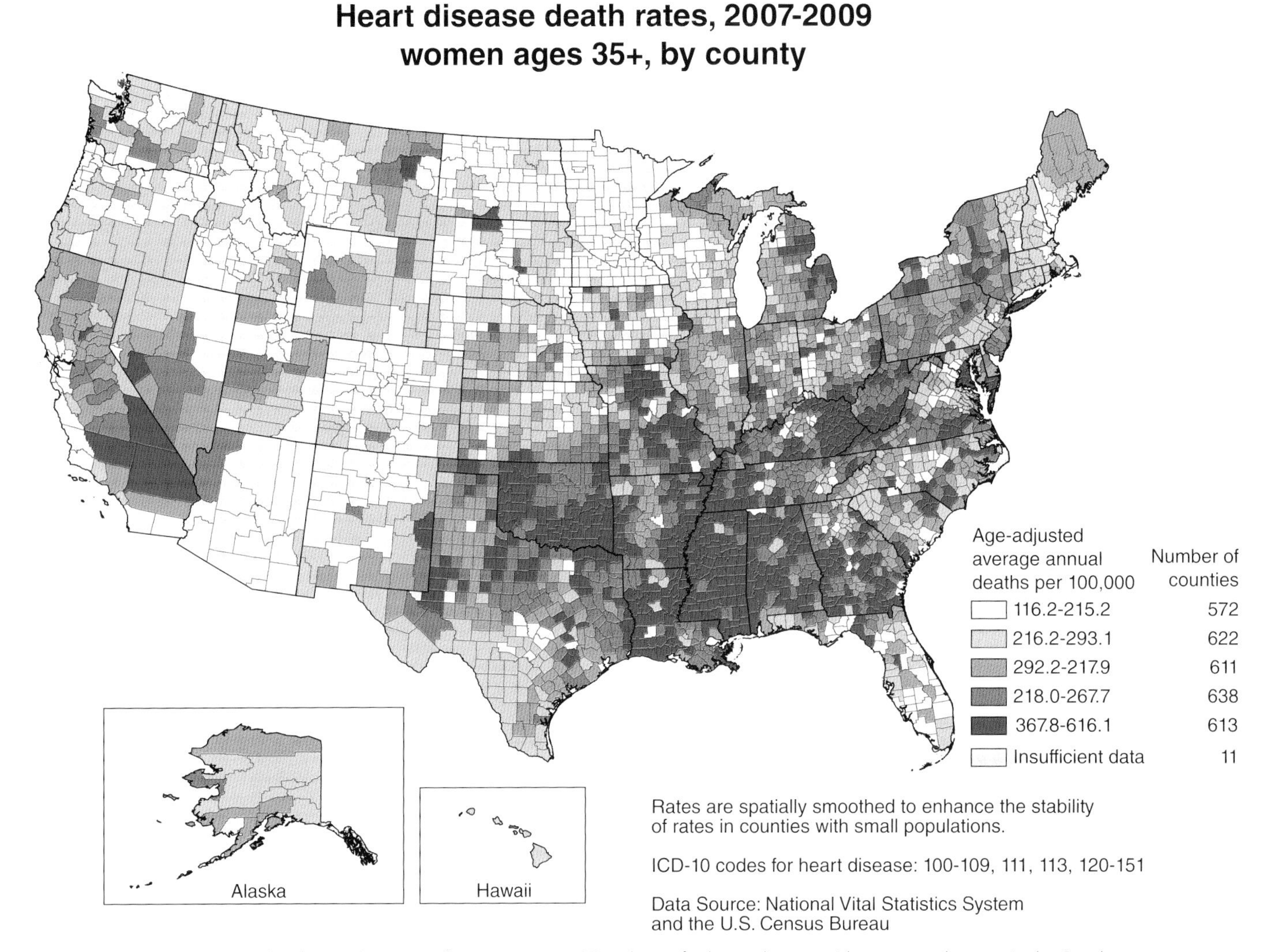

FIGURE 1-3 Demonstrates death rates by county for women ages 35 and over for heart disease with a preponderance in the South. http://www.cdc.gov/dhdsp/data_statistics/fact_sheets/fs_women_heart.htm. Accessed December 26, 2012.

microvascular disease, and in the population covered under the Atherosclerosis Risk in Communities (ARIC) study, a decrease in retinal artery diameter as assessed on retinal photographs corresponded to an increase in CVD incidence in women. This relationship was not seen in men, supporting a more prominent role of microvascular disease in CVD pathophysiology in women as opposed to men.[21] In addition, autopsy data have shown that women have a greater frequency of coronary plaque erosion and distal embolization (Figure 1-9).[22] In the WISE study, approximately half of women with chest pain without obstructive coronary artery disease had microvascular dysfunction.[23] In a study of postmenopausal women, impairment of flow-mediated dilation of the brachial artery predicted the development of cardiovascular events.[24] Hypertensive postmenopausal women were treated with antihypertensive therapy, which resulted in an improvement in flow-mediated vasodilation and an associated improvement in cardiovascular events.[25] Given the occurrence of CVD in women without obstructive coronary artery disease, the term *female-specific ischemic heart disease* has been recommended when discussing disease of the coronary arteries in women.[26]

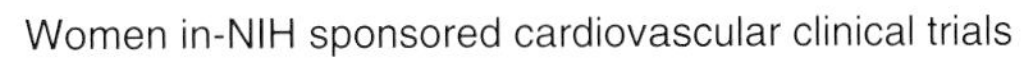

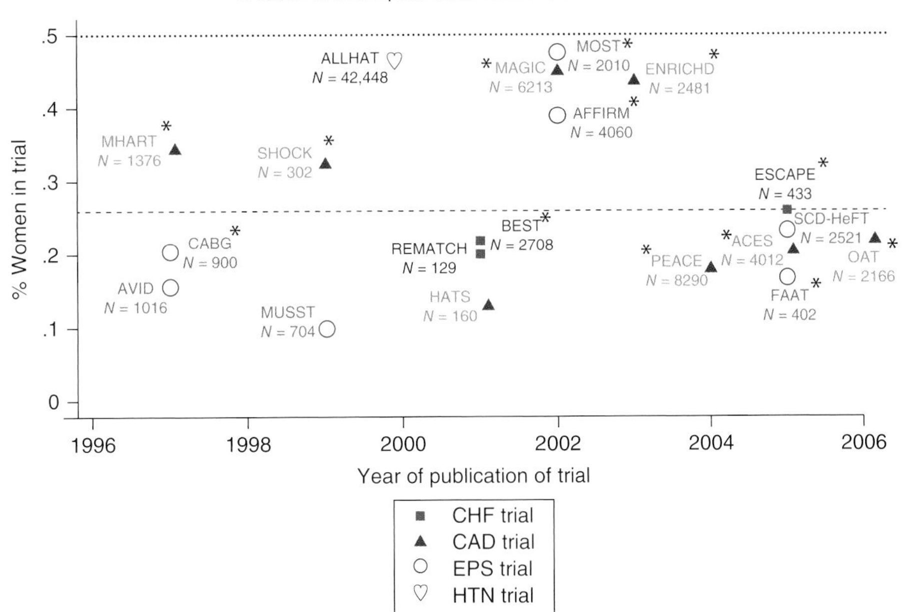

FIGURE 1-4 Enrolment of women in NHLBI-sponsored phase 3 to 4 cardiovascular randomized controlled trials from 1997 to 2006. Each trial is represented by a marker showing the type of cardiovascular disease process it studies (CHF indicates congestive heart failure; CAD, coronary artery disease; EPS, electrophysiological disease; HTN, hypertension). An asterisk by a trial name denotes that the subgroup analyses based on gender were published in the primary paper. The dotted line represents an arbitrarily chosen reference point of 50% enrollment, and the dashed line represents the average enrollment of women over 10 years, 27%.
Reproduced with permission from Kim ES, Carrigan TP, Menon V. Enrollment of women in National Heart, Lung, and Blood Institute-funded cardiovascular randomized controlled trials fails to meet current federal mandates for inclusion. *J Am Coll Cardiol.* 2008;52(8):673.

TABLE 1-1 Comparison of the Mean Proportion of Women in NHLBI-Sponsored Phase 3 to 4 Cardiovascular Randomized Controlled Trials Published between 1997 and 2006 to Proportion of Women Among the General Population with Cardiovascular Disease.

Disease Type	% Women (mean)	% Women Among Those With Disease	Source
Coronary artery disease	29%	46%	AHA
Congestive heart failure	23%	52%	ADHERE
		60%	NHFP
		50%	AHA
Sudden cardiac death	17%	23%	AVID registry
		16%	MUSTT registry
		32%	Seattle/King EMS
Atrial fibrillation	39%	55%	AHA
Hypertension	47%	53%	AHA
Cardiovascular disease	27%	53%	AHA

Abbreviations: ADHERE, Acute Decompensated Heart Failure National Registry; AHA, American Heart Association; NHFP, National Heart Failure Project (patients >65 years old); NHLBI, National Heart, Lung and Blood Institute; Seattle/King EMS, retrospective cohort study of all out-of-pocket arrests in Seattle and King County, WA since 1970s.
Adapted from Kim ES, Menon V. Status of women in cardiovascular clinical trials. *Arterioscler Thromb Vasc Biol.* 2009;29(3):279-283.

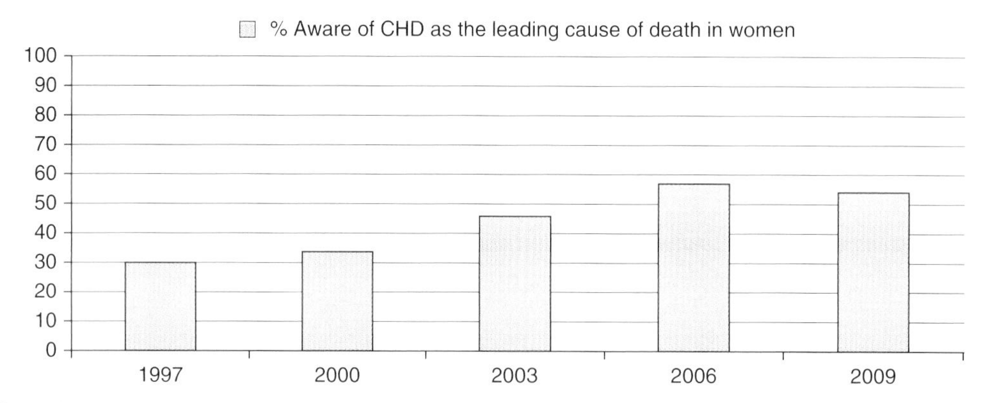

FIGURE 1-5 Overall trends in awareness that coronary heart disease is the leading cause of death in women.
Reproduced with permission from Mosca L, Mochari-Greenberger H, Dolor RJ, Newby LK, Robb KJ. Twelve-year follow-up of American women's awareness of cardiovascular disease risk and barriers to heart health. *Circ Cardiovasc Qual Outcomes.* 2010;3:120-127.

DIAGNOSIS OF MYOCARDIAL ISCHEMIA IN WOMEN

An exercise stress test is used commonly in the evaluation of suspected coronary artery disease. In women, the ST-segment depression noted on exercise stress testing is felt to be less accurate than in men. Also, the sensitivity and specificity of ST-segment depression is lower in women than in men.[27] However, the negative predictive value is high in both.[28] A negative exercise stress test, therefore, can effectively rule out the diagnosis of CAD in women. The Duke Treadmill score, which incorporates exercise time, ST deviation, and an anginal score, is particularly useful in women, and performs better in women than men in predicting significant CVD.[29] Exercise is a powerful predictor

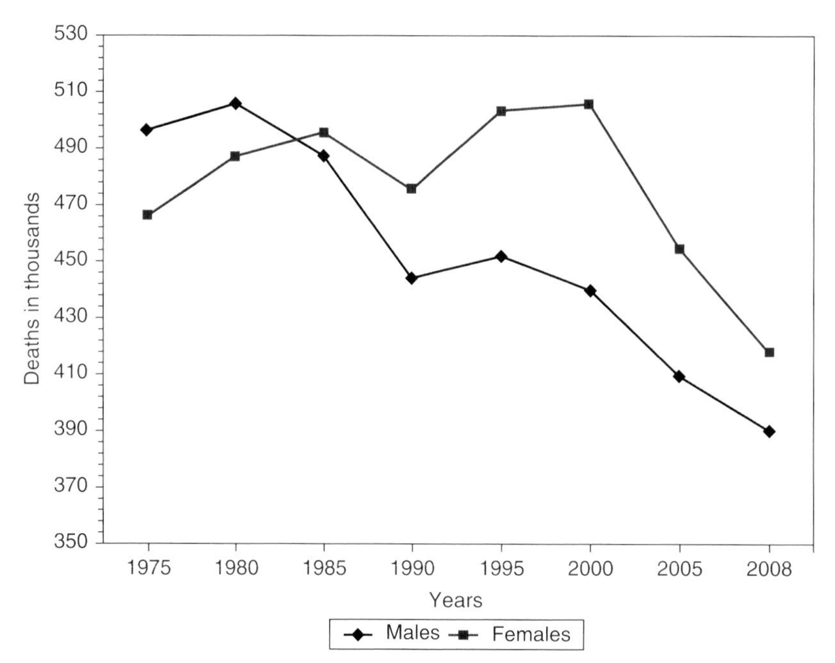

FIGURE 1-6 Cardiovascular disease mortality trends for males and females (United States: 1979-2008). Cardiovascular disease excludes congenial cardiovascular defects [International Classification of Diseases, 10th Revision (ICD-10) codes I00-I99]. The comparability for cardiovascular disease between the International Classification of Diseases, 9th Revision (1979-1998) and ICD-10 (1999-2008) is 0.9962. No comparability ratios were applied. Reproduced with permission from Roger VL, Go AS, Lloyd-Jones DM, et al. Heart disease and stroke statistics—2012 update: a report from the American Heart Association. *Circulation.* 2012;125(1):e2-e220.

of CVD. Importantly, a nomogram has been established defining age-predicted exercise capacity in women.[30] As mentioned earlier, women who are unable to reach 5 metabolic equivalents (METs) or perform <85% of age-predicted fitness level on an exercise stress test have a higher risk of MI and all-cause mortality.[30,31]

Stress echocardiography has similar high levels of sensitivity and specificity in women and men.[32,33] Its lack of radiation is particularly attractive in younger women. Myocardial perfusion imaging utilizing single-photon emission computed tomography (SPECT) has been well studied in women. The incorporation of technetium-99 sestamibi radiotracer and the use of gating technology have improved the sensitivity and specificity of SPECT imaging in women to nearly 90% (Table 1-2).[34,35] SPECT stress imaging effectively risk-stratifies women.[36-38] In a study including women with a normal myocardial perfusion using SPECT imaging, the annual CVD death rate was very low (0.6% per year) in contrast to a much higher event rate (5% per year) in those with abnormal myocardial perfusion.[38]

The use of stress cardiac magnetic resonance (CMR) imaging in the assessment of women is increasing. A recent study of predominantly female patients with chest pain and nonobstructive coronary artery disease who underwent adenosine CMR found that subendocardial ischemia was frequently present when compared to controls (Figure 1-10).[39] In women with ACS and normal coronary arteries who underwent CMR, abnormalities on late gadolinium enhancement consistent with ischemia were frequently noted.[40] In a small substudy from the WISE cohort, women with nonobstructive CAD with an abnormal stress-induced CMR had an increase in adverse cardiovascular events.[41] CMR and its applications to women and CVD are only beginning to be explored; much remains to be learned about CMR's prognostic implications.

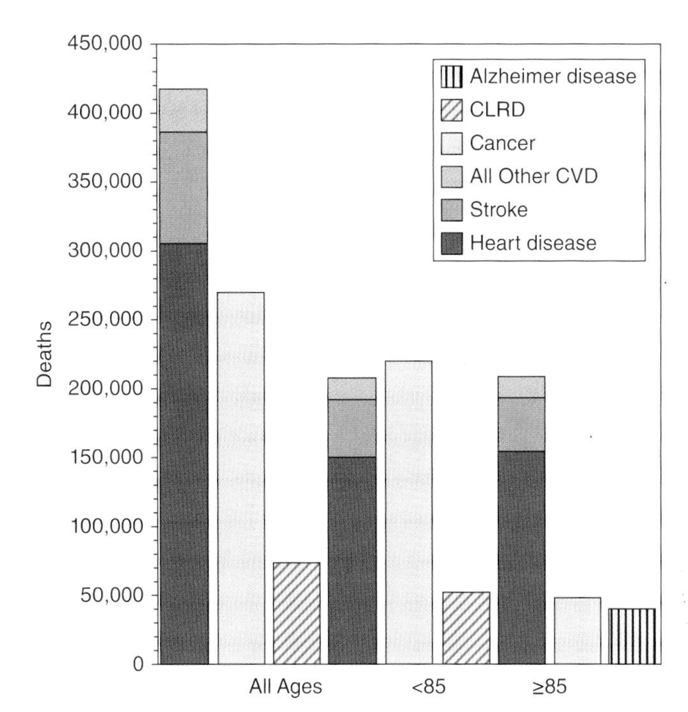

FIGURE 1-7 Cardiovascular disease (CVD) and other major causes of death in females: total, <85 years of age, and ≥85 years of age. Deaths among females, United States, 2008, CLRD indicates chronic lower respiratory disease. Heart disease includes International Classification of Diseases, 10th Revision codes I00-I09, I11, I13, I20-I51; stroke, I60-I69; all other CVD, I10, I12, I70-I99; cancer, C00-C97; CLRD, J40-J47; and Alzheimer disease, G30.
Reproduced with permission from Roger VL, Go AS, Lloyd-Jones DM, et al. Heart disease and stroke statistics—2012 update: a report from the American Heart Association. *Circulation*. 2012;125(1):e2-e220.

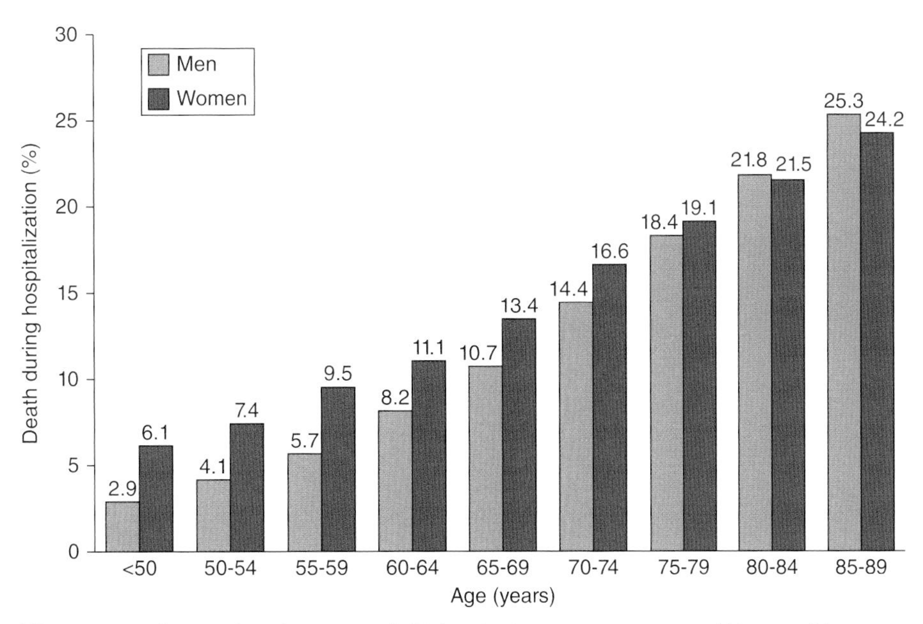

FIGURE 1-8 Shows the difference in early mortality after myocardial infarction in men versus women. Women with premature myocardial infarction (age under 50) have a 2-fold increase in mortality compared to men.
Reproduced with permission from Vaccarino V, Parsons L, Every NR, Barron HV, Krumholz HM. Sex-based differences in early mortality after myocardial infarction. National Registry of Myocardial Infarction 2 Participants. *N Engl J Med*. 1999;341(4):217-225.

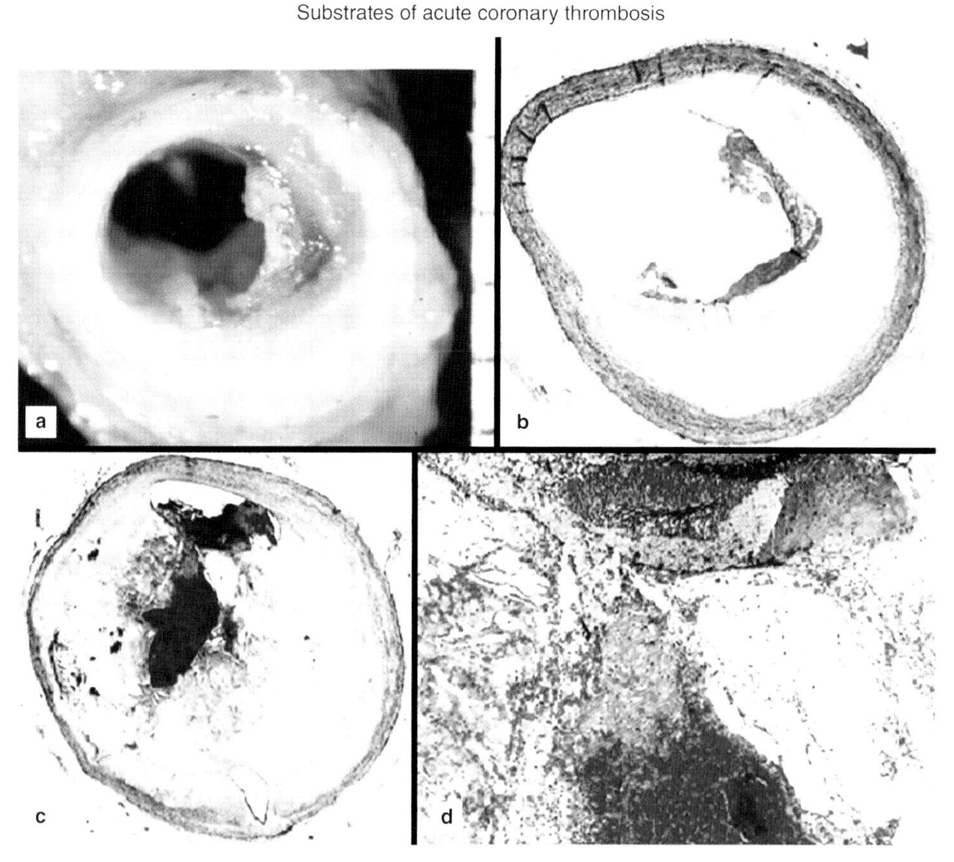

FIGURE 1-9 Substrates of acute coronary thrombosis. A) Plaque erosion: eccentric plaque with overlying subocclusive thrombus. The narrowing is not critical, and disruption of the cap is absent. B) Microscopic illustration demonstrates thrombus overlying intact plaque. The patient was a 58-year-old smoker with a history of emphysema but no heart disease. She recently complained of chest pain but was not extensively evaluated. She had an apparent seizure and developed cardiac arrest from which she could not be resuscitated. C) Plaque rupture: Critical narrowing of this section of left anterior descending artery by atheroma rich in cholesterol crystals. Central hemorrhage into plaque is continuous with the small residual lumen above. Black reflects the postmortem injection of contrast material. D) Higher magnification of "C" demonstrates rupture site. Reproduced with permission from Burke AP, Farb A, Malcom GT, Liang Y, Smialek J, Virmani R. Effect of risk factors on the mechanism of acute thrombosis and sudden coronary death in women. *Circulation*. 1998;97:2110-2116.

TABLE 1-2 Diagnostic Value of Various Stress Testing Modalities in Women

Stress Testing Modality	Sensitivity (%)	Specificity (%)	Negative Predictive Value (NPV)	Positive Predictive Value (PPV)
Exercise ECG [70-76]	31-71	66-78	78	47
Exercise echocardiography [76-78]	80-88	79-86	98	74
Exercise SPECT [79-82]	78-88	64-91	99	87
Pharmacological echocardiography [83-85]	76-90	85-94	68	94
Pharmacological SPECT [87, 88, 86]	80-91	65-86	90	68

Adapted with permission from Kohli P, Gulati M. Exercise stress testing in women: going back to the basics. *Circulation*. 2010;122(24):2570-2580.[25]

MANAGEMENT OF OBSTRUCTIVE CORONARY ARTERY DISEASE IN WOMEN

Mortality due to CVD is higher in women than men.[1] Women with ACS are treated less aggressively than men. In the CRUSADE initiative, women were less likely to receive heparin and GP IIb/IIIa inhibitors and undergo cardiac catheterization and revascularization than men.[42] Women with ACS have also been shown to be less likely to receive early aspirin or β-blocker therapy, and they received less reperfusion therapy and less timely reperfusion.[43]

Strategies for ACS appear to have variable efficacy in women versus men. A meta-analysis of randomized controlled trials of ACS showed that an invasive strategy was more beneficial in women with positive biomarkers than women with negative biomarkers. Such a difference was not seen in men.[5] After percutaneous coronary intervention, women have been shown to have a higher mortality in ST-elevation and non–ST-elevation MI.[44] Furthermore, in ACS patients, women without raised biomarkers did not benefit from GP IIb/IIIa inhibitors, unlike men; when women had raised biomarkers, they did receive a risk reduction with GP IIb/IIIa inhibitors (Table 1-3).[6] Women have been shown to experience higher rates of bleeding with percutaneous intervention; however, this has been shown to be largely attributable to body size and renal function.[45]

Several recent trials have specifically examined drug-eluting stent placement in men and women, and overall, have found similar outcomes after stent placement.[46,47] Among patients undergoing coronary artery bypass grafting (CABG), however, female sex is an independent risk factor for morbidity and mortality. Although women comprise <30% of the CABG population, they have a higher risk of morbidity and mortality and experience less relief from angina than men after CABG.[7,8] Interestingly, this discrepancy appears to be reduced when an off-pump CABG is performed.[48]

MANAGEMENT OF NONOBSTRUCTIVE DISEASE IN WOMEN

Among women with symptoms of myocardial ischemia who are demonstrated to have angiographically nonobstructive coronary artery disease, the prognosis was initially felt to be benign.[49,50] However, more recent data have shown that the prognosis is not benign and the risk of cardiovascular events is higher when compared with asymptomatic women.[19,51] Patients with unstable angina and no critical coronary obstruction still had a 2% risk of death and MI at 30 days post-MI.[52] Among women with persistent chest pain but no obstructive coronary artery disease at cardiac catheterization for suspected ACS, cardiovascular outcomes were worse in those with continued chest pain.[18] Symptomatic women in the WISE study with nonobstructive coronary artery disease (lesions 1%-49%) had a CVD event rate of 16%, compared to only 7.9% in women with no coronary artery disease, and only 2.4% in asymptomatic age- and race-matched controls.[51]

The focus of treatment of nonobstructive coronary artery disease has been on symptom improvement or vascular function response. Statins and angiotensin-converting enzyme inhibitors have been shown to improve endothelial function and symptoms.[53-56]

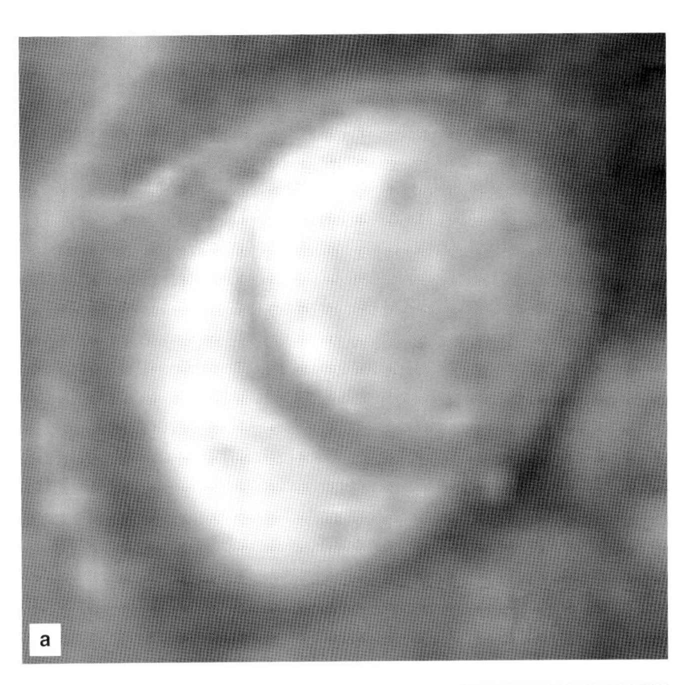

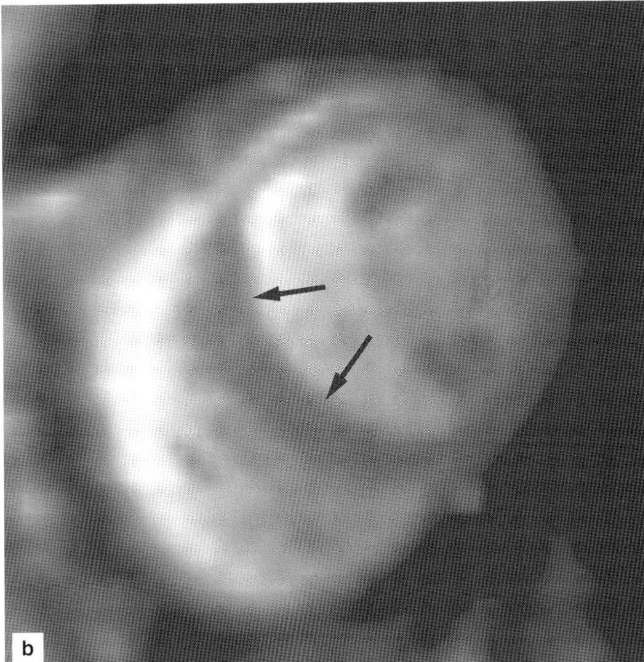

FIGURE 1-10 Stress cardiac magnetic resonance imaging. A) Normal stress imaging with no ischemia. B) Abnormal stress imaging with ischemia.

TABLE 1-3 Efficacy According to Sex and Baseline Cardiac Troponin Concentration.

	Men			Women			
	Glycoprotein IIb/IIa	Control	Odds ratio (95% CI)[†]	Glycoprotein IIb/IIIa	Control	Odds ratio (95% CI)[†]	p for heterogeneity
All patients							
Total	11886	8502		6410	4603		
Death	379 (3.2%)	321 (3.8%)	0.83 (0.71-0.96)	252 (3.9%)	164 (3.6%)	1.08 (0.89-1.33)	0.030
Death or MI	1242 (10.4%)	1070 (12.6%)	0.81 (0.75-0.89)	738 (11.5%)	480 (10.4%)	1.15 (1.01-1.30)	0.0001
Patients with missing data on baseline cardiac troponin							
Total	7617	5769		3923	3033		
Death	241 (3.2%)	224 (3.9%)	0.81 (0.67-0.98)	158 (4.0%)	101 (3.3%)	1.20 (0.93-1.55)	0.011
Death or MI	881 (11.6%)	825 (14.3%)	0.78 (0.70-0.86)	523 (13.3%)	350 (11.5%)	1.18 (1.02-1.36)	0.0001
Patients with data on baseling cardiac troponin[‡]							
Total	4269	2733		2487	1570		
Death	138 (3.2%)	97 (3.5%)	0.85 (0.65-1.11)	94 (3.8%)	63 (4.0%)	0.91 (0.66-1.27)	0.83
Death or MI	361 (8.5%)	245 (9.0%)	0.93 (0.78-1.11)	215 (8.6%)	130 (8.3%)	1.07 (0.85-1.83)	0.38
Patients with baseline cardiac troponin T or I <0.1 μg/L							
Total	2095	1449		1548	1003		
Death	48 (2.3%)	30 (2.1%)	1.07 (0.67-1.71)	36 (2.3%)	20 (2.0%)	1.20 (0.69-2.10)	0.84
Death or MI	159 (7.6%)	100 (6.9%)	1.10 (0.84-1.43)	96 (6.2%)	53 (5.3%)	1.29 (0.91-1.83)	0.65
Patients with baseline cardiac troponin T or I <0.1 μg/L							
Total	2174	1284		939	567		
Death	90 (4.1%)	67 (5.2%)	0.75 (0.54-1.04)	58 (6.2%)	43 (7.6%)	0.80 (0.53-1.21)	0.88
Death or MI	202 (9.3%)	145 (11.3%)	0.82 (0.65-1.03)	119 (12.7%)	77 (13.6%)	0.93 (0.68-1.28)	0.48

Data represent outcome at 30 days. Information on sex was not available for one patient. Glycoprotein IIb/IIIa, glycoprotein IIb/IIIa receptor blocker; MI, myocardial infarction. [‡]Represents level of statistical evidence for heterogeneity in treatment effect between men and women; p corresponds with sex x treatment interaction term in a logistic regression model, with adjustment for between-trial outcome differences. [†]Pooled trial-specific odds ratios by the method of Cochrane Mantel-Haenszel. [‡]Cardiac troponin data were available in 69% of patients enrolled in PRISM, 6% in PRISM=PLUS, 4% in PURSUIT, 23% in PARAGON-B, and 91% in GUSTO-IV. In PRISM, these data were not strictly baseline values, but were obtained a median of 8 h after randomization.

Reproduced with permission from Boersma E, Harrington RA, Moliterno DJ, et al. Platelet glycoprotein IIb/IIIa inhibitors in acute coronary syndromes: a meta-analysis of all major randomised clinical trials. *Lancet.* 2002;359(9302):189-198.

TABLE 1-4 Women are Less Likely to have LDL at Goal with Diabetes or CVD than Men.

	Diabetes	CVD
Women	38.5%	46.6%
Men	44.3%	55.1%

Reproduced with permission from Chou AF, Scholle SH, Weisman CS, Bierman AS, Correa-de-Araujo R, Mosca L. Gender disparities in the quality of cardiovascular disease care in private managed care plans. *Women's Health Issues.* 2007;17(3):120-130.

Statins have been demonstrated to improve microcirculation.[57] Chest pain syndromes have been effectively treated with β-blockers.[58] Imipramine has been shown to improve symptoms in women with chest pain and nonobstructive coronary artery disease. This is possibly related to a visceral analgesic effect.[59] L-arginine has been shown to improve endothelial function and symptoms in patients with nonobstructive coronary artery disease,[60] although concerns about its safety have arisen.[61] The effects of ranolazine are promising. A recent pilot study demonstrated that women with angina, myocardial ischemia, and no obstructive coronary artery disease had an improvement in angina with ranolazine.[9] Randomized control data on women with chest pain and nonobstructive coronary artery disease are currently lacking; further research in this area is needed.

THE UNDERTREATMENT OF WOMEN

Awareness of the tremendous effect CVD has on women is slowly increasing. In 1997, only 30% of American women surveyed were aware that CVD is the leading cause of death in women; this increased to 54% in 2009.[3] In a survey performed in 2004, fewer than 1 in 5 physicians recognized that more women than men die each year from CVD.[4] Unfortunately, women are less likely to receive preventive recommendations, such as lipid-lowering therapy, aspirin, and lifestyle advice, than similarly scoring Framingham-risk men.[4,62] Hypertensive women are less likely to have their blood pressure at goal.[63] Also, women are less likely to be treated to achieve the desired LDL cholesterol goals (Table 1-4).[63,64] Female diabetics, the group at highest risk for CVD, have the greatest gender disparity in achieving LDL cholesterol targets.[65] As demonstrated in numerous national studies, cardiac rehabilitation after MI is underused, particularly in women,[66-69] who are 55% less likely to participate in cardiac rehabilitation than men.[66]

CONCLUSION

Women are affected by CVD in large numbers and to a higher degree. CVD is the leading cause of mortality in women and manifests itself among them with unique characteristics. Increasing data demonstrate that some treatment strategies have a gender-specific effectiveness. In this *Atlas and Synopsis of Women's Cardiovascular Health*, we will discuss important topics related to CVD in women.

REFERENCES

1. Roger VL, et al. Heart disease and stroke statistics, 2012. Update: A report from the American Heart Association. *Circulation*. 2012;125(1):e2-e220.
2. Kim ES, Menon, V. Status of women in cardiovascular clinical trials. *Arterioscler Thromb Vasc Biol*. 2009;29(3):279-283.
3. Mosca L, et al. Twelve-year follow-up of American women's awareness of cardiovascular disease risk and barriers to heart health. *Circ Cardiovasc Qual Outcomes*. 2010;3(2):120-127.
4. Mosca L, et al. National study of physician awareness and adherence to cardiovascular disease prevention guidelines. *Circulation*. 2005;111(4):499-510.
5. O'Donoghue M, et al. Early invasive vs conservative treatment strategies in women and men with unstable angina and non-ST-segment elevation myocardial infarction: a meta-analysis. *JAMA*. 2008;300(1):71-80.
6. Boersma E, et al. Platelet glycoprotein IIb/IIIa inhibitors in acute coronary syndromes: a meta-analysis of all major randomised clinical trials. *Lancet*. 2002;359(9302):189-198.
7. Abramov D, et al. The influence of gender on the outcome of coronary artery bypass surgery. *Ann Thorac Surg*. 2000;70(3): 800-805, discussion 806.
8. Edwards FH, et al. Impact of gender on coronary bypass operative mortality. *Ann Thorac Surg*. 1998;66(1):125-131.
9. Mehta PK, et al. Ranolazine improves angina in women with evidence of myocardial ischemia but no obstructive coronary artery disease. *JACC Cardiovasc Imaging*. 2011;4(5):514-522.
10. Ford ES, Capewell S. Coronary heart disease mortality among young adults in the U.S. from 1980 through 2002: concealed leveling of mortality rates. *J Am Coll Cardiol*. 2007;50(22): 2128-2132.
11. Flegal KM, et al. Prevalence and trends in obesity among US adults, 1999-2008. *JAMA*. 2010;303(3):235-241.
12. Wilson PW, et al. Overweight and obesity as determinants of cardiovascular risk: the Framingham experience. *Arch Intern Med*. 2002;162(16):1867-1872.
13. Thom TJ, Kannel WB, Silbershatz H, D'Agostino RB, Sr. Cardiovascular disease in the United States and prevention approaches.In: Fuster V, Alexander RW, Schlant RC, O'Rourke RA, Roberts R, Sonnenblick EH. eds. *Hurst's the Heart*, 10th ed. New York, NY: McGraw-Hill; 2001:5.
14. Vaccarino V, et al. Sex-based differences in early mortality after myocardial infarction. National Registry of Myocardial Infarction 2 Participants. *N Engl J Med*. 1999;341(4):217-225.
15. Dickerson JA, Nagaraja HN, Raman SV. Gender-related differences in coronary artery dimensions: a volumetric analysis. *Clin Cardiol*. 2010;33(2):E44-E49.
16. Sharaf BL, et al. Detailed angiographic analysis of women with suspected ischemic chest pain (pilot phase data from the NHLBI-sponsored Women's Ischemia Syndrome Evaluation [WISE] Study Angiographic Core Laboratory). *Am J Cardiol*. 2001;87(8):937-941, A3.

17. Kennedy JW, et al. The clinical spectrum of coronary artery disease and its surgical and medical management, 1974-1979. The Coronary Artery Surgery study. *Circulation*. 1982;66(5 pt 2): III16-III23.

18. Johnson BD, et al. Persistent chest pain predicts cardiovascular events in women without obstructive coronary artery disease: results from the NIH-NHLBI-sponsored Women's Ischaemia Syndrome Evaluation (WISE) study. *Eur Heart J*. 2006;27(12):1408-1415.

19. Shaw LJ, et al. The economic burden of angina in women with suspected ischemic heart disease: results from the National Institutes of Health—National Heart, Lung, and Blood Institute—sponsored Women's Ischemia Syndrome Evaluation. *Circulation*. 2006;114(9):894-904.

20. Han SH, et al. Sex differences in atheroma burden and endothelial function in patients with early coronary atherosclerosis. *Eur Heart J*. 2008;29(11):1359-1369.

21. Wong TY, et al. Retinal arteriolar narrowing and risk of coronary heart disease in men and women. The Atherosclerosis Risk in Communities Study. *JAMA*. 2002;287(9):1153-1159.

22. Burke AP, et al. Effect of risk factors on the mechanism of acute thrombosis and sudden coronary death in women. *Circulation*. 1998;97(21):2110-2116.

23. Reis SE, et al. Coronary microvascular dysfunction is highly prevalent in women with chest pain in the absence of coronary artery disease: results from the NHLBI WISE study. *Am Heart J*. 2001;141(5):735-741.

24. Rossi R, et al. Prognostic role of flow-mediated dilation and cardiac risk factors in post-menopausal women. *J Am Coll Cardiol*. 2008;51(10):997-1002.

25. Modena MG, et al. Prognostic role of reversible endothelial dysfunction in hypertensive postmenopausal women. *J Am Coll Cardiol*. 2002;40(3):505-510.

26. Shaw LJ, Bugiardini R, Merz CN. Women and ischemic heart disease: evolving knowledge. *J Am Coll Cardiol*. 2009;54(17):1561-1575.

27. Hemingway H, et al. Incidence and prognostic implications of stable angina pectoris among women and men. *JAMA*. 2006;295(12):1404-1411.

28. Barolsky SM, et al. Differences in electrocardiographic response to exercise of women and men: a non-Bayesian factor. *Circulation*. 1979;60(5):1021-1027.

29. Alexander KP, et al. Value of exercise treadmill testing in women. *J Am Coll Cardiol*. 1998;32(6):1657-1664.

30. Gulati M, et al. The prognostic value of a nomogram for exercise capacity in women. *N Engl J Med*. 2005;353(5):468-475.

31. Gulati M, et al. Exercise capacity and the risk of death in women: the St James Women Take Heart Project. *Circulation*. 2003;108(13):1554-1559.

32. Kwok Y, et al. Meta-analysis of exercise testing to detect coronary artery disease in women. *Am J Cardiol*. 1999;83(5):660-666.

33. Kohli P, Gulati M. Exercise stress testing in women: going back to the basics. *Circulation*. 2010;122(24):2570-2580.

34. Taillefer R, et al. Comparative diagnostic accuracy of Tl-201 and Tc-99m sestamibi SPECT imaging (perfusion and ECG-gated SPECT) in detecting coronary artery disease in women. *J Am Coll Cardiol*. 1997;29(1):69-77.

35. Amanullah AM, et al. Adenosine technetium-99m sestamibi myocardial perfusion SPECT in women: diagnostic efficacy in detection of coronary artery disease. *J Am Coll Cardiol*. 1996;27(4):803-809.

36. Mieres JH, et al. Role of noninvasive testing in the clinical evaluation of women with suspected coronary artery disease: Consensus statement from the Cardiac Imaging Committee, Council on Clinical Cardiology, and the Cardiovascular Imaging and Intervention Committee, Council on Cardiovascular Radiology and Intervention, American Heart Association. *Circulation*. 2005;111(5):682-696.

37. Marwick TH, et al. The noninvasive prediction of cardiac mortality in men and women with known or suspected coronary artery disease. Economics of Noninvasive Diagnosis (END) Study Group. *Am J Med*. 1999;106(2):172-178.

38. Shaw LJ, Iskandrian AE. Prognostic value of gated myocardial perfusion SPECT. *J Nucl Cardiol*. 2004;11(2):171-185.

39. Panting JR, et al. Abnormal subendocardial perfusion in cardiac syndrome X detected by cardiovascular magnetic resonance imaging. *N Engl J Med*. 2002;346(25):1948-1953.

40. Reynolds HR, et al. Mechanisms of myocardial infarction in women without angiographically obstructive coronary artery disease. *Circulation*. 2011;124(13):1414-1425.

41. Johnson BD, et al. Prognosis in women with myocardial ischemia in the absence of obstructive coronary disease: results from the National Institutes of Health-National Heart, Lung, and Blood Institute-Sponsored Women's Ischemia Syndrome Evaluation (WISE). *Circulation*. 2004;109(24):2993-2999.

42. Blomkalns AL, et al. Gender disparities in the diagnosis and treatment of non-ST-segment elevation acute coronary syndromes: large-scale observations from the CRUSADE (Can Rapid Risk Stratification of Unstable Angina Patients Suppress Adverse Outcomes With Early Implementation of the American College of Cardiology/American Heart Association Guidelines) National Quality Improvement Initiative. *J Am Coll Cardiol*. 2005;45(6):832-837.

43. Jneid H, et al. Sex differences in medical care and early death after acute myocardial infarction. *Circulation*. 2008;118(25):2803-2810.

44. Lansky AJ. Outcomes of percutaneous and surgical revascularization in women. *Prog Cardiovasc Dis*. 2004;46(4):305-219.

45. Alexander KP, et al. Sex differences in major bleeding with glycoprotein IIb/IIIa inhibitors: results from the CRUSADE (Can Rapid risk stratification of Unstable angina patients Suppress ADverse outcomes with Early implementation of the ACC/AHA guidelines) initiative. *Circulation*. 2006;114(13): 1380-1387.

46. Solinas E, et al. Gender-specific outcomes after sirolimus-eluting stent implantation. *J Am Coll Cardiol*. 2007;50(22):2111-2116.

47. Lansky AJ, et al. Gender-based outcomes after paclitaxel-eluting stent implantation in patients with coronary artery disease. *J Am Coll Cardiol*. 2005;45(8):1180-1185.

48. Puskas JD, et al. Off-pump techniques benefit men and women and narrow the disparity in mortality after coronary bypass grafting. *Ann Thorac Surg*. 2007;84(5):1447-1454, discussion 1454-1456.

49. Kemp HG, et al. Seven year survival of patients with normal or near normal coronary arteriograms: a CASS registry study. *J Am Coll Cardiol*. 1986;7(3):479-483.

50. Kaski JC, et al. Cardiac syndrome X: clinical characteristics and left ventricular function. Long-term follow-up study. *J Am Coll Cardiol*. 1995;25(4):807-814.

51. Gulati M, et al. Adverse cardiovascular outcomes in women with nonobstructive coronary artery disease: a report from the Women's Ischemia Syndrome Evaluation Study and the St James Women Take Heart Project. *Arch Intern Med*. 2009;169(9): 843-850.

52. Diver DJ, et al. Clinical and arteriographic characterization of patients with unstable angina without critical coronary arterial narrowing (from the TIMI-IIIA Trial). *Am J Cardiol*. 1994;74(6):531-537.

53. Pizzi C, et al. Angiotensin-converting enzyme inhibitors and 3-hydroxy-3-methylglutaryl coenzyme A reductase in cardiac Syndrome X: role of superoxide dismutase activity. *Circulation*. 2004;109(1):53-58.

54. Danaoglu Z, et al. Effect of statin therapy added to ACE-inhibitors on blood pressure control and endothelial functions in normolipidemic hypertensive patients. *Anadolu Kardiyol Derg*. 2003;3(4):331-337.

55. Kayikcioglu M, et al. Benefits of statin treatment in cardiac syndrome-X1. *Eur Heart J*. 2003;24(22):1999-2005.

56. Chen JW, et al. Long-term angiotensin-converting enzyme inhibition reduces plasma asymmetric dimethylarginine and improves endothelial nitric oxide bioavailability and coronary microvascular function in patients with syndrome X. *Am J Cardiol*. 2002;90(9):974-982.

57. Manfrini O, et al. Effect of pravastatin on myocardial perfusion after percutaneous transluminal coronary angioplasty. *Am J Cardiol*. 2004;93(11):1391-1393, A6.

58. Lanza GA, et al. Atenolol versus amlodipine versus isosorbide-5-mononitrate on anginal symptoms in syndrome X. *Am J Cardiol*. 1999;84(7):854-856, A8.

59. Cannon RO, 3rd, et al. Imipramine in patients with chest pain despite normal coronary angiograms. *N Engl J Med*. 1994;330(20):1411-1417.

60. Lerman A, et al. Long-term L-arginine supplementation improves small-vessel coronary endothelial function in humans. *Circulation*. 1998;97(21):2123-2128.

61. Dzavik V, et al. Effect of nitric oxide synthase inhibition on haemodynamics and outcome of patients with persistent cardiogenic shock complicating acute myocardial infarction: a phase II dose-ranging study. *Eur Heart J*. 2007;28(9):1109-1116.

62. Abuful A, Gidron Y, Henkin Y. Physicians' attitudes toward preventive therapy for coronary artery disease: is there a gender bias? *Clin Cardiol*. 2005;28(8):389-393.

63. Chou AF, et al. Gender disparities in the quality of cardiovascular disease care in private managed care plans. *Women's Health Issues*. 2007;17(3):120-130.

64. Gu Q, et al. Gender differences in hypertension treatment, drug utilization patterns, and blood pressure control among US adults with hypertension: data from the National Health and Nutrition Examination Survey 1999-2004. *Am J Hypertens*. 2008;21(7):789-798.

65. Bird CE, et al. Does quality of care for cardiovascular disease and diabetes differ by gender for enrollees in managed care plans? *Women's Health Issues*. 2007;17(3):131-138.

66. Witt BJ, et al. Cardiac rehabilitation after myocardial infarction in the community. *J Am Coll Cardiol*. 2004;44(5):988-996.

67. Suaya JA, et al. Use of cardiac rehabilitation by Medicare beneficiaries after myocardial infarction or coronary bypass surgery. *Circulation*. 2007;116(15):1653-1662.

68. Evenson KR, Rosamond WD, Luepker RV. Predictors of outpatient cardiac rehabilitation utilization: the Minnesota Heart Surgery Registry. *J Cardiopulm Rehabil*. 1998;18(3):192-198.

69. Thomas RJ, et al. National Survey on Gender Differences in Cardiac Rehabilitation Programs. Patient characteristics and enrollment patterns. *J Cardiopulm Rehabil*. 1996;16(6):402-412.

70. Jouven X, et al. Heart-rate profile during exercise as a predictor of sudden death. *N Engl J Med*. 2005;352:1951-1958.

71. Vivekananthan DP, Blackstone EH, Pothier CE, Lauer MS. Heart rate recovery after exercise is a predictor of mortality, independent of the angiographic severity of coronary disease. *J Am Coll Cardiol*. 2003;42:831-838.

72. Kardash M, et al. The slope of ST segment/heart rate relationship during exercise in the prediction of severity of coronary artery disease. *Eur Heart J*. 1982;3:449-458.

73. Froelicher VF. Exercise testing in the new millennium. *Prim Care*. 2001;28:1-4.

74. Lachterman B, et al. Comparison of ST segment/heart rate index to standard ST criteria for analysis of exercise electrocardiogram. *Circulation*. 1990;82:44-50.

75. Kligfield P, Lauer MS. Exercise electrocardiogram testing: beyond the ST segment. *Circulation*. 2006;114:2070-2082.

76. Shepherd JT. Circulatory response to exercise in health. *Circulation*. 1987;76:VI3-VI10.

77. Thomson PD, Kelemen MH. Hypotension accompanying the onset of exertional angina: a sign of severe compromise of left ventricular blood supply. *Circulation*. 1975;52:28-32.

78. Morris SN, Phillips JF, Jordan JW, McHenry PL. Incidence and significance of decreases in systolic blood pressure during graded treadmill exercise testing. *Am J Cardiol*. 1978;41:221-226.

79. Sanmarco ME, Pontius S, Selvester RH. Abnormal blood pressure response and marked ischemic ST-segment depression as predictors of severe coronary artery disease. *Circulation*. 1980;61:572-578.

80. Levites R, Baker T, Anderson GJ. The significance of hypotension developing during treadmill exercise testing. *Am Heart J*. 1978;95:747-753.

81. Manolio TA, et al. Exercise blood pressure response and 5-year risk of elevated blood pressure in a cohort of young adults: the CARDIA study. *Am J Hypertens*. 1994;7:234-241.

82. Singh JP, et al. Blood pressure response during treadmill testing as a risk factor for new-onset hypertension: the Framingham Heart Study. *Circulation*. 1999;99:1831-1836.

83. Mark DB, et al. Exercise treadmill score for predicting prognosis in coronary artery disease. *Ann Intern Med*. 1987;106:793-800.

84. Morise AP, Haddad WJ, Beckner D. Development and validation of a clinical score to estimate the probability of coronary artery disease in men and women presenting with suspected coronary disease. *Am J Med*. 1997;102:350-356.

85. Mark DB, et al. Prognostic value of a treadmill exercise score in outpatients with suspected coronary artery disease. *N Engl J Med*. 1991;325:849-853.

86. Alexander KP, et al. Value of exercise treadmill testing in women. *J Am Coll Cardiol*. 1998;32:1657-1664.

87. Libby P, Bonow RO, Mann DL, Zipes DP. *Brauwald's Heart Disease: A Textbook of Cardiovascular Medicine*. Philadelphia, PA: Saunders; 2007.

88. Kwok Y, et al. Meta-analysis of exercise testing to detect coronary artery disease in women. *Am J Cardiol*. 1999;83:660-666.

2 RISK FACTORS FOR CARDIOVASCULAR DISEASE

Khadijah Breathett, MD
Martha Gulati, MD, MS, FACC, FAHA

INTRODUCTION

Cardiovascular disease (CVD) remains the leading cause of death in women.[1] Identification of risk factors is the first step toward the prevention of CVD. The 2011 Effectiveness-Based Guidelines for the Prevention of Cardiovascular Disease in Women classifies a woman's risk status as either **high risk, at risk**, or **ideal cardiovascular health**.[2] The classic *high-risk profile* includes the presence of any of the following: clinical CVD, cerebrovascular disease, peripheral arterial disease, abdominal aortic aneurysm, end-stage or chronic kidney disease, diabetes mellitus, or a 10-year Framingham-predicted CVD risk of ≥10%.[2] The *at-risk profile* includes having any of the following: cigarette use, systolic blood pressure (SBP) ≥120 mm Hg, diastolic blood pressure (DBP) ≥80 mm Hg, treatment for hypertension, total cholesterol ≥200 mg/dL, high-density-lipoprotein cholesterol (HDL-C) <50 mg/dL, treatment for dyslipidemia, obesity, poor diet, physical inactivity, family history of premature CVD in first-degree relative, metabolic syndrome, advanced subclinical atherosclerosis, poor exercise capacity on treadmill test and/or abnormal heart rate recovery after stopping exercise, systemic autoimmune collagen-vascular disease, history of preeclampsia, gestational diabetes, or pregnancy-induced hypertension.[2] *Ideal cardiovascular health* includes having all of the following without treatment: total cholesterol <200 mg/dL, BP <120/80 mm Hg, fasting blood glucose <100 mg/dL, body mass index (BMI) <25 kg/m^2, abstinence from tobacco, physical activity for adults >20 years with ≥150-min/wk moderate intensity or ≥75 min/wk vigorous intensity exercise[2] (see Table 2-1).

The second step of the health care provider should be to acknowledge that not only are there sex-specific risk factors for CVD and coronary heart disease (CHD), but also that the same risk factors in men and women do not affect them equally and similarly. Understanding the sex differences in CVD risk may result in a more aggressive patient education and primary prevention of CHD and CVD. This chapter summarizes the CHD and CVD risk factors that are nonmodifiable, modifiable, emerging, and female specific (see Figure 2-1).

TRADITIONAL NONMODIFIABLE RISK FACTORS

FAMILY HISTORY OF CVD

Genomics impact the risk of developing CVD. The Framingham Heart Study demonstrated an association between the family history of CHD and the risk of developing CHD.[3] This study revealed that having a single parent die from CHD resulted in a 30% increased risk of developing CHD.[3] This effect was more pronounced in women compared to men, although this finding may be influenced by a sampling bias. On average, the age of parental death was younger in the women compared to the men, and additional age-adjusted parental death studies have shown slightly lower rates of CVD in women compared to men.[3,4] Nonetheless, family history of premature heart disease, defined as heart disease in a first-degree relative in a woman <65 years or man <55 years, is considered a risk factor for heart disease development (see Figure 2-2).[4] The 2010 ACCF/AHA (American College of Cardiology Foundation/American Heart Association) Guideline for Assessment of Cardiovascular Risk in Asymptomatic Adults recommends that family history of atherothrombotic CVD should be obtained for cardiovascular risk assessment in all asymptomatic adults.[5]

RACE AND ETHNICITY

African American and Mexican American women have higher risk for CVD compared to Caucasian women largely due to increased prevalence of hypertension, central obesity, and diabetes.[6,7] The average age-adjusted CHD incidence per 1000 person-years in a National Heart, Lung, and Blood Institute study was 4 for Caucasian women and 4.9 for African American women.[8] After adjusting for risk factors, rates of CVD in African American women are similar to Caucasian women (see Figure 2-3).[9] However, disparities in CHD and CVD persist with African American women having the highest morbidity and mortality.[10,11] Some of this may be accounted for by inequality in racial distribution of medical management and advanced interventions as detailed in the Institute of Medicine Unequal Treatment report.[11]

AGE

Age is a powerful predictor of CVD, and specifically CHD. The prevalence of CVD increases with age for both sexes, but CHD events lag at least 10 years in women compared to men.[7] For men, there is a linear increase of CHD prevalence with age, in contrast with the more exponential increase with age in women, where the risk of heart disease in a woman is 1 in 8 for women aged 45 to 64 years, but 1 in 3 for women aged 65 years or older.[7]

TRADITIONAL MODIFIABLE RISK FACTORS

TOBACCO USE

International evaluations of the impact of tobacco usage for both men and women have revealed similar risks for CHD.[12,13] However, there is data showing that in women who use tobacco, the risk for CHD is 25% greater than men for the age group of 60 to 69 years.[12] The INTERHEART study suggests that the odds of a woman or man with

TABLE 2-1 Classification of CVD Risk in Women

Risk Status	Class
High risk (≥1 high-risk states)	Clinically manifest CHD Clinically manifest cerebrovascular disease Clinically manifest peripheral arterial disease Abdominal aortic aneurysm End-stage or chronic kidney disease Diabetes mellitus 10-year predicted CVD risk ≥10%
At risk (≥ major risk factor)	Cigarette smoking SBP ≥120 mm Hg, DBP ≥80 mm Hg, or treated hypertension Total cholesterol ≥200 mg/dL, HDL-C <50 mg/dL, or treated for dyslipidemia Obesity, particularly central adiposity Poor diet Physical inactivity Family history of premature CVD occurring in first-degree relative in men <55 y of age or in women <65 y of age Metabolic syndrome Evidence of advanced subclinical atherosclerosis (eg, coronary calcification, carotid plaque, or thickened IMT) Poor exercise capacity on treadmill test and/or abnormal heart rate recovery after stopping exercise Systemic autoimmune collagen-vascular disease (eg, lupus or rheumatoid arthritis) History of preeclampsia, gestational diabetes, or pregnancy-induced hypertension
Ideal cardiovascular health (all of these)	Total cholesterol <200 mg/dL (untreated) BP <120/80 mm Hg (untreated) Fasting blood glucose <100 mg/dL (untreated) Body mass index <25 kg/m^2 Abstinence from smoking Physical activity at goal for adults >20 y of age: >150 min/wk moderate intensity, ≥75 min/wk vigorous intensity, or combination Healthy (DASH-like) diet

CHD, coronary heart disease; DASH, dietary approaches to stop hypertension; DBP, diastolic blood pressure; IMT, intima-media thickness; SBP, systolic blood pressure.
Reproduced with permission from Mosca L et al. Effectiveness-Based Guidelines for the Prevention of Cardiovascular Disease in Women—2011 Update. *J Am Coll Cardiol.* 2011;57:1404-1423.

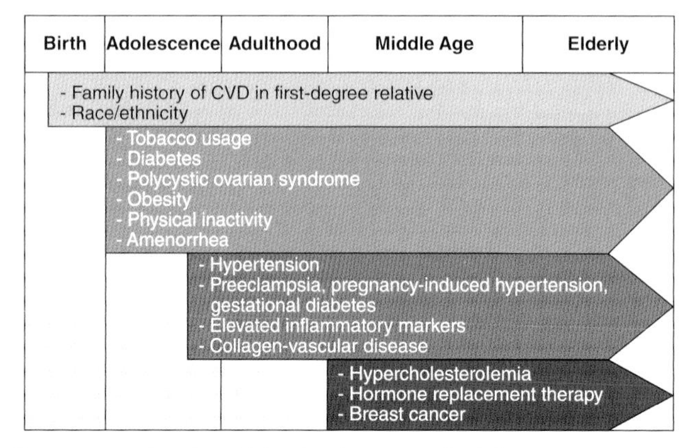

FIGURE 2-1 Risk factor timeline for CVD in women. Timeline of the development of risk factors in a woman's lifetime.
Adapted with permission from Mosca L, et al. Effectiveness-Based Guidelines for the Prevention of Cardiovascular Disease in Women—2011 Update. *J Am Coll Cardiol.* 2011;57:1404-1423.

tobacco usage compared to one without tobacco usage has a 3 times higher risk of developing a myocardial infarction (see Figure 2-4).[13] Furthermore, the overall effects of tobacco usage may be more harmful to women than to men. Female smokers have been reported to die 14.5 years earlier than female nonsmokers, whereas male smokers have been reported to die 13.2 years earlier than male nonsmokers.[14] Education and increased public awareness have assisted in the plight against tobacco usage, particularly among pregnant women.[15] For unclear reasons, the benefit of tobacco cessation has been slightly greater in women than in men with odds of developing a myocardial infarction after tobacco cessation 1½ times higher in men than in women.[13]

HYPERTENSION

The prevalence of hypertension overall was similar in women and men based on the 2009 to 2010 NHANES data, but varies by age.[7,16] Based on the NHANES data, before the age of 45, more men than women have hypertension.[7] As women age, the risk of developing hypertension rises significantly, approaching the level of men from age 45 to 64 and exceeding the rates in men after age 65.[7] During the child-bearing years, women who take oral contraceptive medication are 2 to 3 times more likely to develop hypertension than women who do not take oral contraceptive medications, especially if they are obese.[7,17] Normotensive women who take oral contraceptive medications develop on average 7 to 8 mm Hg increase in systolic blood pressure.[18] In postmenopausal women, risks are heightened with a 10-year incidence of CVD of 3.63% for normotensive women, 7.11% for prehypertensive (systolic blood pressure 120-139 mm Hg or diastolic blood pressure 80-89 mm Hg) women, and 14.16% for hypertensive women[19] (see Figure 2-5). Different target goals will likely be identified in the future installment (eighth report) of the Joint National Committee (JNC) on Prevention, Detection, Evaluation, and Treatment of High Blood Pressure. Improving the public's awareness, prevention, and appropriate treatment would go far in reducing the burden of CHD and CVD.

DIABETES

Diabetes remains a strong risk factor with rising prevalence, affecting 10.8% of US women >20 years of age as of 2010.[20] Diabetes is considered a cardiovascular disease equivalent, given the high risk for the development of CVD. The presence of diabetes is a relatively greater risk factor for CHD in women compared with men, increasing a woman's risk of CHD by 3- to 7-fold with only a 2- to 3-fold increase in diabetic men.[21] Despite advances in care from 1971 to 2000, NHANES reveals that mortality in women with diabetes has doubled compared to women without diabetes whereas the mortality in men with diabetes compared to men without diabetes has declined by 43%.[7]

DYSLIPIDEMIA

Cholesterol levels in women do not follow the same trends as in men. Dyslipidemia is common in women, and more than half of American women have a total cholesterol >200 mg/dL and 36% of them have an LDL cholesterol >130 mg/dL.[7,22] In patients with dyslipidemia, evidence has shown that women on average are 3.5 years older than

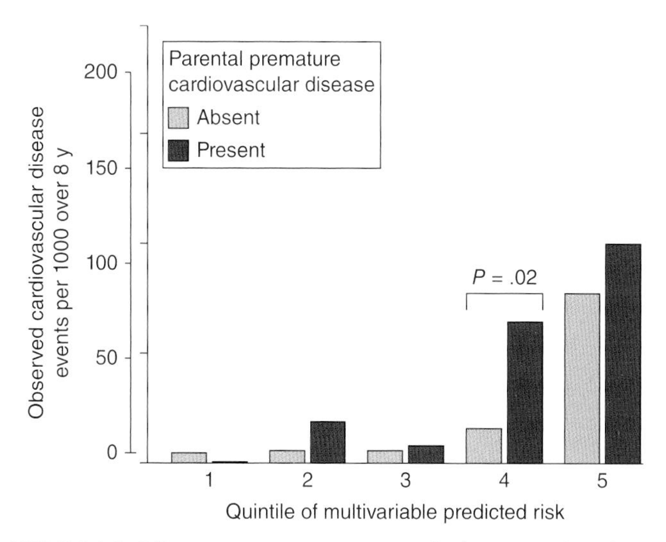

FIGURE 2-2 Offspring participants were stratified into quintiles of predicted risk of cardiovascular disease based on factors: offspring age, systolic blood pressure, total cholesterol to high-density lipoprotein cholesterol ratio, body mass index, diabetes, current smoking, and use of antihypertensive therapy. The risk of CVD based on family history and presence of risk factors are depicted. Study description: Cohort study of 2302 men and women followed an average of 30 years. Reproduced with permission from Lloyd-Jones DM, et al. Parental cardiovascular disease as a risk factor for cardiovascular disease in middle-aged adults: a prospective study of parents and offspring. *JAMA*. 2004;291:2204-2211.

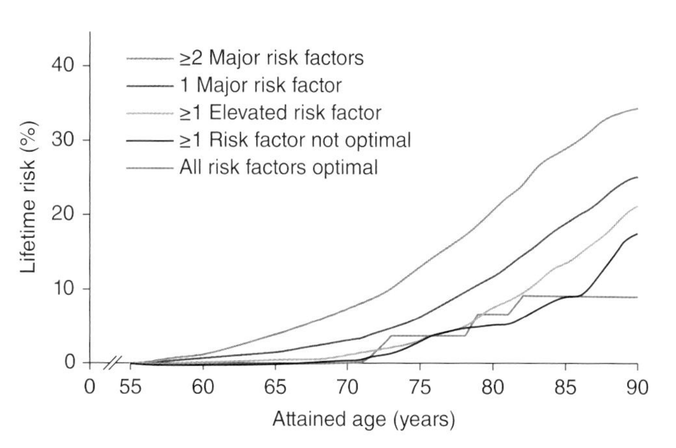

FIGURE 2-3 Lifetime risk of death from cardiovascular disease among African American and Caucasian women at 55 years of age, according to the aggregate burden of risk factors and adjusted for competing risks of death. Optimal indicates nonsmoker, absence of diabetes, total cholesterol <180 mg/dL, untreated systolic blood pressure (SBP) <120 mm Hg, and diastolic blood pressure (DBP) <80 mm Hg; nonoptimal indicates nonsmoker, absence of diabetes, total cholesterol level 180-199 mg/dL, untreated SBP 120-139 mm Hg, or untreated DBP 80-89 mm Hg. Elevated risk indicates nonsmoker, absence of diabetes, total cholesterol level 200-239 mg/dL, untreated SBP 140-159 mm Hg, or untreated DBP 90-99 mm Hg. Major risk factors indicate current smoker, diabetes, treated hypercholesterolemia, untreated total cholesterol level at least 240 mg/dL, treated hypertension, SBP at least 160 mm Hg, or untreated DBP at least 100 mm Hg. Study description: Meta-analysis of 18 cohort studies involving 257,284 African American and Caucasian men and women.
Reproduced with permission from Berry JD, et al. Lifetime risks of cardiovascular disease. *N Engl J Med*. 2012;366:321-329.

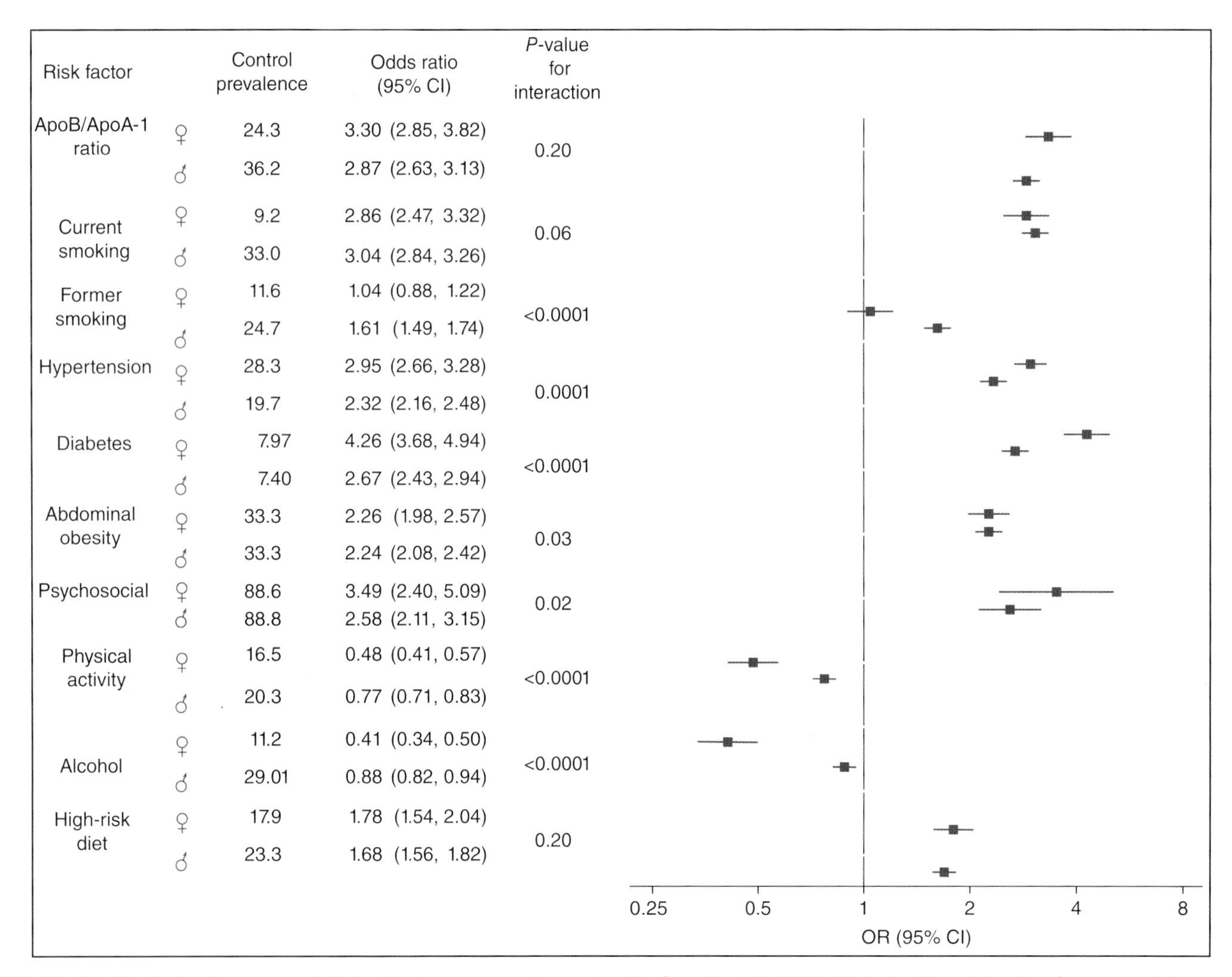

Risk factor		Control prevalence	Odds ratio (95% CI)	*P*-value for interaction
ApoB/ApoA-1 ratio	♀	24.3	3.30 (2.85, 3.82)	0.20
	♂	36.2	2.87 (2.63, 3.13)	
Current smoking	♀	9.2	2.86 (2.47, 3.32)	0.06
	♂	33.0	3.04 (2.84, 3.26)	
Former smoking	♀	11.6	1.04 (0.88, 1.22)	<0.0001
	♂	24.7	1.61 (1.49, 1.74)	
Hypertension	♀	28.3	2.95 (2.66, 3.28)	0.0001
	♂	19.7	2.32 (2.16, 2.48)	
Diabetes	♀	7.97	4.26 (3.68, 4.94)	<0.0001
	♂	7.40	2.67 (2.43, 2.94)	
Abdominal obesity	♀	33.3	2.26 (1.98, 2.57)	0.03
	♂	33.3	2.24 (2.08, 2.42)	
Psychosocial	♀	88.6	3.49 (2.40, 5.09)	0.02
	♂	88.8	2.58 (2.11, 3.15)	
Physical activity	♀	16.5	0.48 (0.41, 0.57)	<0.0001
	♂	20.3	0.77 (0.71, 0.83)	
Alcohol	♀	11.2	0.41 (0.34, 0.50)	<0.0001
	♂	29.01	0.88 (0.82, 0.94)	
High-risk diet	♀	17.9	1.78 (1.54, 2.04)	0.20
	♂	23.3	1.68 (1.56, 1.82)	

FIGURE 2-4 Risk factors for myocardial infarction in women and men: insights from the INTERHEART study. The odds ratio of a myocardial infarction based upon risk factors in men and women are depicted. Study description: Global case-control study including 27,098 participants from 52 countries, of which 6787 were women.
Reproduced with permission from Anand SS, et al. Risk factors for myocardial infarction in women and men: insights from the INTERHEART study. *Eur Heart J.* 2008;29:932-940.

men with higher total cholesterol (TC) and high-density lipoprotein cholesterol (HDL-C) and with lower triglyceride (TG) and TC to HDL-C ratio compared to men.[23] For women, adverse changes in the lipid profile accompany menopause and include increased levels of total cholesterol, LDL-C, and triglycerides and decreased levels of HDL-C, but it remains unclear how much lipid changes are related to aging as opposed to menopause-related hormonal changes.[24-26]

HDL-C is a predictor of CVD in both sexes, but is relatively more predictive in women. The Framingham study showed that in men with the lowest quartile for HDL-C (HDL <36 mg/dL), there was a 70% greater risk of myocardial infarction compared with those in the highest HDL-C quartile (HDL >53 mg/dL). However, this risk was even stronger for women with low HDL-C. Women in the lowest HDL-C quartile (HDL <46 mg/dL) had 6 to 7 times the rate of coronary events compared with those in the highest HDL-C quartile (HDL >67 mg/dL), even after adjustment for other risk factors.[27] For women, HDL-C levels average around 10 mg/dL higher than in men throughout their lives.[27] This is reflected in the Effectiveness-Based

Guidelines for the Prevention of Cardiovascular Disease in Women 2011 Update guidelines and the Adult Treatment Panel III (ATP III) guidelines, as desired HDL-C is recommended to be 50 mg/dL in women as opposed to 40 mg/dL in men.[27]

When deciding upon the best management approach for lipid control in women, we direct the provider to the National Cholesterol Education Program Expert Panel on Detection, Evaluation, and Treatment of High Blood Cholesterol in Adults (NCEP ATP) guideline, which should be updated in the near future.

PHYSICAL ACTIVITY

Physical inactivity is a large contributor to CHD, accounting for 12.2% global burden of CHD.[7] Despite education about the effects of physical inactivity, it continues to worsen. From 2001 to 2006, the proportion of women who exercised >12 bouts a month decreased from 49% to 43.3%.[7] The reliance of self-assessment of activity levels may be insufficient particularly in women. In one study, the women overestimated 138% higher physical activity than actually measured compared to men who overestimated 44% higher physical activity than actually measured.[7] Women and men do not have an equal risk of CHD based on activity levels and corresponding central obesity and waist circumference[13,28] (see Figure 2-4). The Hazard Ratio of future CHD for individuals with inactivity (sedentary job and no recreational physical activity) and increased waist circumference compared to individuals with high activity levels (sedentary job with >1 hour recreational physical activity per day, standing job with >0.5 hours recreational physical activity, physical job with at least some recreational physical activity, or heavy manual job) and decreased waist circumference is 4-fold higher in women and 1.75-fold higher in men.[28] (see Table 2-2) The benefit of physical activity conversely

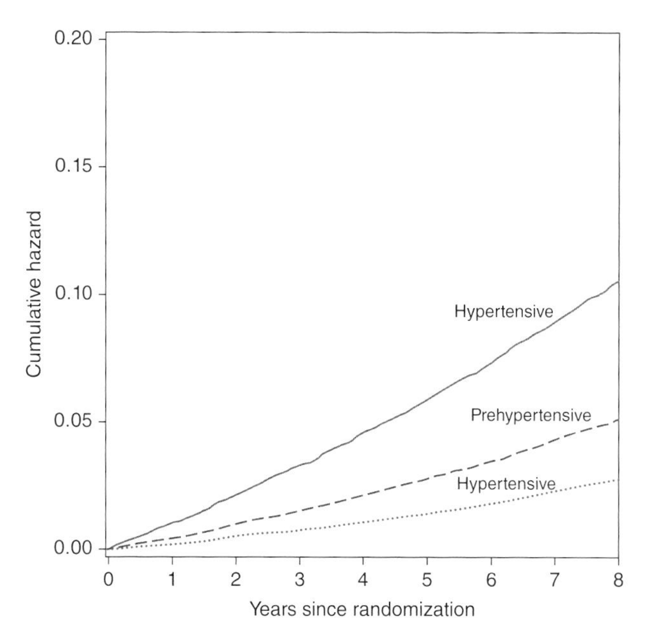

FIGURE 2-5 Cumulative hazard of cardiovascular events by the seventh report of the Joint National Committee on Prevention, Detection, Evaluation, and Treatment of High Blood Pressure. The cumulative hazard of cardiovascular events including myocardial infarction, stroke, hospitalized heart failure, or cardiovascular death is depicted based upon blood pressure levels. Normotensive represents systolic blood pressure <120 mm Hg and diastolic blood pressure <80 mm Hg. Prehypertensive represents systolic blood pressure 120-139 mm Hg or diastolic blood pressure 80-89 mm Hg. Hypertensive represents systolic blood pressure ≥140 mm Hg or diastolic blood pressure ≥90 mm Hg. Study description: Cohort study of Women's Health Initiative with 60,785 postmenopausal women followed for 7.7 years.
Adapted with permission from Hsia, J et al. Prehypertension and cardiovascular disease risk in the Women's Health Initiative. *Circulation*. 2007;115:855-860.

TABLE 2-2 Hazard Ratios[a] for Future Coronary Heart Disease in Men and Women Classified on the Basis of Physical Activity and Waist Circumference

	Active	Moderately Active	Moderately Inactive	Inactive
Men				
Waist <91.0 cm (<35.8 in)	1.00	1.04(0.75-1.45)	1.08(0.77-1.51)	2.18(1.62-2.93)
Waist 91.0-97.9 cm (35.8-38.5 in)	1.39(1.01-1.93)	1.58(1.16-2.15)	1.50(1.10-2.05)	2.05(1.54-2.72)
Waist >98.0 cm (>38.6 in)	1.71(1.26-2.33)	2.32(1.74-3.10)	2.25(1.71-2.98)	3.04(2.35-3.94)
Women				
Waist <76.0 cm (29.9 in)	1.00	2.70(1.29-5.66)	2.58(1.24-5.36)	4.48(2.18-9.19)
Waist 76.0-84.9 cm (29.9-33.4 in)	4.51(2.17-9.37)	4.09(2.00-8.38)	4.37(2.19-8.73)	9.35(4.75-18.4)
Waist >85.0 cm (>33.5 in)	5.34(2.53-11.3)	6.34(3.14-12.79)	9.44(4.81-18.56)	11.38(5.83-22.20)

[a]Coronary heart disease hazard ratios based upon waist circumference and activity levels are listed with 95% confidence intervals in parenthesis. Active is defined as sedentary job with >1 h recreational activity per day, standing job with >0.5 h recreational physical activity per day, physical job with at least some recreational physical activity, or heavy manual job. Moderately active is defined as sedentary job with 0.5-1 h recreational physical activity per day, standing job with 0.5 h recreational activity, physical job with no recreational physical activity. Moderately inactive is defined as sedentary job with <0.5 h recreational physical activity per day, standing job with no recreational physical activity. Inactive is defined as sedentary job and no recreational physical activity. Study description: Prospective, population-based study 21,729 men and women aged 45-79 years living in Norfolk, United Kingdom. Adapted with permission from Arsenault BJ, et al. Physical inactivity, abdominal obesity and risk of coronary heart disease in apparently healthy men and women. *Int J Obes (Lond)*. 2010;34:340-347.

may be higher in women than in men. In a study with young adults followed through middle-age, women with high activity levels gained 6.1 kg less in weight and 3.8 cm less in waist circumference than women with little physical activity, while the corresponding data in men with high activity levels were a gain of 2.6 kg less and 3.1 cm less when compared to men with little physical activity.[7]

Physical fitness, also known as exercise capacity, has been shown to be a strong independent predictor of all-cause mortality in asymptomatic women.[29] In the St. James Women Take Heart Project, asymptomatic women who were unable to achieve 5 metabolic equivalents (METs) on a Bruce protocol had a 3-fold greater risk of death compared with women who achieved >8 METs.[29] In addition, the risk of death among asymptomatic and symptomatic women whose exercise capacity was <85% of the predicted value for age was at least twice that of women whose exercise capacity was at least 85% of their age-predicted value.[29] Assessment of age-predicted fitness can be estimated using the validated nomogram (see Figure 2-6). In the Effectiveness-Based Guidelines for the Prevention of Cardiovascular Disease in Women 2011 Update, physical inactivity or poor physical fitness is criteria for placing a woman in the at-risk group.[2]

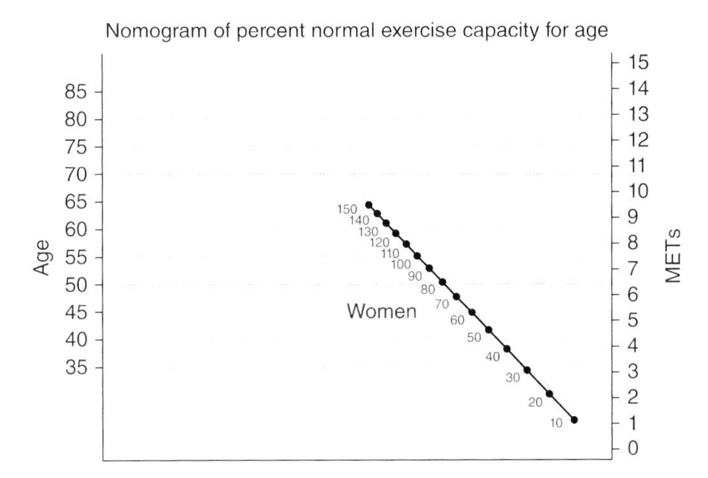

FIGURE 2-6 Nomogram of the percentage or predicted exercise capacity for age in asymptomatic women. A line drawn from the patient's age on the left-hand scale to the MET value on the right-hand scale will cross the percentage line corresponding to the patient's percentage of predicted exercise capacity for age.
Reproduced with permission from Gulati M, et al: The prognostic value of a nomogram for exercise capacity in women. *N Engl J Med.* 2005;353:468.

EMERGING RISK FACTORS

OBESITY

Obesity, defined as a body mass index (BMI) of >30 kg/m^2, is an epidemic in the United States and had equal prevalence in women and men in 2010.[30] However, women are still becoming more obese as they age.[30] Over 42% of women aged ≥60 are obese.[30] In 2004, obesity contributed to 13% of CVD deaths.[7] It was the most powerful predictor of diabetes in the Nurses' Health Study, which compared women with BMI ≥35 kg/m^2 and women with BMI <23 kg/m^2.[7] The same study also revealed a 4 times higher risk of death from CVD for nonsmoking women with BMI ≥32 kg/m^2 compared to women with BMI <19 kg/m^2.[31] Improved health literacy has shown increased awareness of obesity and the CHD risks, but many women have incorrect perceptions of their weight.[32] The health care provider must champion the importance of appropriate weight control and assist with awareness of this disease.

METABOLIC SYNDROME

Metabolic syndrome is defined as having at least 3 of the following: fasting plasma glucose ≥100 mg/dL, HDL<50 mg/dL in women (<40 mg/dL in men) or receiving treatment for low HDL, triglycerides >150 mg/dL or receiving treatment for elevated triglycerides, waist circumference ≥35 in. in women (≥40 in. in men), and systolic blood pressure ≥130 mm Hg or diastolic blood pressure ≥85 mm Hg or receiving treatment for hypertension.[7] NHANES data from 2003 to 2006 revealed that the age-adjusted prevalence of metabolic syndrome in women was 32.6%, rising to 54.4% in women aged ≥60 and also persistently higher in ethnic minority women.[7] In addition, the risk of CVD has been noted to be 1.3 times higher in women than in men.[7] After identifying the population with metabolic syndrome, aggressive prevention measures will help reduce the burden of CHD.

HIGH-SENSITIVITY C-REACTIVE PROTEIN

High-sensitivity C-reactive protein (hsCRP) has an association with risk of future CVD.[33,34] Although other markers of inflammation including fibrinogen, leukocyte count, albumin, and erythrocyte sedimentation rate have shown linear correlation with CRP, the preponderance of data for CVD exists with CRP.[34] Often CRP levels are higher in women than in men.[34] High-sensitivity CRP is additive in predicting risk of CVD with corresponding higher levels of non-HDL, apolipoprotein B100, TC/HDL-C ratio, and apolipoprotein B100/apolipoprotein A1.[33] In many cases, CRP is a better predictor of CVD in women with a goal LDL level.[35,36] An elevated CRP, >3, becomes particularly helpful in determining an accurate CVD risk even after using the Framingham risk score and is utilized in the Reynolds risk score which is described in the next chapter[36] (see Figure 2-7). Nonetheless, measuring hsCRP is not recommended in routine risk assessment among women, but rather as an option in those persons in the intermediate risk range based on the Framingham risk score.[36,37] The benefits of assessing hsCRP or any treatment based on this strategy remain uncertain.

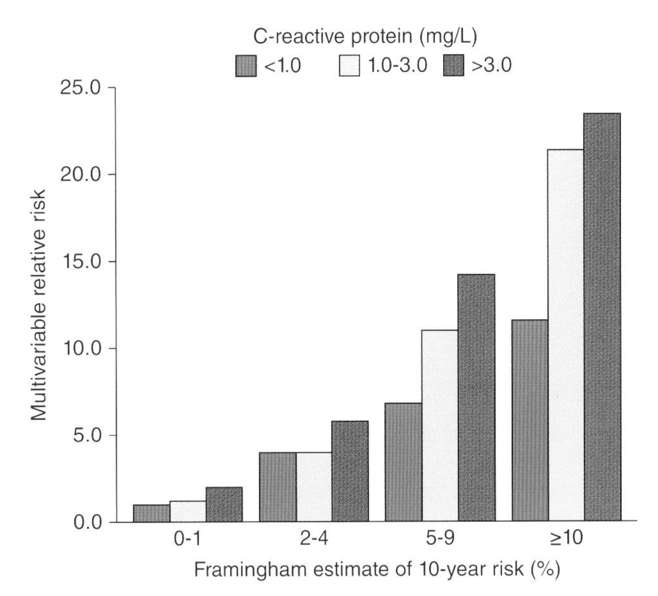

FIGURE 2-7 Multivariate adjusted relative risk of CVD in the Women's Health Study, according to levels of CRP and the estimated 10-year risk based on the Framingham cardiovascular risk score. Study description: Prospective study of 27,939 women with initial average age of 55 years from the Woman's Health Study.
Reproduced with permission from Albert MA, Ridker PM. C-reactive protein as a risk predictor: do race/ethnicity and gender make a difference? *Circulation.* 2006;114:e67-e74.

SYSTEMIC AUTOIMMUNE COLLAGEN-VASCULAR DISEASE (LUPUS OR RHEUMATOID ARTHRITIS)

Systemic lupus erythematosus (SLE) and rheumatoid arthritis (RA) are known inflammatory diseases which inordinately affect women, and the risk for coronary artery disease (CAD) increases up to 50 times the risk of the general population in patients with SLE.[2,38-40] Increased proinflammatory HDL, increased production of asymmetric dimethyl arginine (ADMA), and endogenous inhibitor of nitrous oxide have all been implicated in worsening risk of CAD for patients with inflammatory disease.[41,42] RA has been shown to increase the number of diseased coronary vessels as well as mortality from CAD.[40] The odds ratio of having RA for each diseased coronary vessel is 1.73 times higher, and the hazard ratio for CAD with RA versus CAD alone is doubled[40] (see Figure 2-8). Upon diagnosis of a systemic autoimmune collagen-vascular disease, aggressive primary prevention is indicated throughout the patient's life.

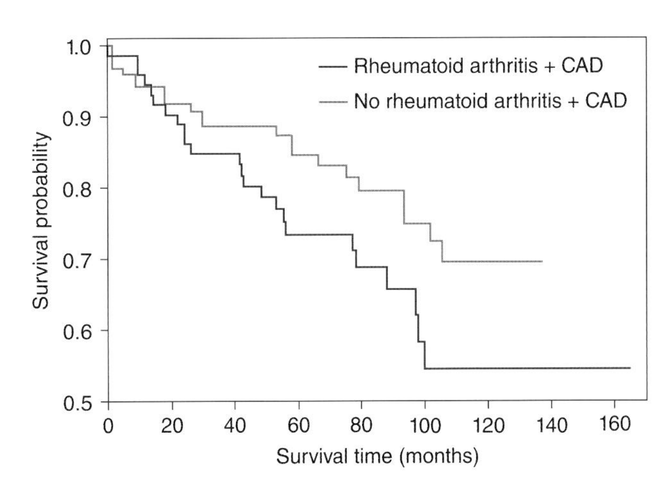

FIGURE 2-8 Kaplan-Meier survival curves in CAD patients with and without rheumatoid arthritis. Kaplan-Meier survival curves for patients with rheumatoid arthritis + CAD and without rheumatoid arthritis + CAD are depicted with $p = .097$. Study description: Retrospective matched cohort of 75 patients with rheumatoid arthritis and new diagnosis of CAD and 128 patients with new diagnosis of CAD alone.
Adapted with permission from Warrington KJ, et al. Rheumatoid arthritis is an independent risk factor for multi-vessel coronary artery disease: a case control study. *Arthritis Res Ther.* 2005;7:R984-R991.

SUBCLINICAL ATHEROSCLEROSIS

Subclinical atherosclerosis remains a threat for future CVD mortality, particularly in women. The asymptomatic nature of this disease requires a high level of suspicion to diagnose and is worth the effort to do so. The prognostic capabilities of diagnosing CVD mortality is significantly higher with measurements like coronary calcium in women compared to men.[43] There have also been differences in disease patterns of carotid plaque and thickened intima-media, although in general women compared to men have less mortality and less need for intervention.[44,45]

FEMALE-SPECIFIC RISK FACTORS

PREECLAMPSIA AND PREGNANCY-INDUCED HYPERTENSION

Preeclampsia, the development of new-onset hypertension and proteinuria (urinary excretion ≥300 mg protein in 24 hours) after 20 weeks gestation, and pregnancy-induced hypertension or gestational

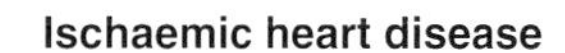

Study	Ischaemic heart disease: Total No of cases/women who had preeclampsia	Ischaemic heart disease: Total No of cases/women who did not have preeclampsia	Relative risk (random) (95% CI)
Hannaford 1997[w8]	69/2371	216/14 831	1.65 (1.26-2.16)
Irgens 2001[w15]	27/24 155	325/602 117	3.61 (0.76-17.18)*
Smith 2001[w16]	12/22 781	31/106 509	1.70 (0.86-3.35)
Wilson 2003[w13]	26/1043	10/796	1.95 (0.90-4.22)
Kestenbaum 2003[W14]	35/20 552	64/92 902	2.55 (1.70-3.83)†
Funai 2005[W17]	41/1070	269/35 991	3.01 (2.18-4.33)
Ray 2005[W18]	228/36 982‡	1262/950 885	2.10 (1.82-2.42)
Wirkstrom 2005[W19]	176/12 533	2306/383 081	2.21 (1.56-3.31)†
Total (95% CI)	614/121 487	4483/2 187 112	2.16 (1.86-2.52)

Test for heterogeneity: $\chi^2 = 9.60$, df = 7, P = 0.21, $I^2 = 27.1\%$

Test for overall effect: z = 10.00, P = 0.001

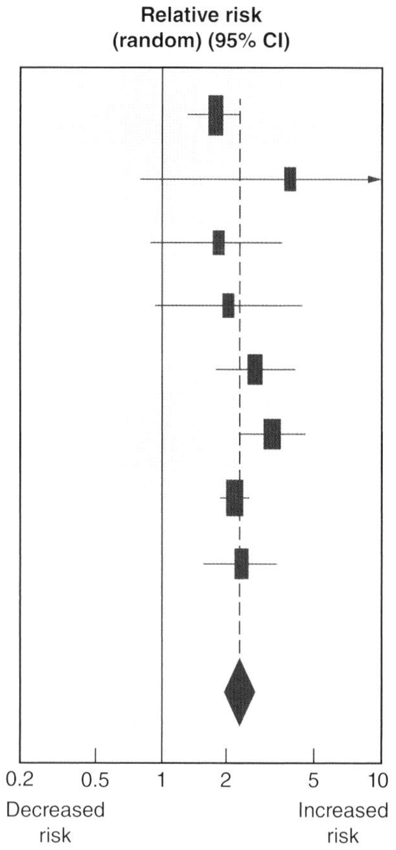

FIGURE 2-9 The risk of fatal and nonfatal ischemic heart disease events in later life based upon history of preeclampsia is depicted from a systematic review of the evidence. Study description: Systematic review and meta-analysis including 198,252 women with preeclampsia.
Reproduced with permission from Bellamy L, Casas J-P, Hingorani AD, Williams DJ. Preeclampsia and risk of cardiovascular disease and cancer in later life: systematic review and meta-analysis. *BMJ*. 2007;335:974.

hypertension are all associated with CVD.[46-49] Many times the health care providers are not aware of this association and are, therefore, unable to appropriately counsel the patients.[47] There are ongoing studies to assess if patients are even asked about a history of preeclampsia during a new patient visit. This is a great misfortune given that the relative risk of developing CVD after preeclampsia is 2-fold higher after 11.7 years[46] (see Figure 2-9). A recent Finnish study has also suggested that any form of hypertension including gestational hypertension, diastolic hypertension, chronic hypertension, and superimposed preeclampsia/eclampsia have been associated with increased risk of future development of ischemic heart disease.[49] Gestational hypertension has also been associated with increased risk of heart failure, diabetes, chronic kidney disease, as well as general CVD.[49] In addition, further risk of CVD by elevated blood pressure and BMI is passed on to the offspring of preeclamptic mothers.[50] Currently there are no specific guidelines for CVD management in women with a history of preeclampsia. Yet, recognizing that these patients are in higher risk and require aggressive care will go far in helping reduce the CVD risk in women.

GESTATIONAL DIABETES MELLITUS

Gestational diabetes increases a woman's risk of CVD by impairing glucose metabolism, contributing to obesity, dyslipidemia, and increased inflammatory markers.[51] Effects have been noted as short as 2 years after delivery with 57% of women developing diabetes or impaired glucose tolerance.[51] After 11 years, the hazard ratio of CAD in women with a history of gestational diabetes compared to women without a history of gestational diabetes is nearly double[52] (see Figure 2-10). The Avon Longitudinal Study of Parents and Children in England has shown that gestational diabetes increases the 10-year risk of developing CVD by 26%.[53] The Effectiveness-Based Guidelines for the Prevention of Cardiovascular Disease in Women 2011 Update incorporated a history of gestational diabetes as an "at risk" criterion, requiring attention to cardiovascular risk factors and the implementation of therapeutic lifestyle changes in these women throughout their life.[2]

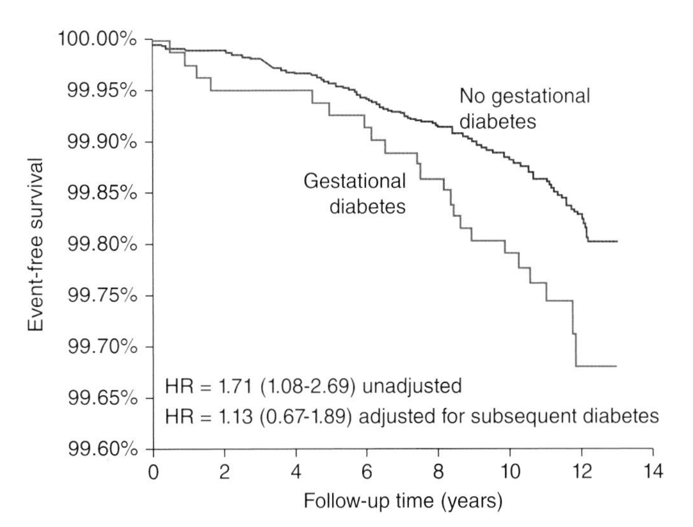

FIGURE 2-10 Kaplan-Meier survival curves for CVD and CAD events in women with and without a history of gestational diabetes. Study description: Matched cohort 8191 women with gestational diabetes and 81,262 women without gestational diabetes followed for an average of 11.5 years.
Adapted with permission from Shah BR, Retnakaran R, Booth GL. Increased risk of cardiovascular disease in young women following gestational diabetes mellitus. *Dia Care.* 2008;31:1668-1669.

POLYCYSTIC OVARIAN SYNDROME

Polycystic ovarian syndrome (PCOS) is defined as hyperandrogenemia with a history of irregular menses and affects 5% to 7% of reproductive-aged women.[54,55] PCOS has been associated with a 3-fold higher risk of CVD.[54] After adjusting for age and basal metabolic index, it has been shown to increase the odds ratio of CVD by 1.71.[54] The cumulative 5-year cardiovascular event-free survival for a woman with PCOS is 78.9% and 88.7% without PCOS.[54] This may be secondary to obvious hormonal reasons as well as higher levels of CD40 ligand, homocysteine.[54] Although high-sensitivity CRP does not consistently correlate with the presence of PCOS, the presence of both greatly increases the risk of CVD by 12.2%.[54,55] Subsequently coronary calcification is more prevalent in young women with PCOS aged 30 to 45 years.[54]

AMENORRHEA

Amenorrhea secondary to both hypothalamic changes and hysterectomy is associated with CVD of varying degrees.[56,57] Functional hypothalamic amenorrhea, hypoestrogenemia in the absence of menses, is generally due to stress, weight loss, or exercise.[56] Early CVD has been seen in this population, and psychogenic stress has been shown to be a risk factor for angiographic CAD.[56,58] Endothelial dysfunction and abnormal response to stress are perceived to be etiologies.[56,58] Hysterectomy with and without oophorectomy, however, have little impact on CVD after adjusting for traditional risk factors[57] (see Table 2-3).

REPRODUCTIVE HORMONES/HORMONE REPLACEMENT THERAPY

Oral Contraceptive Therapy

The American College of Obstetricians and Gynecologists (ACOG) and the World Health Organization (WHO) have published guidelines on medical eligibility for contraceptive use.[59,60] For most women, who are healthy and free of cardiovascular disease and cardiovascular risk factors, the use of combination estrogen-progestin oral contraceptives is associated with low relative and absolute risks of CVD.[59,60] Women who are smokers, >35 years of age, have uncontrolled hypertension, and have a history of ischemic heart disease have an

TABLE 2-3 Combined Models[a] of Incident Cardiovascular Disease by Hysterectomy/Oophorectomy Status

Model No. and Variables		HR	95% CI	P	Adjustments
1	Hysterectomy only	1.23	(1.11-1.36)	<0.001	None
	Hysterectomy plus oophorectomy	1.28	(1.16-1.42)	<0.001	
	All hysterectomies	1.26	(1.16-1.36)	<0.001	
2	Hysterectomy only	1.14	(1.02-1.27)	0.021	Demographics (age, ethnicity, family history of early MI, education, income)
	Hysterectomy plus oophorectomy	1.19	(1.07-1.33)	0.002	
	All hysterectomies	1.16	(1.07-1.27)	<0.001	
3	Hysterectomy only	1.11	(0.99-1.25)	0.064	Above plus body measures (waist, BMI, WBC, physical activity, dietary saturated fat)
	Hysterectomy plus oophorectomy	1.16	(1.04-1.30)	0.009	
	All hysterectomies	1.14	(1.04-1.25)	0.006	
4	Hysterectomy only	1.10	(0.98-1.23)	0.118	Above plus baseline conditions (smoking, hypertension, diabetes, high cholesterol, PAD ever, DVT ever)
	Hysterectomy plus oophorectomy	1.11	(0.99-1.24)	0.086	
	All hysterectomies	1.10	(1.00-1.21)	0.042	

BMI, body mass index; DVT, deep venous thrombosis; PAD, peripheral arterial disease;WBC, white blood cell.
[a]Combined models of CVD hazard ratio based upon hysterectomy and oophorectomy status combined with risk factors are depicted. Study description: Cohort study from the Women's Health Initiative 89,914 women.
Adapted with permission from Howard BV, et al. Risk of cardiovascular disease by hysterectomy status, with and without oophorectomy: the Women's Health Initiative Observational Study. *Circulation*. 2005;111:1462-1470.

unacceptable level of risk associated with oral contraceptives and as such, should not be prescribed oral contraceptives.[59,60]

Postmenopausal Hormone Therapy

The majority of CVD occurs after menopause in women, which is associated with an increased burden of established cardiac risk factors. Because of this, it was hypothesized that postmenopause hormone therapy would reduce the CVD risk, and initial observational data supported this hypothesis. Nonetheless, to date, randomized trials such as Heart and Estrogen/Progestin Replacement Study (HERS) I, HERS II, Women's Health Initiative (WHI), and Raloxifene Use for The Heart (RUTH) did not find hormone therapy or selective estrogen receptor modulators (SERMs) to prevent CVD, in terms of either primary or secondary prevention.[61-63] However, there is new data that perhaps hormone replacement therapy may be less detrimental to middle-aged women, aged 50 to 59.[19,62,64,65] The AHA Effectiveness-Based Guidelines for the Prevention of Cardiovascular Disease in Women 2011 Update states that hormone replacement therapy and SERMS should not be used for the primary or secondary prevention of cardiovascular disease and are a Class III, level of evidence A, intervention.[2]

BREAST CANCER/BREAST CANCER TREATMENT

Chemotherapy

The classes of anthracycline and trastuzumab are commonly used in the treatment of breast cancer. For over 30 years, anthracycline has also been associated with alarming rates of cardiotoxicity and heart failure that may not be reversible.[66-69] Anthracyclines are thought to cause myocardiocyte cell death, and trastuzumab causes myocardiocyte cell injury which may make the latter more reversible with evidence-based heart failure medications.[67] Women who receive these forms of therapy warrant regular cardiac assessment for prompt dose adjustment and management of heart failure.[67]

Radiation Treatment

Although a great risk for CVD stems from radiation therapy, some of the risk may also be initiated pretherapy.[70-72] Higher coronary artery calcium scores have been seen in women aged 55 to 64 years with breast cancer compared to those without cancer.[70] Radiation therapy has shown increased vascular deaths and higher incidence of CHD with radiation of the left breast[72,73] (see Figure 2-11). However in one cohort analysis, radiation therapy has shown no significant risk for CHD from 1980 to 1986 compared to the period from 1970 to 1979, perhaps owing to technical advances in breast cancer therapy[71] (see Figure 2-12). Women with a history of breast cancer should be monitored closely for the development of CHD.

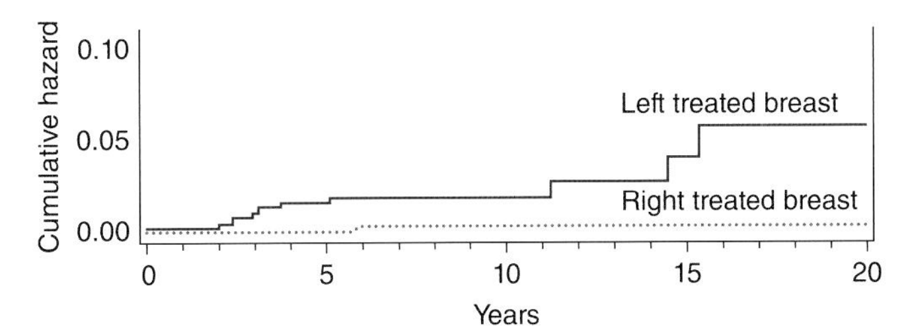

FIGURE 2-11 Cumulative incidence of first posttreatment myocardial infarction following breast-conserving surgery and radiotherapy for breast cancer, stratified by the laterality of the treated breast. Study description: Cohort of 828 patients with breast-conserving surgery and radiation therapy.
Adapted with permission from Jagsi R, Griffith KA, Koelling T, Roberts R, Pierce LJ. Rates of myocardial infarction and coronary artery disease and risk factors in patients treated with radiation therapy for early-stage breast cancer. *Cancer* 2007;109:650-657.

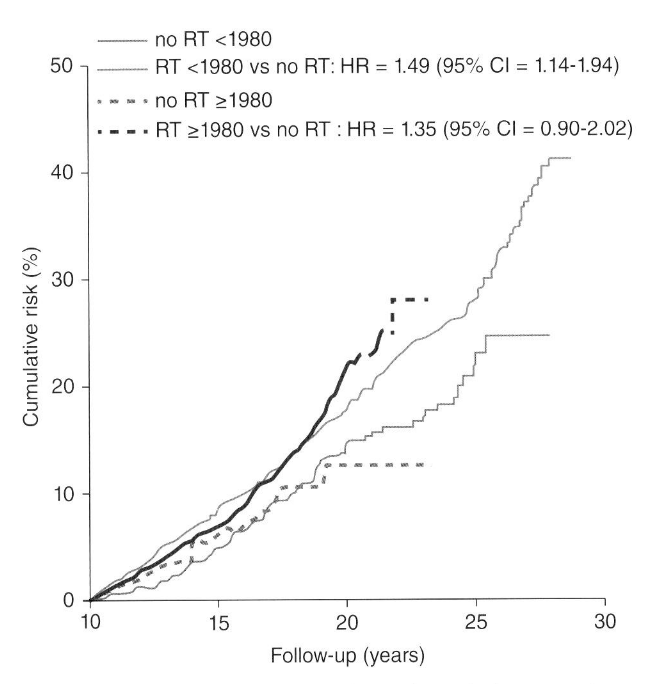

FIGURE 2-12 Risk of cardiovascular disease by radiotherapy and treatment period, adjusted for age. This is done to assess for the difference that may be impacted by higher dosage levels with more archaic forms of radiation pre 1980. Study description: Cohort of 4414 ten-year survivors of breast cancer over median follow-up for 18 years. *Abbreviation*: RT, radiation therapy.
Reproduced with permission from Hooning MJ, et al. Long-term risk of cardiovascular disease in 10-year survivors of breast cancer. *J Natl Cancer Inst.* 2007;99:365-375.

CONCLUSION

The health care provider has a prominent role in the prevention of CHD in women which can present at varied times throughout a woman's life span. Attention to the risk factors that are nonmodifiable, modifiable, emerging, and female specific at each visit will help the provider keep the patient aware of her CHD risk and assist with appropriate management. It is also imperative that the health care provider takes a direct role in promoting lifestyle modification. Although lifestyle modification is one of the most difficult goals for patients to achieve and thus for providers to instruct and lead, it is one of the most beneficial modes of primary and secondary prevention of CHD. Tobacco cessation and reduction of metabolic syndrome disease profile alone lead to noticeable benefit in risk reduction of CHD, more so in women than in men. The AHA 2011 prevention guidelines recommend assessing for evaluation of CVD risk and implementing lifestyle recommendations for all patients which include tobacco cessation, diet high in vegetables/fruit and low in sodium/saturated fats, engaging in regular physical activity, and maintaining an appropriate weight.[10] Further medicinal goals should be based upon specific risk factors which can be guided by the JNC for hypertension, NCEP ATP for lipids, and supplemented by Effectiveness-Based Guidelines for the Prevention of Cardiovascular Disease in Women (see Figure 2-13).

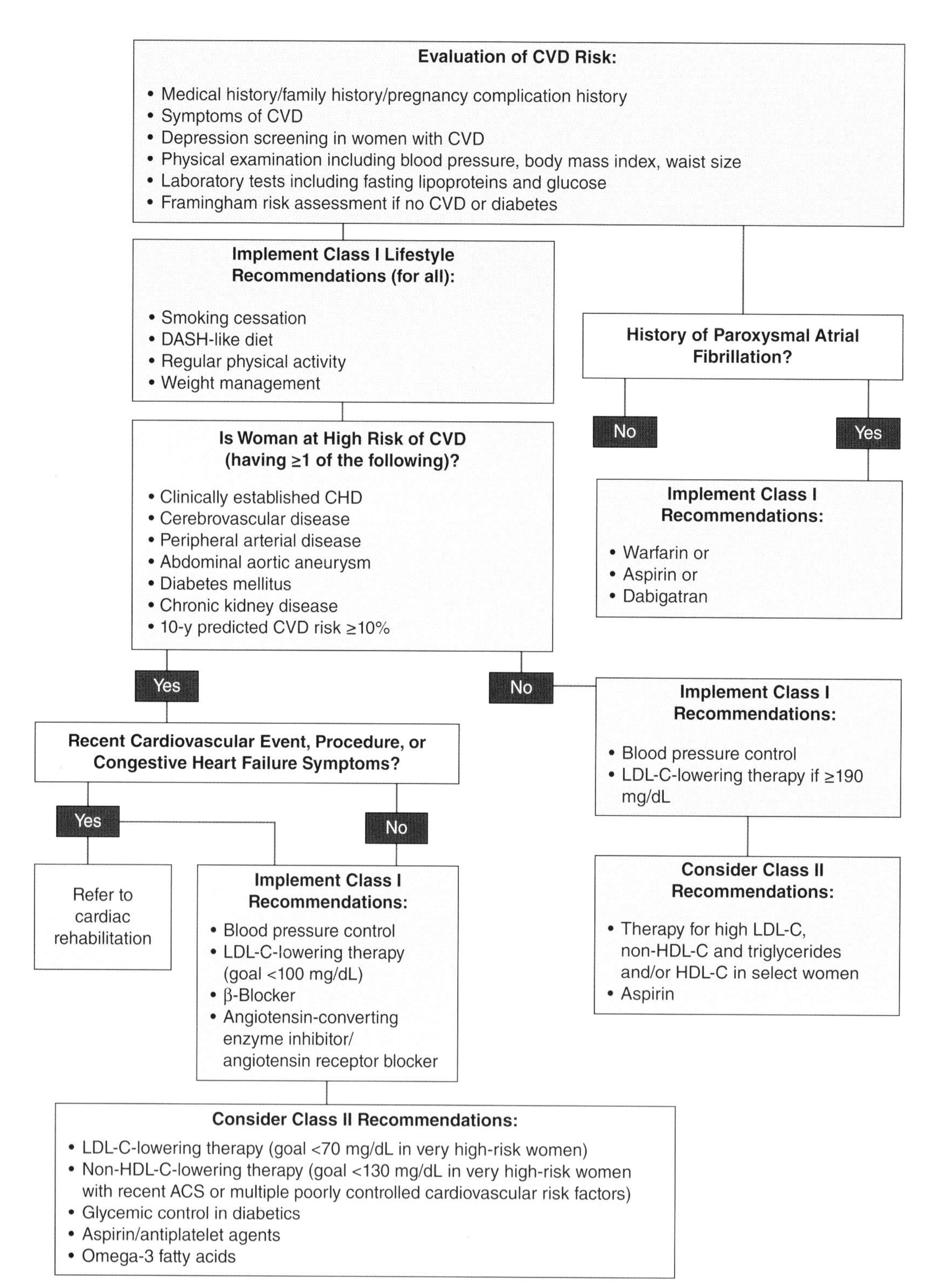

FIGURE 2-13 Flow diagram for CVD prevention in women. *Abbreviations*: ACS, acute coronary syndrome; CHD, coronary heart disease; DASH, dietary approaches to stop hypertension.
Reproduced with permission from Mosca L, et al. Effectiveness-Based Guidelines for the Prevention of Cardiovascular Disease in Women—2011 Update. *J Am Coll Cardiol.* 2011;57:1404-1423.

REFERENCES

1. CDC-DHDSP Fact Sheets. Women and Heart Disease Fact Sheet. http://www.cdc.gov/dhdsp/data_statistics/fact_sheets/fs_women_heart.htm. Accessed on 29 Dec 2012.
2. Mosca L, et al. Effectiveness-Based Guidelines for the Prevention of Cardiovascular Disease in Women—2011 Update. *J Am Coll Cardiol.* 2011;57:1404-1423.
3. Schildkraut JM, Myers RH, Cupples LA, Kiely DK, Kannel WB. Coronary risk associated with age and sex of parental heart disease in the Framingham Study. *Am J Cardiol.* 1989:64;555-559.
4. Lloyd-Jones DM, et al. Parental cardiovascular disease as a risk factor for cardiovascular disease in middle-aged adults: a prospective study of parents and offspring. *JAMA.* 2004;291:2204-2211.
5. Greenland P, et al. 2010 ACCF/AHA guideline for assessment of cardiovascular risk in asymptomatic adults: a report of the American College of Cardiology Foundation/American Heart Association Task Force on Practice Guidelines. *J Am Coll Cardiol.* 2010;56:e50-e103.
6. Sundquist J, et al. Cardiovascular disease risk factors among older black, Mexican-American, and white women and men: an analysis of NHANES III, 1988-1994. Third National Health and Nutrition Examination Survey. *J Am Geriatr Soc.* 2001;49:109-116.
7. Go AS, et al. Heart disease and stroke statistics—2013 update: a report from the American Heart Association. *Circulation.* 2013;127:e6-e245.
8. Roger VL, et al. Heart Disease and Stroke Statistics—2011 Update.: A Report from the American Heart Association. *Circulation.* 2011;123:e18-e209.
9. Berry JD, et al. Lifetime risks of cardiovascular disease. *N Engl J Med.* 2012;366:321-329.
10. Mosca L, et al. Twelve-year follow-up of American women's awareness of cardiovascular disease risk and barriers to heart health. *Circ Cardiovasc Qual Outcomes.* 2010;3:120-127.
11. Unequal Treatment: Confronting Racial and Ethnic Disparities in Health Care: Institute of Medicine. http://www.iom.edu/Reports/2002/Unequal-Treatment-Confronting-Racial-and-Ethnic-Disparities-in-Health-Care.aspx. Accessed on 21 Aug 2012.
12. Huxley RR, Woodward M. Cigarette smoking as a risk factor for coronary heart disease in women compared with men: a systematic review and meta-analysis of prospective cohort studies. *The Lancet.* 2011;378:1297-1305.
13. Anand SS, et al. Risk factors for myocardial infarction in women and men: insights from the INTERHEART study. *Eur Heart J.* 2008;29:932-940.
14. Annual smoking-attributable mortality, years of potential life lost, and economic costs—United States, 1995-1999. *MMWR Morb Mortal Wkly Rep.* 2002;51:300-303.
15. Lloyd-Jones D, et al. Executive summary: heart disease and stroke statistics—2010 update: a report from the American Heart Association. *Circulation.* 2010;121:948-954.
16. Guo F, et al. Trends in prevalence, awareness, management, and control of hypertension among United States adults, 1999 to 2010. *J Am Coll Cardiol.* 2012;60:599-606.
17. Chobanian AV, et al. Seventh report of the Joint National Committee on Prevention, Detection, Evaluation, and Treatment of High Blood Pressure. *Hypertension.* 2003;42:1206-1252.
18. Shufelt CL, Noel Bairey Merz C. Contraceptive hormone use and cardiovascular disease. *J Am Coll Cardiol.* 2009;53:221-231.
19. Hsia J, et al. Prehypertension and cardiovascular disease risk in the Women's Health Initiative. *Circulation.* 2007;115:855-860.
20. CDC: 2011 National Estimates. 2011 National Diabetes Fact Sheet: Publications: Diabetes DDT. http://www.cdc.gov/diabetes/pubs/estimates11.htm. Accessed on 30 Dec 2012.
21. Huxley R. Excess risk of fatal coronary heart disease associated with diabetes in men and women: meta-analysis of 37 prospective cohort studies. *BMJ.* 2006;332:73-78.
22. Vital Signs: Prevalence, Treatment, and Control of High Levels of Low-Density Lipoprotein Cholesterol—United States, 1999-2002 and 2005-2008. http://www.cdc.gov/mmwr/preview/mmwrhtml/mm6004a5.htm#tab.
23. Kolovou GD, et al. Gender differences in the lipid profile of dyslipidemic subjects. *Eur J Intern Med.* 2009;20:145-151.
24. Polotsky HN, Polotsky AJ. Metabolic implications of menopause. *Semin Reprod Med.* 2010;28:426-434.
25. Jensen J, et al. Influence of menopause on serum lipids and lipoproteins. *Maturitas.* 1990;12:321-331.
26. Gierach GL, et al. Hypertension, menopause, and coronary artery disease risk in the Women's Ischemia Syndrome Evaluation (WISE) Study. *J Am Coll. Cardiol.* 2006;47:S50-S58.
27. Abbott RD, et al. High-density lipoprotein cholesterol, total cholesterol screening, and myocardial infarction. The Framingham Study. *Arterioscler Thromb Vasc Biol.* 1988;8:207-211.
28. Arsenault BJ, et al. Physical inactivity, abdominal obesity and risk of coronary heart disease in apparently healthy men and women. *Int J Obes* (Lond) 2010;34:340-347.
29. Gulati M, et al. Exercise Capacity and the Risk of Death in Women The St James Women Take Heart Project. *Circulation.* 2003;108:1554-1559.
30. Products: Data Briefs: Number 82—January 2012. http://www.cdc.gov/nchs/data/databriefs/db82.htm. Accessed on 17 May 2013.
31. Manson JE, et al. Body weight and mortality among women. *N Engl J Med.* 1995;333:677-685.
32. Darlow S, et al. Weight perceptions and perceived risk for diabetes and heart disease among overweight and obese women, Suffolk County, New York, 2008. *Prev Chronic Dis.* 2012. doi:10.5888/pcd9.110185. Accessed on 17 May 2013.
33. Ridker PM, et al. Non-HDL cholesterol, apolipoproteins A-I and B100, standard lipid measures, lipid ratios, and CRP as risk factors for cardiovascular disease in women. *JAMA.* 2005;294:326-333.
34. Kaptoge S, et al. C-reactive protein concentration and risk of coronary heart disease, stroke, and mortality: an individual participant meta-analysis. *Lancet.* 2010;375:132-140.
35. Ridker PM, et al. C-reactive protein and other markers of inflammation in the prediction of cardiovascular disease in women. *N Engl J Med.* 2000;342:836-843.

36. Albert MA, Ridker PM. C-reactive protein as a risk predictor: do race/ethnicity and gender make a difference? *Circulation.* 2006;114:e67-e74.

37. Third report of the National Cholesterol Education Program (NCEP) Expert Panel on Detection, Evaluation, and Treatment of High Blood Cholesterol in Adults (Adult Treatment Panel III): Final Report. *Circulation.* 2002;106:3143-3421.

38. CDC. Arthritis: Basics: Definition: Lupus. http://www.cdc.gov/arthritis/basics/lupus.htm#2. Accessed on 31 Dec 2012.

39. CDC. Arthritis: Basics: Definition: Rheumatoid Arthritis. http://www.cdc.gov/arthritis/basics/rheumatoid.htm. Accessed on 31 Dec 2012.

40. Warrington KJ, et al. Rheumatoid arthritis is an independent risk factor for multi-vessel coronary artery disease: a case control study. *Arthritis Res Ther.* 2005;7:R984-R991.

41. McMahon M, et al. Proinflammatory high-density lipoprotein as a biomarker for atherosclerosis in patients with systemic lupus erythematosus and rheumatoid arthritis. *Arthritis Rheum.* 2006;54:2541-2549.

42. Turiel M, et al. Non-invasive assessment of coronary flow reserve and ADMA levels: a case-control study of early rheumatoid arthritis patients. *Rheumatology.* 2009;48:834-839.

43. Raggi P, et al. Gender-based differences in the prognostic value of coronary calcification. *J Womens Health (Larchmt).* 2004;13:273-283.

44. Ebrahim S, et al. Carotid plaque, intima media thickness, cardiovascular risk factors, and prevalent cardiovascular disease in men and women: the British regional heart study. *Stroke.* 1999;30:841-850.

45. Mughal MM, et al. Symptomatic and asymptomatic carotid artery plaque. *Expert Rev Cardiovasc Ther.* 2011;9:1315-1330.

46. Bellamy L, et al. Pre-eclampsia and risk of cardiovascular disease and cancer in later life: systematic review and meta-analysis. *BMJ.* 2007;335:974.

47. Young B, et al. Physicians' knowledge of future vascular disease in women with preeclampsia. *Hypertens Pregnancy.* 2012;31:50-58.

48. Hutcheon JA, et al. Epidemiology of pre-eclampsia and the other hypertensive disorders of pregnancy. *Best Pract Res Clin Obstet Gynaecol.* 2011;25:391-403.

49. Männistö T, et al. Elevated blood pressure in pregnancy and subsequent chronic disease risk. *Circulation.* 2013;127:681-690.

50. Davis EF, et al. Cardiovascular risk factors in children and young adults born to preeclamptic pregnancies: a systematic review. *Pediatrics.* 2012;129:e1552-e1561.

51. Rivero K, et al. Prevalence of the impaired glucose metabolism and its association with risk factors for coronary artery disease in women with gestational diabetes. *Diabetes Res Clin Pract.* 2008;79:433-437.

52. Shah BR, et al. Increased risk of cardiovascular disease in young women following gestational diabetes mellitus. *Dia Care.* 2008;31:1668-1669.

53. Fraser A, et al. Associations of Pregnancy Complications With Calculated Cardiovascular Disease Risk and Cardiovascular Risk Factors in Middle Age clinical perspective: The Avon Longitudinal Study of Parents and Children. *Circulation.* 2012;125:1367-1380.

54. Shaw LJ, et al. Postmenopausal women with a history of irregular menses and elevated androgen measurements at high risk for worsening cardiovascular event-free survival: results from the National Institutes of Health—National Heart, Lung, and Blood Institute sponsored Women's Ischemia Syndrome Evaluation. *J Clin Endocrinol Metab.* 2008;93:1276-1284.

55. Oktem M, et al. Polycystic ovary syndrome is associated with elevated plasma soluble CD40 ligand, a marker of coronary artery disease. *Fertil Steril.* 2009;91:2545-2550.

56. O'Donnell E, et al. Clinical review: cardiovascular consequences of ovarian disruption: a focus on functional hypothalamic amenorrhea in physically active women. *J Clin Endocrinol Metab.* 2011;96:3638-3648.

57. Howard BV, et al. Risk of cardiovascular disease by hysterectomy status, with and without oophorectomy: the Women's Health Initiative Observational Study. *Circulation.* 2005;111:1462-1470.

58. Bairey Merz CN, et al. Hypoestrogenemia of hypothalamic origin and coronary artery disease in premenopausal women: a report from the NHLBI-sponsored WISE study. *J Am Coll Cardiol.* 2003;41:413-419.

59. ACOG practice bulletin No. 73: Use of hormonal contraception in women with coexisting medical conditions. *Obstet Gynecol.* 2006;107:1453-1472.

60. WHO. Medical eligibility criteria for contraceptive use. http://www.who.int/reproductivehealth/publications/family_planning/9789241563888/en/. Accessed on 17 May 2013.

61. Grady D, et al. Cardiovascular disease outcomes during 6.8 years of hormone therapy: Heart and Estrogen/progestin Replacement Study follow-up (HERS II). *JAMA.* 2002;288:49-57.

62. Rossouw JE, et al. Risks and benefits of estrogen plus progestin in healthy postmenopausal women: principal results From the Women's Health Initiative randomized controlled trial. *JAMA.* 2002;288:321-333.

63. Collins P, et al. Effects of the selective estrogen receptor modulator raloxifene on coronary outcomes in the Raloxifene Use for The Heart trial: results of subgroup analyses by age and other factors. *Circulation.* 2009;119:922-930.

64. Miller VM, Manson JE. Women's Health Initiative hormone therapy trials: new insights on cardiovascular disease from additional years of follow up. *Curr Cardiovasc Risk Rep.* 2013;7:196-202.

65. Schierbeck LL, et al. Effect of hormone replacement therapy on cardiovascular events in recently postmenopausal women: randomized trial. *BMJ.* 2012;345:e6409.

66. Romond EH, et al. Seven-year follow-up assessment of cardiac function in NSABP B-31, a randomized trial comparing doxorubicin and cyclophosphamide followed by paclitaxel (ACP) with ACP plus trastuzumab as adjuvant therapy for patients with node-positive, human epidermal growth factor receptor 2-positive breast cancer. *J Clin Oncol.* 2012;30:3792-3799.

67. Bird BRJH, Swain SM. Cardiac toxicity in breast cancer survivors: review of potential cardiac problems. *Clin Cancer Res.* 2008;14:14-24.

68. Mackey JR, et al. Adjuvant docetaxel, doxorubicin, and cyclophosphamide in node-positive breast cancer: 10-year follow-up of the phase 3 randomised BCIRG 001 trial. *Lancet Oncol.* 2013;14:72-80.

69. Bowles EJA, et al. Risk of heart failure in breast cancer patients after anthracycline and trastuzumab treatment: a retrospective cohort study. *JNCI J Natl Cancer Inst.* 2012;104:1293-1305.

70. Mast ME, et al. Preradiotherapy calcium scores of the coronary arteries in a cohort of women with early-stage breast cancer: a comparison with a cohort of healthy women. *Int J Radiat Oncol Biol Phys.* 2012;83:853-858.

71. Hooning MJ, et al. Long-term risk of cardiovascular disease in 10-year survivors of breast cancer. *J Natl Cancer Inst.* 2007;99:365-375.

72. Jagsi R, et al. Rates of myocardial infarction and coronary artery disease and risk factors in patients treated with radiation therapy for early-stage breast cancer. *Cancer.* 2007;109:650-657.

73. Favourable and unfavourable effects on long-term survival of radiotherapy for early breast cancer: an overview of the randomised trials. Early Breast Cancer Trialists' Collaborative Group. *Lancet.* 2000;355:1757-1770.

3 ASSESSMENT OF RISK OF CARDIOVASCULAR DISEASE IN WOMEN

Priya Kohli, MD, MPH
JoAnne Foody, MD, FACC, FAHA

INTRODUCTION

Age, gender, hypertension, tobacco use, hypercholesterolemia, and diabetes have long been recognized as risk factors for cardiovascular disease (CVD) in women.[1,2] These factors often act together to increase this risk. Multiple algorithms utilizing these and other risk factors have been developed for assessment of CVD risk in women.[1-7] Traditionally, these algorithms have focused on short term, or risk of CVD in a 10-year time frame. These risk scores are used to identify women who may benefit from early aggressive interventions, including diet and lifestyle modifications and lipid-lowering and antihypertensive medications. More recently, focus has shifted to assessment of lifetime risk of CVD as well as use of measures of subclinical atherosclerosis in risk assessment in women. This chapter will discuss risk assessment for CVD in women, including global risk assessment algorithms, use of nontraditional risk factors, and markers of subclinical atherosclerosis and risk factors for CVD that are unique to women.

RISK ASSESSMENT ALGORITHMS

FRAMINGHAM RISK SCORE (ATP III)

Of these scores, the Framingham risk score, as it is incorporated into the Third Report of the Expert Panel on Detection, Evaluation, and Treatment of High Blood Cholesterol (Adult Treatment Panel III) (ATP III),[3] is the most commonly used. For each risk factor (age, total cholesterol, smoking status, HDL, and systolic blood pressure) a point value is assigned (see Table 3-1) and an absolute 10-year risk for coronary heart disease can be determined (see Table 3-2). An online ATP III risk score calculator can be found at: http://hp2010.nhlbihin.net/atpIII/calculator.asp?usertype=prof. Based on the risk factor profiles and calculated 10-year risk of CVD, patients are stratified into 3 risk categories with different goal of low-density lipoprotein (LDL) and non–high-density lipoprotein (non-HDL) levels (see Table 3-3).

PREDICTION OF LIFETIME RISK

When compared to men, the 10-year predicted risk of CHD by the ATP III risk score is lower across all age groups (Figure 3-1).[8] Despite this, up to 50% of women will subsequently develop CVD.[9] In the Cardiovascular Lifetime Risk Pooling Project, presence of traditional risk factors, such as diabetes, current tobacco use, elevated cholesterol, and elevated systolic blood pressure, at age 55 years accurately predicted lifetime risk of death from cardiovascular disease (Figure 3-2).[5] When identifying women who might benefit from more prevention-aggressive measures, consideration of lifetime risk of CVD may help guide therapy. As an example, the ATP III 10-year risk of CVD for a 50-year-old nonsmoking, nondiabetic woman with risk factors of elevated cholesterol and systolic blood pressure is only 2%, whereas her lifetime risk of CVD is closer to 50%.[5,9] A 30-year risk calculator from the Framingham study has been developed.[10]

USE OF NONTRADITIONAL RISK FACTORS, INCLUDING MARKERS OF SUBCLINCAL ATHEROSCLEROSIS

Given the limitations of traditional risk assessment for CVD in women, numerous other parameters have proposed to further risk-stratify women. These include family history of coronary disease,[2] diet and lifestyle habits, alternative lipid measures and inflammatory biomarkers,[6] and markers of subclinical atherosclerosis.[11,12]

AMERICAN HEART ASSOCIATION GUIDELINES FOR THE PREVENTION OF CVD IN WOMEN: CLASSIFICATION OF CVD RISK

One such alternative risk classification system is detailed in the 2011 Update to the Guidelines for Prevention of CVD in Women (Table 3-4).[2] Expanding on the traditional risk factors included in the ATP III score; this classification method has been validated in the Women's Health Initiative cohort. Women classified as high risk, at risk, and optimal risk had rates of myocardial infarction, CVD death, or stroke of 19.0%, 5.5%, and 2.2%, respectively.[13]

REYNOLDS RISK SCORE

Development of the Reynolds risk score included consideration of alternative lipid measures like apolipoproteins and lipoprotein(a) (Lp[a]) in addition to inflammatory biomarkers such as high-sensitivity C-reactive protein (hsCRP) and markers of glycemic control. The final simplified Reynolds risk score includes these parameters, except the alternative lipid measures (Figure 3-3).[6] Currently, routine use of hsCRP and alternative lipids measures is not recommended, although these tests may be useful in women who require further risk stratification.

MEASUREMENT OF SUBCLINICAL ATHEROSCLEROSIS

Similar to biomarkers and alternative lipid measures, routine assessment of subclinical atherosclerosis is not recommended. However, it has been shown that among women who are classified as "low risk" by the ATP III risk score, some will have evidence of coronary subclinical atherosclerosis, which is associated with increased CVD events. Coronary artery calcium (CAC), as detected by computed

TABLE 3-1 Estimate of 10-Year Risk for Women (Framingham Point Scores)[3]

Age (years)	Points
20-34	−7
35-39	−3
40-44	0
45-49	3
50-54	6
55-59	8
60-64	10
65-69	12
70-74	14
75-79	16

	Points				
Total Cholesterol (mg/dL)[a]	**Age 20-39 y**	**Age 40-49 y**	**Age 50-59 y**	**Age 60-69 y**	**Age 70-79 y**
<160	0	0	0	0	0
160-199	4	3	2	1	1
200-239	8	6	4	2	1
240-279	11	8	5	3	2
≥280	13	10	7	4	2

	Points				
	Age 20-39 y	**Age 40-49 y**	**Age 50-59 y**	**Age 60-69 y**	**Age 70-79 y**
Nonsmoker	0	0	0	0	0
Smoker[b]	9	7	4	2	1

HDL (mg/dL)[a]	Points
≥60	−1
50-59	0
40-49	1
<40	2

	Points	
Systolic BP (mm Hg)[c]	**If Untreated**	**If Treated**
<120	0	0
120-129	1	3
130-139	2	4
140-159	3	5
≥160	4	6

[a]Total cholesterol and HDL cholesterol values should be the average of at least 2 measurements.
[b]"Smoker" is defined as any cigarette smoking in the past month.
[c]Blood pressure measurement made at the time of assessment.

tomography, is one such assessment of subclinical atherosclerosis. In the Multi-Ethnic Study of Atherosclerosis, 32% of women classified as "low risk" were found to have a CAC score >0 (Table 3-5), which was associated with a higher incidence of CVD events (Figure 3-4).

CVD RISK FACTORS UNIQUE TO WOMEN

Complications of pregnancy, like preeclampsia and gestational diabetes, have been associated with worse CVD outcomes.[14-17] Women who suffer from these complications during pregnancy should be referred for more careful monitoring of risk factors postpartum.

TABLE 3-2 Determination of 10-Year Risk of CVD

Point Total	10-Year Risk (%)
<9	<1
9	1
10	1
11	1
12	1
13	2
14	2
15	3
16	4
17	5
18	6
19	8
20	11
21	14
22	17
23	22
24	27
≥25	≥30

Points for each risk factor are determined from Table 3-1 and summed for a total. This total of all the points corresponds to a 10-year risk.[3]

TABLE 3-3 Comparison of LDL Cholesterol and Non-HDL Cholesterol Goals for 3 Risk Categories[3]

Risk Category	LDL Goal (mg/dL)	Non-HDL Goal (mg/dL)
CHD and CHD risk equivalent (10-year risk for CHD >20%)	<100	<130
Multiple (2+) risk factors and 10-year risk ≤20%	<130	<160
0-1 risk factor	<160	<190

CHD, coronary heart disease; including myocardial infarction and death from coronary heart disease.

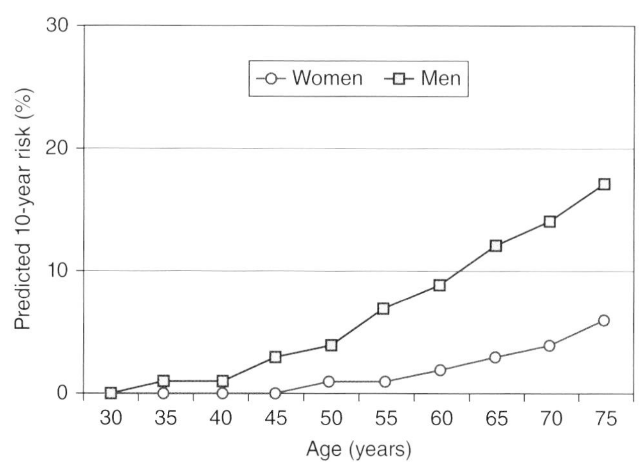

FIGURE 3-1 Ten-year predicted risks, using the ATP-III Assessment Tool, for men and women at selected ages, with risk factors held constant at approximate age-adjusted average values.[8]
Reproduced with permission from Cavanaugh-Hussey MW, Berry JD, Lloyd-Jones DM. Who exceeds ATP-III risk thresholds? Systematic examination of the effect of varying age and risk factor levels in the ATP-III risk assessment tool. *Prev Med.* 2008;47:619-623.

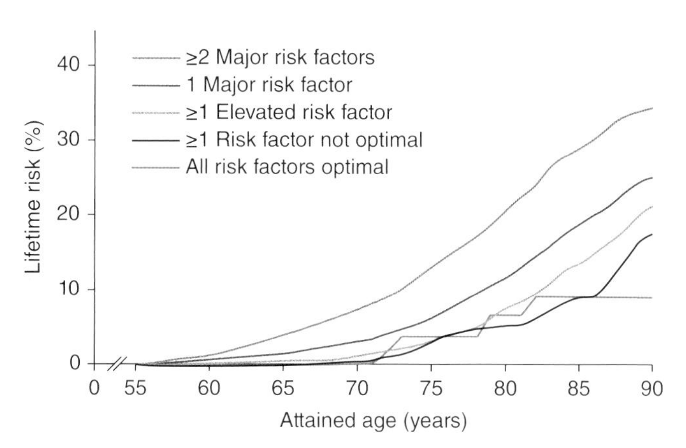

FIGURE 3-2 Lifetime risk of death from cardiovascular disease among black women and white women at 55 years of age, according to the Aggregate Burden of Risk Factors and Adjusted for Competing Risks of Death.
Reproduced with permission from Berry JD, Dyer A, Cai X, et al. Lifetime risks of cardiovascular disease. *N Engl J Med.* 2012;366:321-329.
All risk factors optimal: total cholesterol <180 mg/dL, untreated blood pressure <120 mm Hg systolic, and <80 mm Hg diastolic, nonsmoker, nondiabetic.
≥1 risk factor not optimal: nonsmoker, nondiabetic with total cholesterol 180-199 mg/dL, untreated blood pressure 120-139 mm Hg systolic or 80-89 mm Hg diastolic.
≥1 risk factor elevated: nonsmoker, nondiabetic with total cholesterol 200-239 mg/dL, untreated blood pressure 140-159 mm Hg systolic or 90-99 mm Hg diastolic.
Major risk factors: current smoker, diabetic, treated hypercholesterolemia, untreated total cholesterol ≥240 mg/dL, treated hypertension, untreated blood pressure ≥160 mm Hg diastolic, or ≥100 mm Hg diastolic.

TABLE 3-4 Classification of CVD Risk in Women

Risk Status	Criteria
High risk (≥1 high-risk states)	Clinically manifest CVD
	Clinically manifest cerebrovascular disease
	Clinically manifest peripheral arterial disease
	Abdominal aortic aneurysm
	End-stage or chronic kidney disease
	Diabetes mellitus
	10-year predicted CVD risk ≥10% (by ATP III)
At risk (≥1 major risk factors)	Cigarette smoking
	Systolic blood pressure ≥120 mm Hg, diastolic blood pressure ≥80 mm Hg, or treated hypertension
	Total cholesterol ≥200 mg/dL, HDL <50 mg/dL, or treated dyslipidemia
	Obesity
	Poor diet
	Physical inactivity
	Family history of premature CVD occurring in first-degree relatives in men <55 years old or in women <65 years old
	Metabolic syndrome
	Evidence of advanced subclinical atherosclerosis
	Poor exercise capacity on treadmill test and/or abnormal heart rate recovery after stopping exercise
	Systemic autoimmune collagen vascular disease
	History of preeclampsia, gestational diabetes, or pregnancy-induced hypertension
Ideal cardiovascular health (all of these)	Total cholesterol <200 mg/dL (untreated)
	BP <120/80 (untreated)
	Fasting blood glucose <100 mg/dL (untreated)
	Body mass index <25 kg/m^2
	Abstinence from smoking
	Physical activity at goal for adults >20 years of age: ≥150 min/wk moderate intensity, ≥75 min/wk vigorous intensity, or combination
	Healthy (DASH-like) diet

Adapted from Mosca L, Benjamin EJ, Berra K, et al. Effectiveness-based guidelines for the prevention of cardiovascular disease in women—2011 update: a guideline from the American Heart Association. *Circulation.* 2011;123:1243-1262.
DASH, dietary approaches to stop hypertension.

Model B, the Reynolds Risk Score

10-year cardiovascular disease risk (%) = $[1 - 0.98634^{(\exp[B - 22.325])}] \times 100\%$, where B = 0.0799 × age + 3.137 × natural logarithm (systolic blood pressure) + 0.180 × natural logarithm (high-sensitivity C-reactive protein) + 1.382 × natural logarithm (total cholesterol) − 1.172 × natural logarithm (high-density lipoprotein cholesterol) + 0.134 × hemoglobin A_{1c} (%) (if diabetic) + 0.818 (if current smoker) + 0.438 (if family history of premature myocardial infarction).

FIGURE 3-3 Reynolds risk score equation.
Reproduced with permission from Ridker PM, Buring JE, Rifai N, Cook NR. Development and validation of improved algorithms for the assessment of global cardiovascular risk in women: the Reynolds risk score. *JAMA.* 2007;297:611-619.

CONCLUSION

Assessment of CVD risk in women begins with assessment of traditional risk factors as outlined earlier. For women who are classified as "low risk," consideration of lifetime risk of CVD and nontraditional CVD risk factors may identify a subgroup that can benefit from early aggressive interventions.

TABLE 3-5 Percentage of Women Classified as "Low Risk" Based on ATP III With Prevalent CAC

	CAC Score	
Race/Ethnicity	0	>0
White	694 (63)	412 (37)
Asian	207 (66)	107 (34)
African American	513 (71)	210 (29)
Hispanic	400 (74)	140 (26)
Overall	**1814 (68)**	**870 (32)**

Adapted with permission from Lakoski SG, Greenland P, Wong ND, et al. Coronary artery calcium scores and risk for cardiovascular events in women classified as "low risk" based on Framingham risk score: the multi-ethnic study of atherosclerosis (MESA). *Arch Int Med.* 2007;167(22):2437-2442. Data is given as number (percentage) of women.

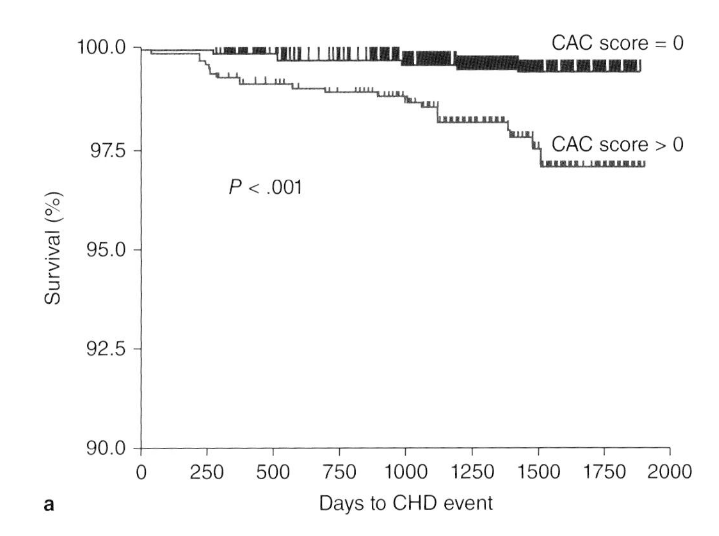

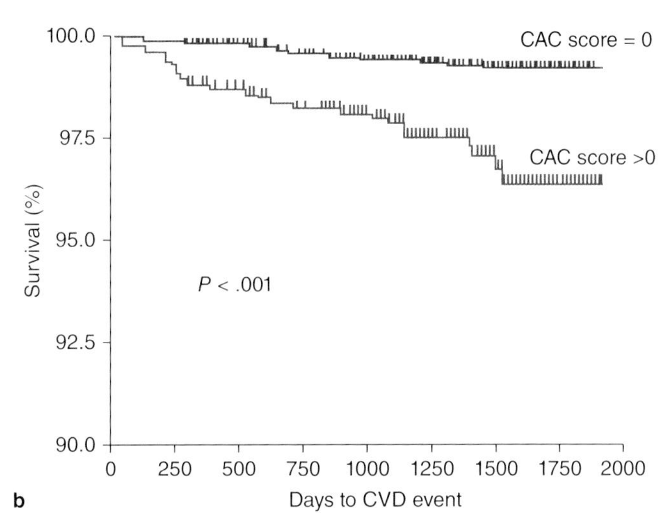

FIGURE 3-4 The cumulative incidence of coronary heart disease (A) and cardiovascular disease (B) events according to the presence or absence of CAC.
Reproduced with permission from Lakoski SG, Greenland P, Wong ND, et al. Coronary artery calcium scores and risk for cardiovascular events in women classified as "low risk" based on Framingham risk score: the multi-ethnic study of atherosclerosis (MESA). *Arch Int Med.* 2007;167(22): 2437-2442.

REFERENCES

1. D'Agostino RB, Sr, Vasan RS, Pencina MJ, et al. General cardiovascular risk profile for use in primary care: the Framingham Heart Study. *Circulation*. 2008;117: 743-753.
2. Mosca L, Benjamin EJ, Berra K, et al. Effectiveness-based guidelines for the prevention of cardiovascular disease in women—2011 update: a guideline from the American Heart Association. *Circulation*. 2011;123:1243-1262.
3. Expert Panel on Detection, Evaluation, and Treatment of High Blood Cholesterol in Adults. Executive summary of the third report of the National Cholesterol Education Program (NCEP) expert panel on detection, evaluation, and treatment of high blood cholesterol in adults (Adult Treatment Panel III). *JAMA*. 2001;285:2486-2497.
4. Assmann G, Cullen P, Schulte H. Simple scoring scheme for calculating the risk of acute coronary events based on the 10-year follow-up of the prospective cardiovascular Münster (PROCAM) study. *Circulation*. 2002;105:310-315.
5. Berry JD, Dyer A, Cai X, et al. Lifetime risks of cardiovascular disease. *N Engl J Med*. 2012;366:321-329.
6. Ridker PM, Buring JE, Rifai N, et al. Development and validation of improved algorithms for the assessment of global cardiovascular risk in women: the Reynolds risk score. *JAMA*. 2007;297:611-619.
7. Hippisley-Cox J, Coupland C, Vinogradova Y, et al. Derivation and validation of QRISK, a new cardiovascular disease risk score for the United Kingdom: prospective open cohort study. *BMJ*. 2007;335:136.
8. Cavanaugh-Hussey MW, Berry JD, Lloyd-Jones DM. Who exceeds ATP-III risk thresholds? Systematic examination of the effect of varying age and risk factor levels in the ATP-III risk assessment tool. *Prev Med*. 2008;47:619-623.
9. Lloyd-Jones DM, Leip EP, Larson MG, et al. Prediction of lifetime risk for cardiovascular disease by risk factor burden at 50 years of age. *Circulation*. 2006;113:791-798.
10. Pencina MJ, D'Agostino RB, Sr, Larson MG, et al. Predicting the 30-year risk of cardiovascular disease: the Framingham Heart Study. *Circulation*. 2009;119:3078-3084.
11. Lakoski SG, Greenland P, Wong ND, et al. Coronary artery calcium scores and risk for cardiovascular events in women classified as "low risk" based on Framingham risk score: the multi-ethnic study of atherosclerosis (MESA). *Arch Intern Med*. 2007;167:2437-2442.

12. Polonsky TS, McClelland RL, Jorgensen NW, et al. Coronary artery calcium score and risk classification for coronary heart disease prediction. *JAMA*. 2010;303:1610-1616.
13. Hsia J, Rodabough RJ, Manson JE, et al. Evaluation of the American Heart Association cardiovascular disease prevention guideline for women. *Circ Cardiovasc Qual Outcomes*. 2010;3:128-134.
14. Ray JG, Vermeulen MJ, Schull MJ, et al. Cardiovascular health after maternal placental syndromes (CHAMPS): population-based retrospective cohort study. *Lancet*. 2005;366:1797-1803.
15. Smith GC, Pell JP, Walsh D. Spontaneous loss of early pregnancy and risk of ischaemic heart disease in later life: retrospective cohort study. *BMJ*. 2003;326:423-424.
16. Wilson BJ, Watson MS, Prescott GJ, et al. Hypertensive diseases of pregnancy and risk of hypertension and stroke in later life: results from cohort study. *BMJ*. 2003;326:845.
17. Bellamy L, Casas JP, Hingorani AD, et al. Pre-eclampsia and risk of cardiovascular disease and cancer in later life: systematic review and meta-analysis. *BMJ*. 2007;335:974.

4 CORONARY ARTERY DISEASE IN WOMEN

Christina Salazar, MD
Martha Gulati, MD, MS, FACC, FAHA

INTRODUCTION

Cardiovascular disease (CVD) remains the leading cause of death in women.[1] Nearly half-a-million women die each year in the United States from ischemic heart disease (IHD) and its related conditions with the most recent annual statistics on mortality reporting that CVD accounted for 421,918 deaths among women in the United States.[2] In fact, current projections indicate this number will continue to rise with our aging population[2-4] (Figure 4-1). Since 1982 more women than men have died annually from IHD[2] (Figure 4-2), which is the leading killer of women with annual mortality rates exceeding those due to breast cancer in women of any age[2,5] (Figure 4-3). Although in the last decade, there have been significant declines in female mortality due to coronary heart disease, these reductions lag behind those seen in men[1] (see Figure 4-2). In addition, women under 65 suffer the highest relative sex-specific cardiovascular heart disease mortality (Figure 4-4). A study from the Journal of American Clinical Cardiology in 2007 noted that although mortality from coronary heart disease (CHD) in men across all age groups has decreased, there has been a notable increase in mortality among women belonging to youngest age group (<55 years).[6] This group of women, in particular, also have increased risk factors for CHD.[6] Additionally, women were more likely to die of cardiac arrest before hospital arrival compared to men, 52% and 42% respectively.[3] This prehospital death rate represents a worsening trend among women and a significant change from prior decades.[7,8] Though there have been declines in sudden cardiac deaths in men, the condition of women has changed little[9] (Figure 4-5), even those who are living with cardiovascular disease suffer greater morbidity and mortality than men. Upon examination of the specific diagnoses of CVD and comparison of their effects on gender, it has been proved that women not only suffer greater mortality, but greater morbidity as well. When compared with men, women suffer 2 times greater mortality and morbidity from angina and coronary artery bypass graft surgery (CABG).[10] There is a 2 times greater incidence of congestive heart failure (CHF) and 1½ times greater 1-year mortality from myocardial infarction (MI) in women than men.[10] Lastly, women with proven coronary artery disease (CAD) but stable angina have a higher probability of death or MI than men[11] (Figure 4-6).

There are differences in the prevalence, symptoms, and pathophysiology of myocardial ischemia in women when compared to men.[1] This chapter reviews the sex-specific issues related to myocardial ischemia in women in relation to traditional and novel risk factors, presentation, diagnosis, treatment, and outcomes.

Discussion of CAD in women, with focus on gender differences in diagnosis.

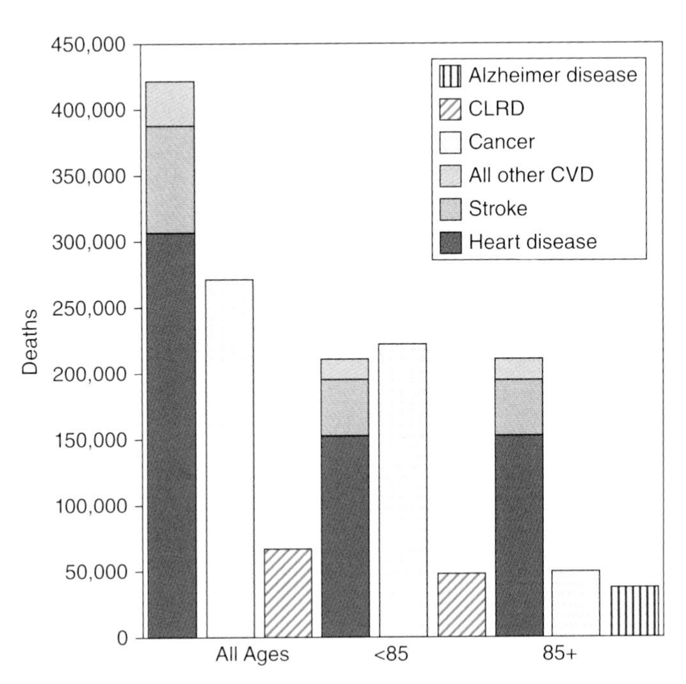

FIGURE 4-1 Cardiovascular disease (CVD) and other major causes of death: total, <85 years, and ≥85 years. Deaths among women, United States, 2007. *Abbreviations:* CLRD, chronic lower respiratory disease.[2] National Center for Health Statistics and National Heart, Lung, and Blood Institute.

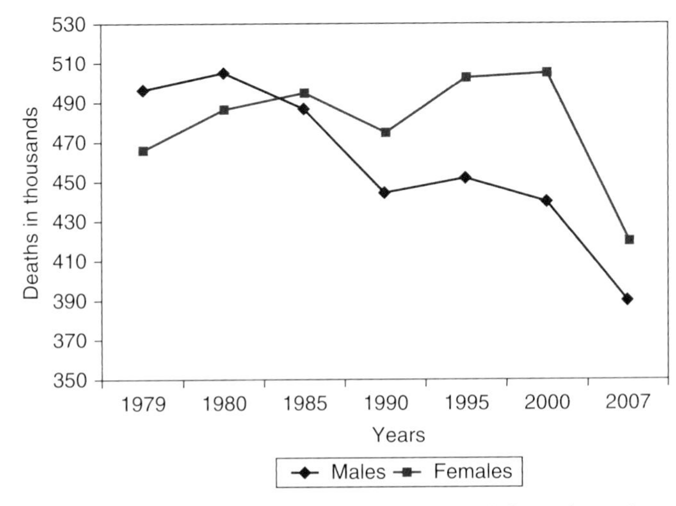

FIGURE 4-2 Cardiovascular disease mortality trends for males and females (United States: 1979-2007). The overall comparability for cardiovascular disease between the International Classification of Diseases, 9th Revision (1979-1998) and International Classification of Diseases, 10th Revision (1999-2007) is 0.9962. No comparability ratios were applied.[2]

Based on the sex-specific differences it may be easier to identify women who are at risk and those who are diagnosed with ischemic heart disease under a female pattern of disease versus our traditional understanding of male-pattern disease as women can have both patterns.

The graph in Figure 4-7 shows a cumulative change (in percentage) in mortality rate for males versus black and white females. It shows that the trend is decreasing more rapidly in men and there are more deaths in women from IHD than men despite the overall decrease in mortality over the past 3 decades (Figure 4-7).

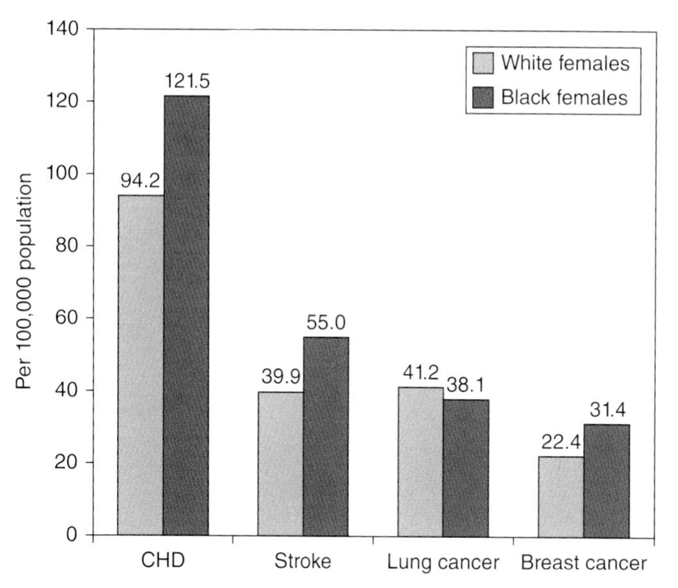

FIGURE 4-3 Age-adjusted death rates for coronary heart disease (CHD), stroke, and lung and breast cancer for white and black women (United States: 2007).[2]
National Center for Health Statistics.

MALE-PATTERN DISEASE

Traditionally, evaluation and management of IHD has been approached by defining and treating a "culprit" lesion. There are a vast array of diagnostic tools specifically designed to determine the likelihood of a "culprit" obstructive coronary lesion as well as evidence-based guidelines for treatment traditionally applied to both men and women. However, there is a greater prevalence of nonobstructive disease in women than men.[1] The prevalence of obstructive CAD in women is relatively low before menopause and equal to the prevalence in men in the seventh decade. In general, the comparable incidence rates are achieved with women who are 10 years older than men, so women at age 65 have the same incidence of CAD as men at age 55. As a result, there is lower likelihood of obstructive coronary disease in the women we evaluate.

Overall, the prevalence and incidence of all forms of ischemic heart disease are lower in women compared to men, and the age at presentation is delayed (Figure 4-8). However, after 75 years of age, women outnumber men and the total number of elderly female IHD patients is greater than men[12] (Figure 4-9).

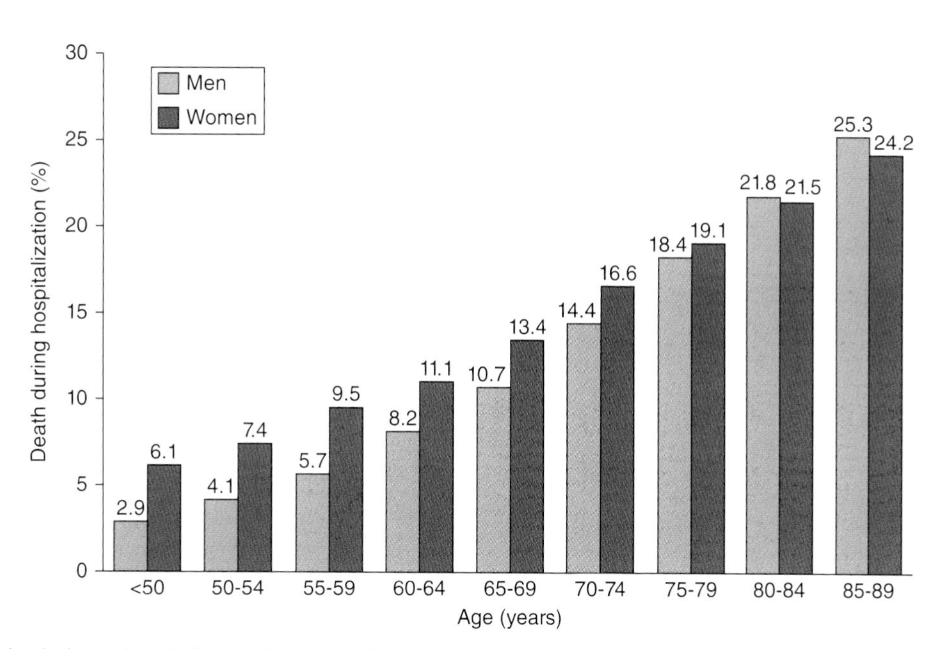

FIGURE 4-4 Rates of death during hospitalization for myocardial infarction among women and men according to age. The interaction between sex and age was significant ($P < 0.001$).[68]

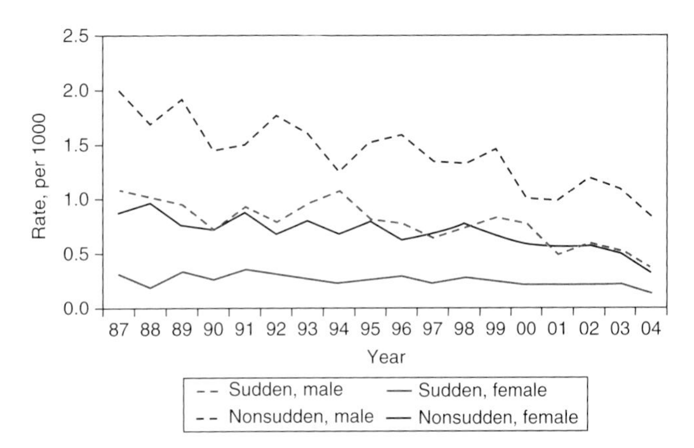

FIGURE 4-5 Age- and race-adjusted rate of sudden and nonsudden deaths from coronary artery disease, by gender.
ARIC Community Surveillance Study 1987-2004.[9]

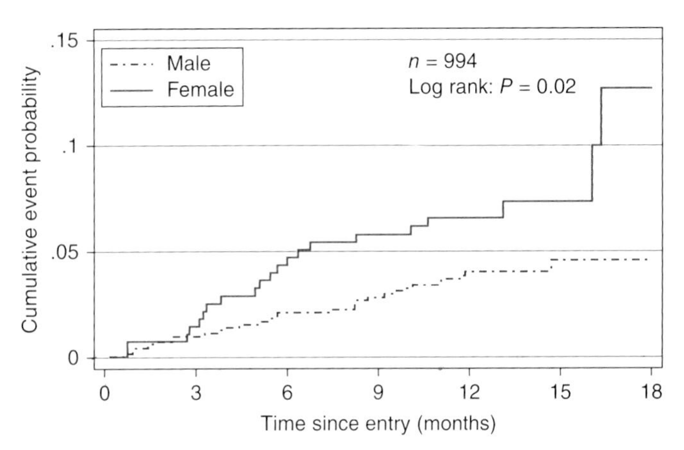

FIGURE 4-6 Cumulative probability of death or MI in patients with confirmed coronary disease and stable angina according to gender.[11]

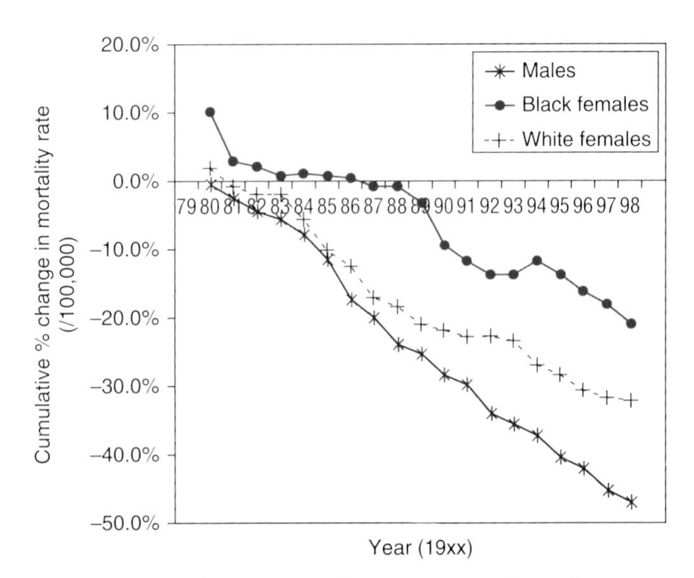

FIGURE 4-7 Cumulative percent change in coronary heart disease mortality in black and white women as compared with men in the United States from 1979 to 1998.[3]

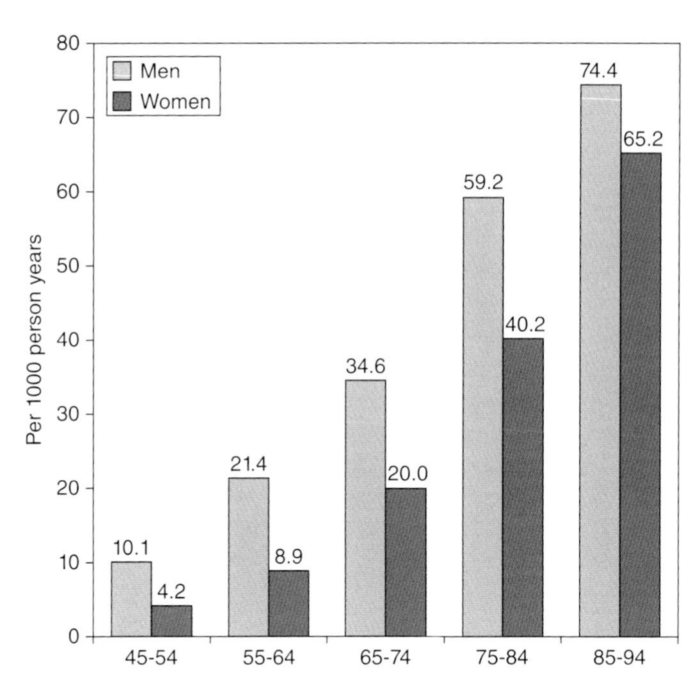

FIGURE 4-8 Incidence of cardiovascular disease* by age and sex (FHS, 1980-2003).[2]
*Coronary artery disease, heart failure, stroke, or intermittent claudication.

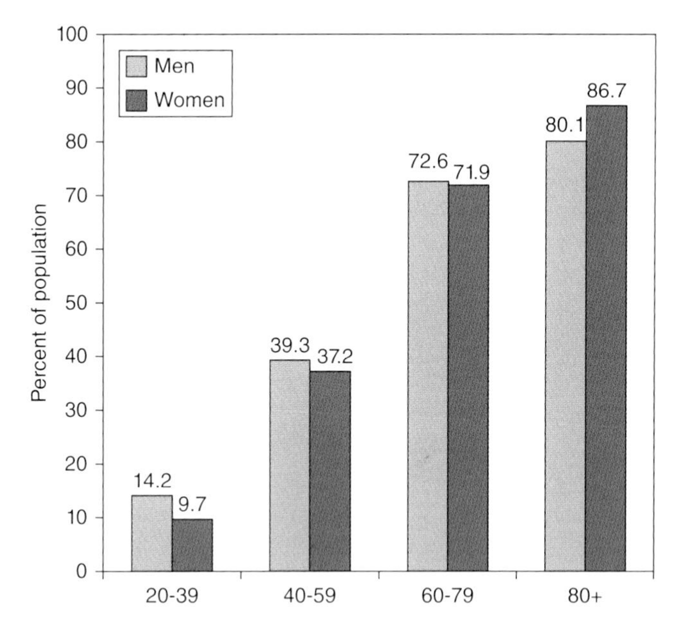

FIGURE 4-9 Prevalence of cardiovascular disease in adults ≥20 years of age by age and sex (National Health and Nutrition Examination Survey: 2005-2008).[2]
National Center for Health Statistics and National Heart, Lung, and Blood Institute. These data include coronary heart disease, heart failure, stroke, and hypertension.

TRADITIONAL RISK FACTORS

The presence of any cardiovascular risk factor increases the lifetime risk of developing IHD[13,14] (Figure 4-10) and >80% of women have >1 cardiac risk factor present.[15] It is possible that many of the traditional cardiac risk factors in women have a greater impact or higher prevalence.[1] In regards to specific risk factors, women have higher cholesterol levels than men after their fifth decade of life and elevation in their triglycerides is a more potent risk factor in women compared with men.[15-18] In women, diabetes and hypertension appear to confer a higher risk of coronary events, as diabetes is more prevalent in women.[15,19] This could potentially be secondary to smaller coronaries in women and the more aggressive nature of coronary disease in diabetics or, alternatively, because women may require a greater risk factor burden compared to men before developing IHD, or the "higher risk factor burden" hypothesis.[12] As seen in Figure 4-11, men and women who present with unstable ischemic syndrome have similar high-risk profiles based on the Thrombolysis in Myocardial Infarction (TIMI) risk scores, but women have a different cardiovascular risk profile. Specifically, women were more likely to present with a history of cardiovascular risk factors (including hypertension and diabetes mellitus), prior angina episodes, ST depression on their ECGs, and increased age, whereas men were more likely to present with prior coronary artery disease and elevated markers of myonecrosis ($P < 0.001$ for each; see Figure 4-11).[20] But, certainly, the reason why the CHD death rates in US women aged 35 to 54 appears to be increasing is likely because of the obesity epidemic, which is more prevalent in women than men[21,22] (Figure 4-12). With nearly 2 of every 3 US women >20 years of age now overweight or obese (Figure 4-13), the rate of diabetes is more than double in Hispanic women compared to non-Hispanic white women.[22] Lastly, metabolic syndrome is more common after menopause and women with the combination of central obesity, glucose intolerance,

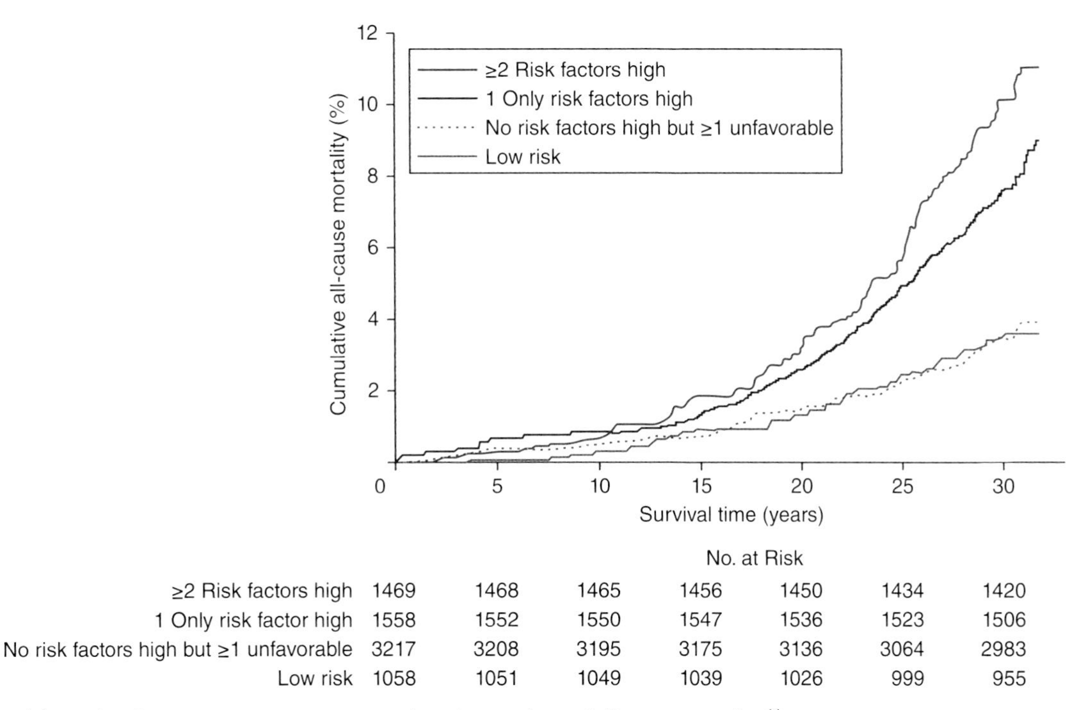

FIGURE 4-10 Risk factor burden in young women increased cardiovascular and all-cause mortality.[14]

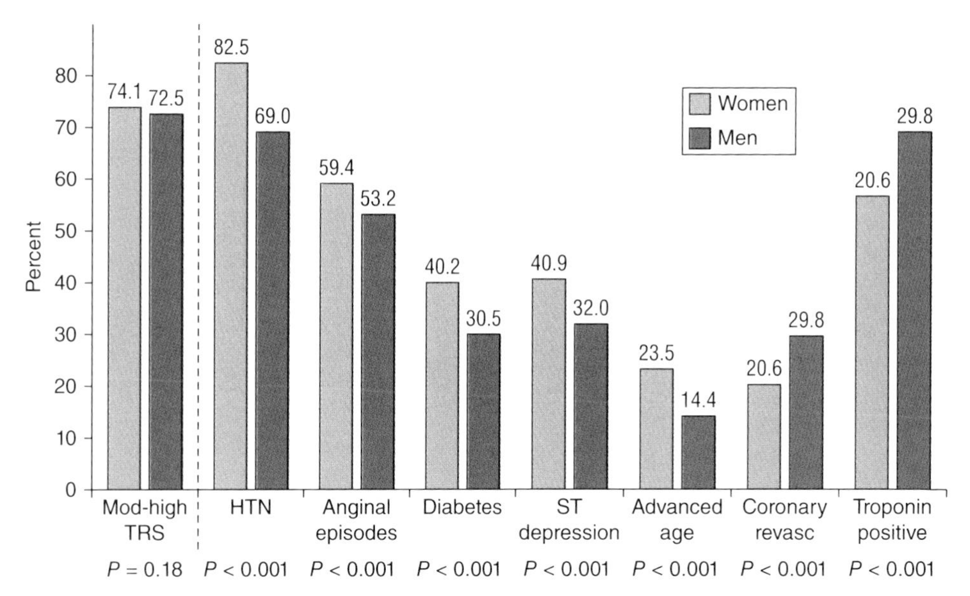

FIGURE 4-11 Features of women and men presenting with unstable ischemic heart disease. Moderate to high TRS indicates a Thrombolysis in Myocardial Infarction (TIMI) risk score ≥3.[20] *Abbreviations:* HTN, hypertension; Revasc, revascularization; troponin positive, troponin I ≥0.04 ng/mL.

hypertension, and dyslipidemia are at the highest risk of developing IHD compared to men.[23] From a 2007 meta-analysis, the data demonstrated that the cardiovascular risk conferred by the metabolic syndrome was three times higher in women than it was in men.[23]

WOMEN WHO PRESENT WITH ACS

In 60% of cases, the initial presentation of IHD in women is acute MI or sudden cardiac death (SCD).[2,16,22,24] For those women who do present with an initial fatal ischemic event, there are morphologic differences in the etiology by age and gender.[25-28] The postmortem examination reveals plaque rupture in men and older women. There is usually a large necrotic core and disrupted fibrous cap infiltrated by macrophages and lymphocytes.[29] In younger women, however, there is a greater tendency toward plaque erosion. In this scenario, the fibrous cap is absent and the exposed intima consists mostly of smooth muscle and proteoglycans (Figure 4-14). Other unique pathophysiologic features in women with ischemic heart disease include adverse coronary reactivity,[30] microvascular dysfunction,[31] and distal microembolization[32] in addition to the plaque erosion. This is unlike men who are more likely to have obstructive coronary disease.[1]

SYMPTOMS

The definition of "typical" or male-pattern symptoms has been established from mostly male populations.[33] However, women suffer as much or more from angina than men,[34] and they have fewer "typical" symptoms than men. But the majority of women still present with these typical symptoms.[35] In a recent report there appeared to be no difference in diagnosing acute coronary syndromes in men and women presenting with typical symptoms, including chest pain or discomfort, dyspnea, diaphoresis, and arm or shoulder pain.[36] However, women often present with a different symptom complex than men. Women generally report more acute than prodromal symptoms and up to half of women with acute myocardial infarction had no chest pain prior to the event.[37] Among Acute Coronary Syndrome (ACS) patients, women have more frequent unstable

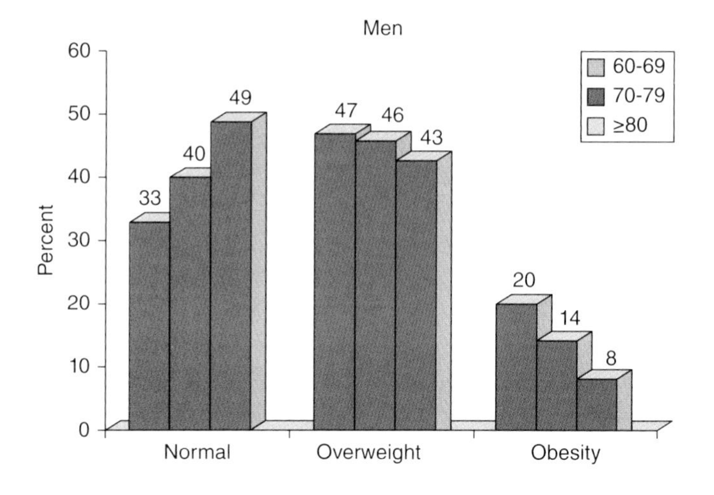

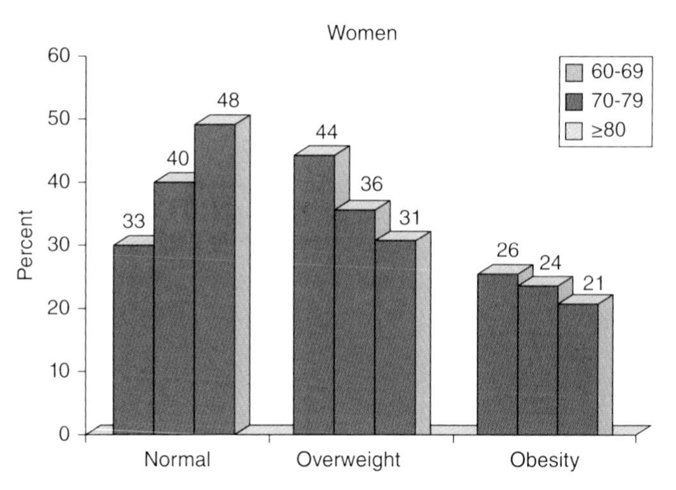

FIGURE 4-12 Prevalence of normal weight, overweight, and obesity by age and gender in a Mexican population.
Reproduced with permission from Ruiz-Arregui L, Castillo-Martínez L, Orea-Tejeda A, et al. Prevalence of self-reported overweight-obesity and its association with socioeconomic and health factors among older Mexican adults. *Salud Publica Mex.* 2007;49 (suppl 4):S482-S487.

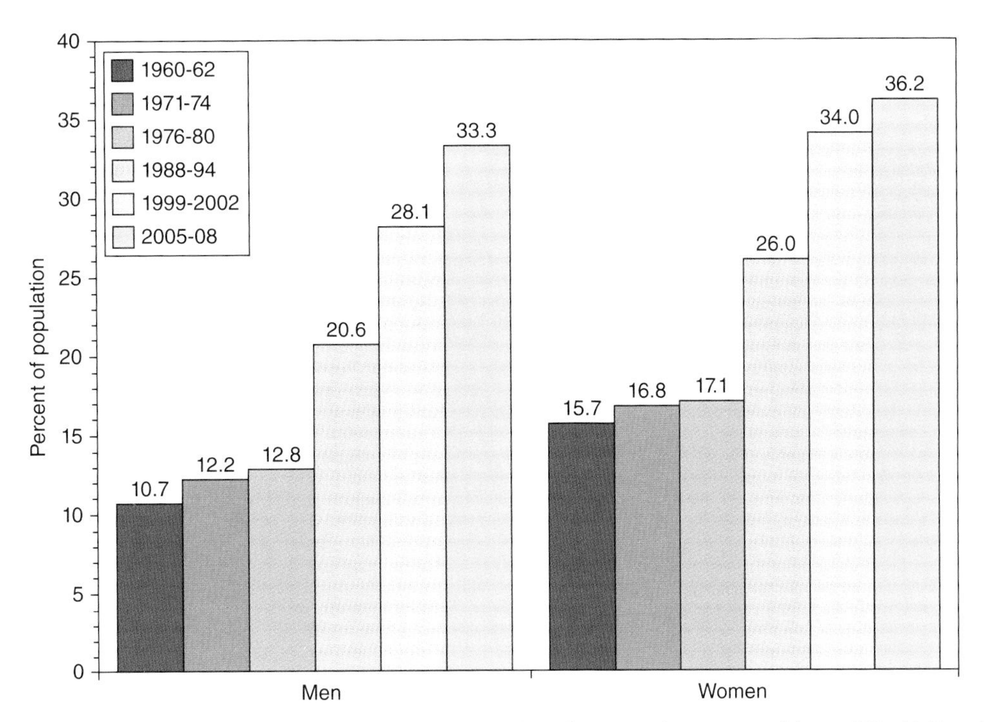

FIGURE 4-13 Age-adjusted prevalence of obesity in adults 20 to 74 years of age by sex and survey year (National Health Examination Survey: 1960-1962; National Health and Nutrition Examination Survey: 1971-1974, 1976-1980, 1988-1994, 1999-2002, and 2005-2008). Obesity is defined as a body mass index of 30.0 kg/m^2.[2]
Data derived from Health, United States, 2010 (National Center for Health Statistics).

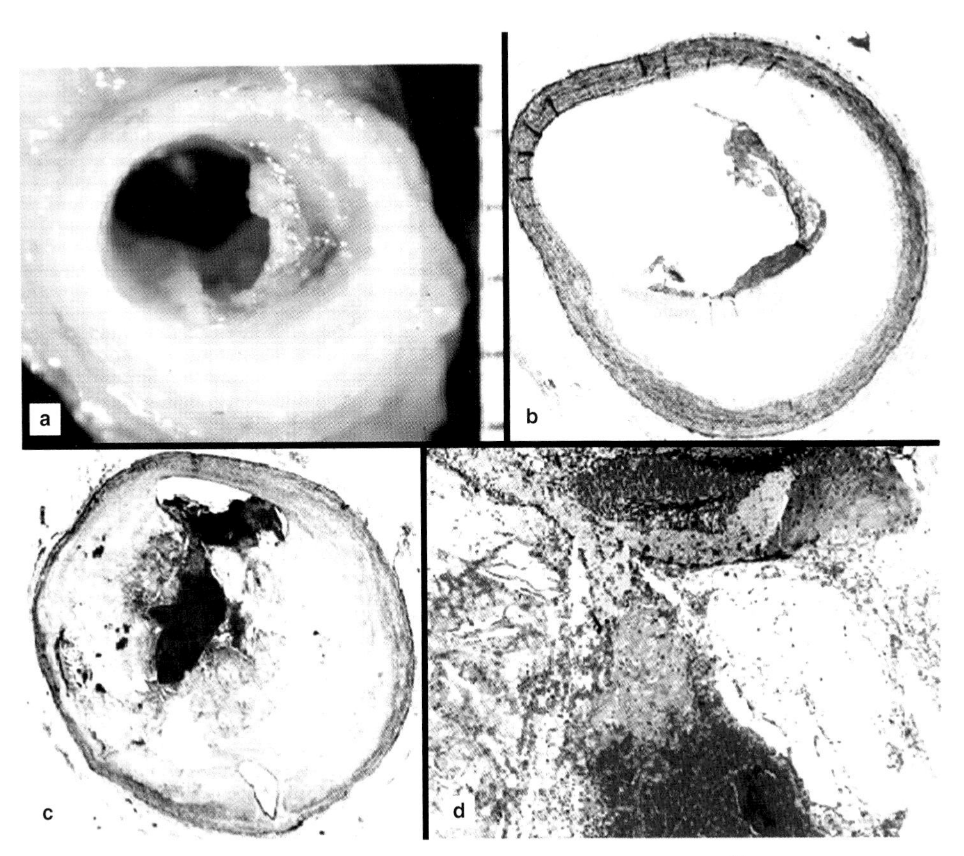

FIGURE 4-14 Plaque erosion, the typical presentation for sudden cardiac death in younger women.[29]

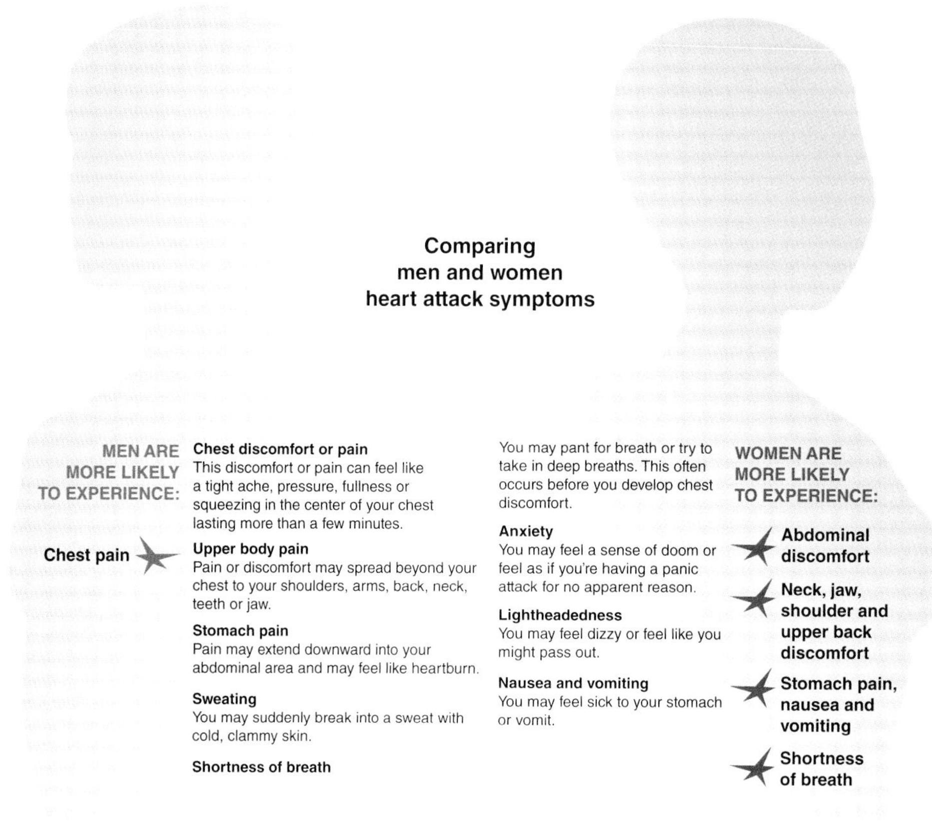

FIGURE 4-15 There are differences in risk factors and symptoms in those women who present with ischemic heart disease when compared to men. Used with permission from The Florida Times Union.

angina and "atypical" symptoms (Figure 4-15). After sudden cardiac death (SCD), the most common presentation is atypical including fatigue, shortness of breath, and atypical chest pain.[33,38-41] Even though women are more likely than men to have "atypical" symptoms, they present almost 2 times as frequently than men for evaluation and hospitalization of chest pain (4 million versus 2.4 million).[4]

GENDER DIFFERENCES IN DIAGNOSIS

In cardiovascular medicine, an exercise stress test is often the initial test to diagnose CAD in both men and women. The exercise ECG is the recommended first test of choice in the evaluation of symptomatic, intermediate-risk women who are able to exercise and have a normal baseline ECG.[42] Stress ECG has lower accuracy (60%-70%) compared to men (80%) (Table 4-1). The sensitivity

TABLE 4-1 Diagnostic value of various stress testing modalities in women.[42]

Stress-Testing Modality	Sensitivity	Specificity	NPV	PPV
Exercise ECG	31-71	66-78	78	47
Exercise echocardiography	80-88	79-86	98	74
Exercise SPECT	78-88	64-91	99	87
Pharmacological echocardiography	76-90	85-94	68	94
Pharmacological SPECT	80-91	65-75	90	68

Values are percentages. PPV indicates positive predictive value.

and specificity of ST-segment depression are lower in men[43] but given the lower incidence of obstructive CAD in women, this influences the accuracy of the stress ECG. To better predict the presence of CAD and IHD mortality in women, the Duke Treadmill score should be used.[44,45] This takes into account exercise duration and symptoms during the stress test. The DTS has been shown to have a good diagnostic and prognostic value in both men and women.[44-47] Overall, survival for women appears to be better at all levels of the DTS compared with men.[44,47] The DTS is a valuable tool to predict the risk of future myocardial infarction, revascularization, cardiac survival, and all-cause mortality in both genders, but it does not appear effective at assessing prognosis in the elderly (those aged ≥75 years).[48] For asymptomatic women, the Women Take Heart Project showed that the DTS was an independent predictor of all-cause and cardiac mortality.[49]

Exercise capacity can be estimated during an exercise stress test. Predictors of MI, IHD death, and all-cause mortality in women can be determined from an exercise capacity <5 metabolic equivalents (METs) or inability to achieve >85% age-predicted fitness level.[42,50,51] Although the focus of stress exercise ECG has centered mainly on ST-segment depression as a method of diagnosing CAD, the use of additional exercise parameters in women improves the diagnostic accuracy of the exercise stress test, as well as the prognostic assessment. In women, exercise capacity, percentage of age-predicted exercise capacity, chronotropic response, heart rate recovery (HRR), blood pressure response, and the DTS can all be used to enhance the diagnostic and prognostic value of exercise ECG [42] (Table 4-2). Even in asymptomatic women, METs can be a predictor of annual mortality rate. Importantly, women who are referred for pharmacologic stress test have the highest annual mortality rate (Figure 4-16) compared to those symptomatic or asymptomatic women who undergo an exercise stress test.

For the women with an abnormal ECG, stress testing may lead to cardiac imaging. Stress-induced perfusion abnormality assessment detects reductions in myocardial perfusion that occur prior to ECG or wall motion abnormalities seen on ECG. Most commonly, myocardial perfusion single-photon emission computed tomography (SPECT) is a nuclear-based technology that is most commonly used for women and men presenting with chest pain. Large observational series have noted similar abilities to risk-stratify women and men with chest pain symptoms.[52-57]

Stress-induced wall motion abnormality assessment by echocardiography has been associated with high diagnostic specificity, seen in Table 4-2. This testing assesses for wall motion abnormalities that appear after perfusion abnormalities. In women who cannot exercise, pharmacologic stress can be used in both SPECT and stress echocardiography. SPECT imaging has been effective in risk-stratifying women. Women who have a normal myocardial perfusion study have a low annual IHD event rate (0.6% per year) and those with an abnormal myocardial perfusion have a much higher event rate of (5% per year).[57] However, there are several limitations to SPECT in women including reduced sensitivity because of severe multi-vessel disease, "balanced ischemia" or as a result of microvascular disease, limited resolution where smaller abnormalities are not detected because of a smaller heart, breast attenuation, and radiation exposure.[58]

This figure summarizes the work-up algorithm for noninvasive testing in symptomatic women as discussed in more detail in testing chapter of this atlas (Figure 4-17).

Table 4-1 lists the sensitivity and specificity of exercise ECG, stress Echo, and stress SPECT in women.

TREATMENT AND OUTCOMES

According to the first Evidence-Based Guidelines for Cardiovascular Disease Prevention in Women in 2004 and update in 2007, there are similar recommendations to prevent cardiovascular disease in women as men with few exceptions.[22] The most notable exception is that aspirin is not routinely recommended for the primary prevention of MI in women as it is in men. The difference for the most recent guidelines in 2011 for cardiovascular disease prevention in women is a switch in focus from evidence-based to effectiveness-based guidelines. The Class III guidelines did not change, see Table 4-3. In regards to CVD risk assessment, the 2007 guidelines adopted an optimal risk category that is discussed elsewhere in this book. It should be noted that since 2007 the body of evidence supporting this category of risk has increased, so the 2011 guidelines included the risk category and changed the name to "Ideal Cardiovascular Health" which includes specific ranges for total cholesterol, blood pressure, fasting blood glucose, BMI, abstinence from smoking, healthy diet, and physical activity goal. It is discussed in detail in the risk assessment section of this atlas. Refer to Figure 4-18 from Effectiveness-Based Guidelines for Prevention of Cardiovascular Disease in Women for a flow diagram of Class I and II recommendations.[22]

For secondary prevention of IHD, the evidence-based benefits of the cardiovascular drugs including ASA, thienopyridines like Plavix, statins, angiotensin-converting enzyme inhibitors (ACEI), angiotensin receptor blockers, and β-blockers are similar in both genders.[11,59-64] Optimal medical therapy for women with IHD is no different than for men.[1] There are differences in the intensity of medical therapy or counseling, which can ultimately influence outcomes.[11,61-64] Even though the secondary guideline therapies are the same in women and men, there is evidence from the Canadian Registry of ACS of underutilization of these evidence-based treatments in women[65] (Table 4-4).

In regards to invasive strategies for ACS, gender differences are also demonstrated. In a meta-analysis of multiple ACS trials, an invasive strategy resulted in a reduction of the composite endpoint of death, MI, or repeat ACE in men and women, but it was more beneficial in women with positive biomarkers. There was no reduction of the composite endpoint in women with negative biomarkers. This difference was not seen in men.[66] Based on Get With The Guidelines,[63] an in-hospital program for improving care by promoting consistent adherence to the latest scientific treatment guidelines, women's clinical performance after MI based on multiple measures, treatments, and outcomes was significantly worse. Compared with men, women with AMI were less likely to undergo a cardiac catheterization procedure during their index hospitalization (45.6% vs 56.2%; P <0.0001), PCI (36.1% vs 52.3%; P <0.0001), CABG (5.4% vs 9.2%; P <0.0001), and any revascularization (40.9% vs 60.2%; P <0.0001) (Table 4-5). These sex differences in invasive procedures persisted after multivariable adjustment (Table 4-6).[63] In-hospital mortality post-STEMI is greater for women than men (Figure 4-19).[63]

TABLE 4-2 Non-ECG exercise test variables of diagnostic and prognostic value in women.[42]

Exercise Variable	Method of Assessment	High-Risk Values	Remarks
Exercise capacity	Estimated by the stress protocol (in METs)	<5 METs; <85% of predicted value (predicted METs = 14.7–(0.13 × age)	Predictive of mortality and cardiovascular events in both asymptomatic and symptomatic women
Chronotropic response	Achievement of age-predicted HR	<85% of age-predicted HR	Predictive of survival in symptomatic women
	Chronotropic index: chronotropic index = HR*/metabolic reserve; metabolic reserve = $(MET_{stage} - 1)/(MET_{peak} - 1)$; HRR = $(HR_{stage} - HR_{rest})$/(100% age-predicted peak HR – HR_{rest})	Chronotropic index ≤ 0.80	Predictive of mortality and cardiovascular events in asymptomatic and symptomatic women
HRR	Difference between HR at peak exercise and HR after 1-minute recovery	≤12 bpm after 1-minute recovery (upright cool-down period)	Predictive of mortality in asymptomatic and symptomatic women
DTS	DTS = exercise time–(5 × ST deviation) – (4 × angina score index)	Low-risk DTS, ≥5; moderate-risk DTS, > −11, <5; high-risk DTS, ≤ −11	Predictive of all-cause mortality and cardiac mortality in asymptomatic and symptomatic women; in symptomatic women, moderate- and high-risk DTS indicate more severe CAD
ΔST/ΔHR index	Maximum change in ST-segment depression/change in HR	Abnormal, >1.6 μV/bpm	Increases the sensitivity for detection of CAD in asymptomatic women
ST/HR slope	Greatest statistically significant slope by linear regression relating ST-segment depression to HR during exercise	Abnormal, >2.4 μV/bpm; markedly abnormal, >6.0 μV/bpm	Increases the sensitivity for detection of CAD in asymptomatic women
BP response	Assessment of BP response to exercise, change in SBP and DBP from rest with maximal stress	Decrease in SBP >10 mm Hg from baseline	High likelihood of ischemia/detection of CAD in left main coronary artery and/or 3-vessel disease
		SBP >190 mm Hg with exercise testing	Increased risk of developing hypertension
		Exaggerated DBP response to exercise	increased risk of developing hypertension

BP, blood pressure; DBP, diastolic blood pressure; SBP, systolic blood pressure.
Source: American Heart Association, Inc.
*Using peak age-predicted HR = 206 – 0.88 (age) in asymptomatic women for chronotropic index calculation.

In the setting of acute or chronic obstructive coronary disease, women have an overall worse prognosis than men.[2,16,67-73] The prognosis is significantly worse in younger women. As noted in Figure 4-20,[29] there is a significantly higher rate across all age groups in men compared with women of annual rate of first MI. However, younger women aged 45 to 54 years were at a significantly higher risk of mortality post-MI. This has been explained in part due to comorbidity, infarct severity, and medical management differences, but this does not fully explain the high-risk younger female cohort.[68] On a positive note, women have overall superior cardiac survival to men if they are evaluated for stable chest pain symptoms.[44,74,75] However, the 1-year death and reinfarction rates are higher in women presenting with acute MI.[2]

In addition, women are more likely to be admitted for CHF with preserved LV function than men and they are more likely to die irrespective of whether they have obstructive or nonobstructive coronary disease.[2] After CABG, operative mortality is higher for women, which is similar to data on angioplasty.[71,72,76-80] However, the long-term outcome after PCI and CABG appears similar by gender.[71,72,78-81]

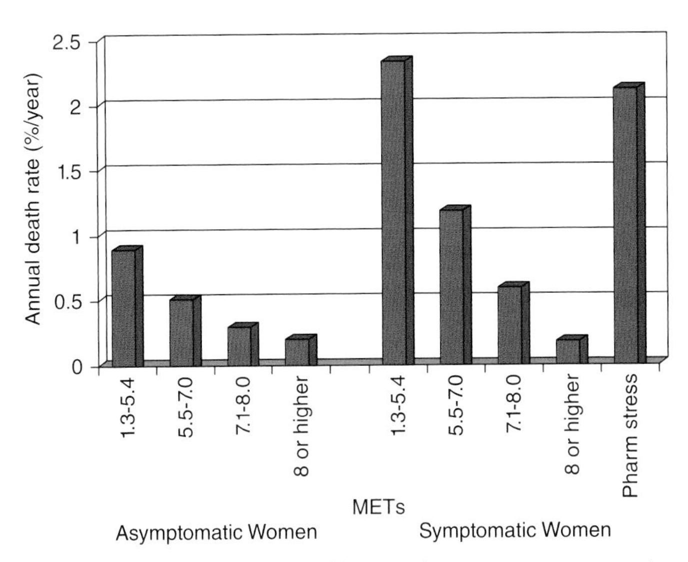

FIGURE 4-16 Prognostic value of functional capacity in asymptomatic (*N* = 8715) and symptomatic (*n* = 8214) women as synthesized from published reports and available data.[58]

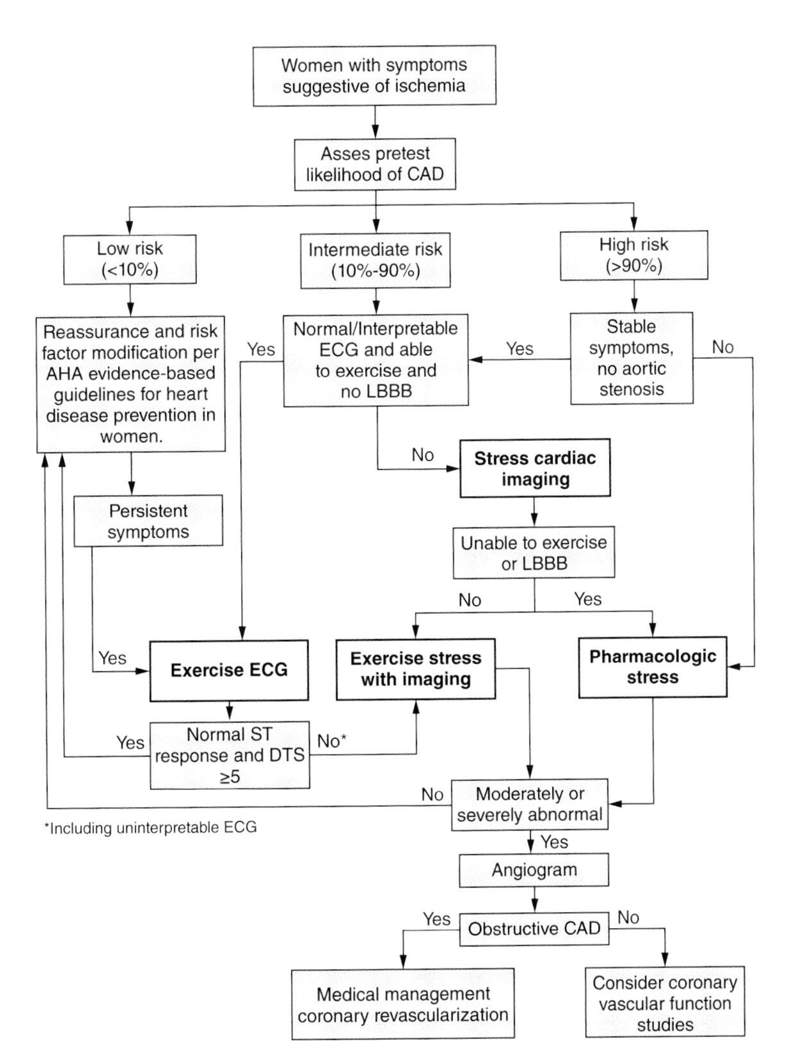

FIGURE 4-17 Algorithm for stress testing in the evaluation of a symptomatic woman at low, intermediate, and high risk is determined by the patient's pretest probability of CAD.[42] *Abbreviations:* LBBB indicates left bundle branch block.

FEMALE-PATTERN DISEASE

NOVEL RISK FACTORS

The traditional cardiac risk factors in male-pattern disease rely on the Framingham Risk Calculator to give an estimate of individual risk for IHD; however, this can often underestimate the risk in women.[82-84] Biomarkers such as highly specific C-reactive protein (hs-CRP), troponin I, *N*-terminal probrain natriuretic peptide, and cystatin C may improve risk assessment of IHD.[85] Hs-CRP is higher in women compared with men even in women with inflammatory disease.[86,87] An elevation in this biomarker predicts a higher risk of IHD than traditional risk factors.[86-90] The role that hs-CRP should play in risk assessment for IHD in women is not well defined and not currently routinely recommended in the 2011 effectiveness-based guidelines for prevention of cardiovascular disease in women.[22] However, the AHA has recommended use of novel modalities to refine risk assessment in intermediate-risk patients when there is uncertainty about starting a statin drug.[91,92] Hormonal changes are unique to women and these changes make women prone to IHD. Specifically ovulation dysfunction is associated with an increased risk of IHD and adverse CVD events.[1] Premature coronary atherosclerosis has been associated with one cause of ovarian dysfunction called functional hypothalamic amenorrhea.[93] As stated earlier, metabolic syndrome and diabetes put a woman at increased risk of developing IHD and polycystic ovarian syndrome is strongly associated with those risk factors.[94] Problems during pregnancy, including preeclampsia and gestational diabetes, infer elevated risk for women and development of IHD.[1] Preeclampsia doubles the risk of IHD and gestational diabetes increases risk for development of diabetes later in life, leading to increased risk of IHD.[95,96]

Lastly, the therapies used in the treatment of breast cancer should be considered. There has been improved survival but an elevated risk of IHD in women who receive the breast cancer treatment,[97] however, it is unclear whether the increased risk comes from the disease or specific treatments.

TABLE 4-3 Class III interventions (not useful/effective and may be harmful) for the prevention of CVD in women. CVD indicates cardiovascular disease; MI, myocardial infarction.[22]

Class III interventions
Menopausal Therapy
Hormone therapy and selective estrogen-receptor modulators (SERMs) should not be used for the primary or secondary prevention of CVD (*Class III, Level of Evidence A*).
Antioxidant Supplements
Antioxidant vitamin supplements (eg, vitamin E, C, and β-carotene) should not be used for the primary or secondary prevention of CVD (*Class III, Level of Evidence A*).
Folic Acid*
Folic Acid, with or without B_6 and B_{12} supplementation, should not be used for the primary or secondary prevention of CVD (*Class III, Level of Evidence A*).
Aspirin for MI in Women < 65 years of Age
Routine use of aspirin in healthy women <65 years of age is not recommended to prevent MI (*Class III, Level of Evidence B*).

*Folic acid supplementation should be used in the childbearing years to prevent neural tube defects.

PRESENTATION

It is not infrequent for women who present with ACS and undergo coronary angiography to have either "normal" coronaries or nonobstructive CAD.[1] There were 50% lower odds for women compared to men to have obstructive CAD, according to a registry that includes 600 hospitals.[98] Other registries that include ACS patients have demonstrated an increased frequency of nonobstructive CAD in women compared to men.[77,99] However, even in those women who present with angina, according to the Women Ischemia Syndrome Evaluation (WISE) data, 57% will not have obstructive coronary disease but more than half of those patients with nonobstructive disease will continue to have the same signs and symptoms of ischemia with repeated hospitalizations and coronary angiography.[1] This is not a benign prognosis. From the WISE data, women with symptoms of ischemia and no obstructive CAD had higher mortality and adverse cardiovascular events compared with asymptomatic women[100] (Figures 4-21 and 4-22).

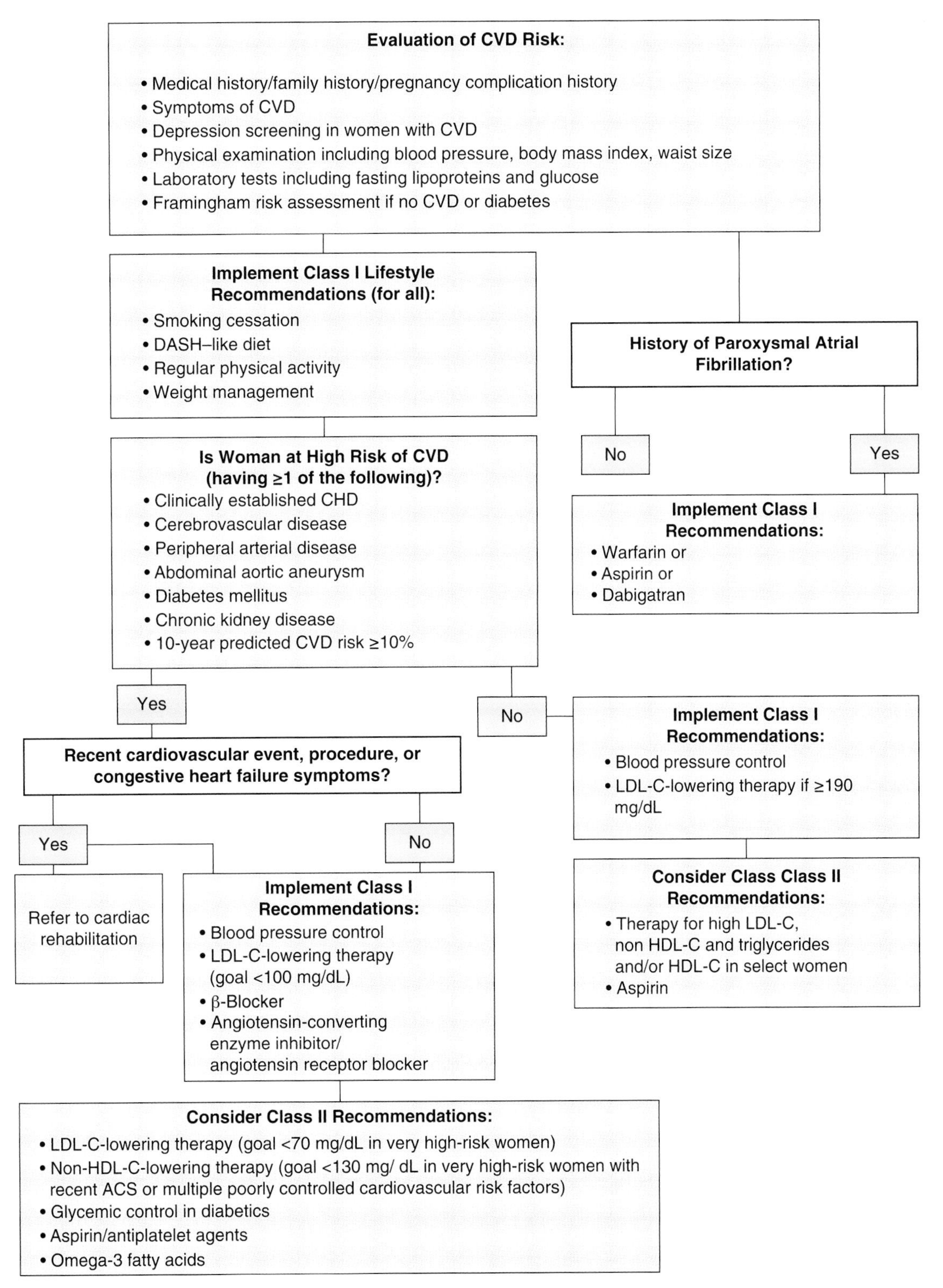

FIGURE 4-18 Flow diagram for CVD prevention care in women.[22] *Abbreviations*: ACS, acute coronary syndrome; CHD, coronary heart disease; CVD indicates cardiovascular disease; DASH, Dietary Approaches to Stop Hypertension; HDL-C, high-density lipoprotein cholesterol; LDL-C, low-density lipoprotein cholesterol.

DIAGNOSIS

From a diagnostic standpoint it is known that women have a lower pretest probability of IHD based on the prevalence of the disease compared to men. This is associated with a higher probability of "false-positive" test results and thus a lower specificity of noninvasive testing in women (Bayes theorem).[12] Additionally, there is a greater prevalence of nonobstructive disease and higher frequency of myocardial ischemia in women.[29] The approach to patient management of IHD has been to determine the likelihood of a "culprit" obstructive coronary lesion with our vast array of diagnostic tools. This "culprit" lesion is then usually felt to be the etiology of patient symptoms and ischemia. However, given the greater prevalence of nonobstructive disease in women, this method becomes less effective[29] (Figure 4-23).

Cardiovascular MR imaging is clinically important in assessing for subendocardial ischemia, more precise assessment of left ventricular function, and a detailed evaluation of the myocardium and peripheral vasculature.[101-104] In those women who have absence of obstructive coronary artery disease by coronary angiography, cardiac MR may provide evidence to the etiology of chest pain symptoms if subendocardial perfusion is noted.[102] In a small study of 20 patients (comprising 80% women) and in another study, women with abnormal

TABLE 4-4 Underutilization of Evidence-Based Treatments in Women. Canadian Registry of ACS.[65]

	Male (*n* = 4471)	Female (*n* = 2087)	*P*-Value
Medications at Discharge			
Antiplatelet	93%	93%	0.49
β-Blocker	79%	76%	0.0015
Lipid-lowering	65%	56%	<0.0001
ACE inhibitors	60%	56%	0.006
Procedures			
Angiography	50%	42%	<0.0001
PCI	23%	18%	<0.0001
CABG	0.08%	0.04%	<0.0001
Outcomes			
Death	2%	3%	0.0078
Death/MI	8%	8%	0.36
Death 1 year	8%	11%	0.0017
Death/MI 1 year	16%	17%	0.095

TABLE 4-5 Sex-based differences in clinical performance measures and invasive procedures.[63]

Measure/Treatment	Overall (*n* = 78,254), % (*n*)	Men (*n* = 47,556), % (*n*)	Women (*n* = 30,698), % (*n*)	*p*
Early medical therapy				
Aspirin within <24 h	92.4 (65,018)	93.3 (40,332)	91.0 (24,686)	<0.0001
β-Blockers within <24 h	86.2 (55,777)	87.2 (34,653)	84.7 (21,124)	<0.0001
Invasive procedures				
Cardiac catheterization	52.1 (40,745)	56.2 (26,733)	45.6 (14,012)	<0.0001
PCI	45.9 (32,323)	52.3 (22,253)	36.1 (10,070)	<0.0001
CABG	7.7 (5,394)	9.2 (3,893)	5.4 (1,501)	<0.0001
Revascularization	52.6 (37,023)	60.2 (25,614)	40.9 (11,409)	<0.0001
Timeliness of reperfusion*				
DTN time, median (25th-75th), min	40.0 (25.0-70.0)	39.0 (24.0-66.0)	47.0 (27.0-83.0)	<0.0001
DTB time, median (25th-75th), min	97.0 (70.0-140.0)	95.0 (69.0-135.0)	103.0 (74.0-154.0)	<0.0001
DTN ≤30 min, % (*n*)	33.2 (933)	35.2 (711)	28.3 (222)	0.0005
DTB ≤90 min, % (*n*)	43.2 (3,316)	44.8 (2,510)	39.0 (806)	<0.0001
Acute reperfusion*				
Any reperfusion therapy	67.3 (17,058)	73.0 (12,184)	56.3 (4,874)	<0.0001
Reperfusion therapies				<0.0001
Primary PCI	56.4 (14,292)	61.1 (10,196)	47.3 (4096)	
Fibrinolytic therapy	5.8 (1,467)	6.2 (1,028)	5.1 (439)	
Fibrinolytic therapy+PCI	5.1 (1,299)	5.8 (960)	3.9 (339)	

*STEMI sub population.

TABLE 4-6 Adjusted odds ratios (ORs) for clinical performance measures, invasive procedures, and in-hospital death.[63]

Measure/Treatment/Outcome	*n*	Adjusted OR (95% CI) (Women vs Men)	*P*
Early medical therapy			
Aspirin within 24 h	70,360	0.86 (0.81-0.90)	<0.0001
β-Blocker within 24 h	64,681	0.90 (0.86-0.93)	<0.0001
Invasive procedures			
Cardiac catheterization	74,769	0.91 (0.88-0.94)	<0.0001
PCI	67,477	0.78 (0.74-0.81)	<0.0001
CABG	67,477	0.60 (0.55-0.65)	<0.0001
Revascularization	67,477	0.68 (0.65-0.71)	<0.0001
Acute reperfusion and timeliness of reperfusion[†]			
DTN ≤30 min	2,807	0.78 (0.65-0.92)	0.004
DTB ≤90 min	7,673	0.87 (0.79-0.95)	0.004
Reperfusion therapy	24,742	0.75 (0.70-0.80)	<0.0001
Primary PCI	24,742	0.83 (0.78-0.87)	<0.0001
Fibrinolytic therapy	24,742	0.87 (0.81-0.93)	<0.0001
In-hospital death			
Overall AMI cohort	70,105	1.04 (0.99-1.10)	0.1
STEMI subpopulation	23,015	1.12 (1.02-1.23)	0.015

*ORs, which are for women vs men, were adjusted for age, race, BMI, insurance type, systolic blood pressure, cardiac diagnosis, initial ECG with diagnostic ST-segment elevation or left bundle-branch block, diabetes, hypertension, hyperlipidemia, heart failure, previous MI, peripheral vascular disease, renal insufficiency, stroke, chronic obstructive pulmonary disease, and adult history of smoking. The generalized estimation equations approach was also employed to adjust for clustering within hospitals.
[†]STEMI subpopulation.

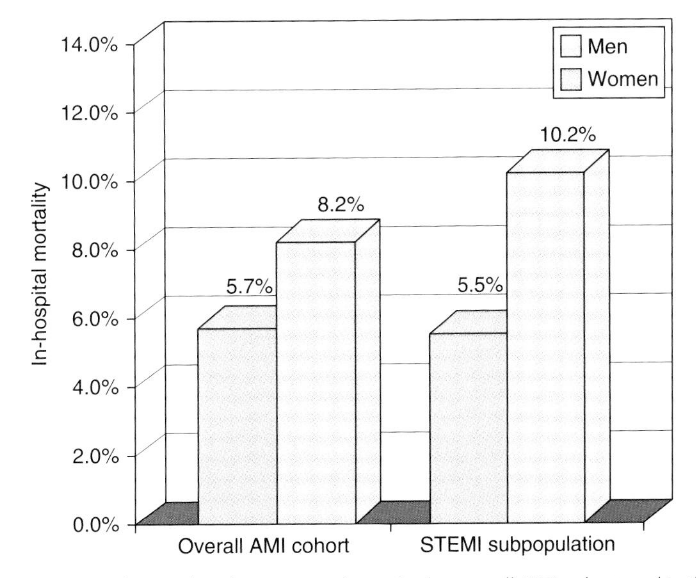

FIGURE 4-19 In-hospital mortality rates among hospitalized women and men in the overall AMI cohort and in the STEMI subpopulation.[63]

stress tests and normal coronary arteries underwent adenosine CMR. Besides, subendocardial ischemia was frequently present.[102,105] In women who present with ACS and have a coronary angiogram with normal coronaries, subendocardial ischemia on CMR was the most common finding.[32]

CORONARY REACTIVITY TESTING

Coronary reactivity testing done during coronary angiography is the gold standard for diagnosing microvascular disease and endothelial wall dysfunction. It allows for direct measurement of blood flow characteristics in response to vasoactive agents for the diagnoses of microvascular coronary dysfunction.[106] It can be useful in differentiating a woman's chest pain symptoms. Current evidence suggests its associated risk is relatively low when compared with adverse prognosis associated with microvascular coronary dysfunction[107] (Figures 4-24 and 4-25). Prinzmetal angina was thought to be vasospasm of the epicardial arteries causing coronary reactivity.[108] However, more recently, microvascular coronary dysfunction involving both the endothelial and nonendothelial pathways can be responsible for ischemia in women.[109]

MICROVASCULAR CORONARY DYSFUNCTION

In women who present with persistent chest pain, no obstructive CAD, and ischemic evidenced by stress testing, microvascular coronary dysfunction (MCD) is the predominant etiological mechanism of ischemia.[110] MCD is defined as limited coronary flow reserve (CFR) and/or coronary endothelial dysfunction.[110] MCD patients face a 2.5% annual adverse cardiac event rate, which includes myocardial infarction, congestive heart failure, stroke, and sudden cardiac death.[111] Currently, the gold standard for the diagnosis of MCD requires the exclusion of obstructive CAD by coronary angiography,[112] followed by evaluation of microvascular coronary function by Doppler guide wire in the cardiac catheterization laboratory for endothelial function testing in response to intra-coronary acetylcholine (Figure 4-24), and CFR testing in response to adenosine (Figure 4-25) by CRT.[110]

OUTCOMES

The WISE study reported that 34% of the women studied had normal coronary arteries and 57% had nonobstructive disease with lesions <50% (Figure 4-26). However, the prognosis of women with "normal" coronary arteries who tested positive for ischemia was worse than women who were tested negative for ischemia. One could conclude that the absence of angiographic coronary lesions does not necessarily represent "normal" coronary arteries. The same women who are more likely than men to have normal angiographic coronary arteries are 4 times more likely to be readmitted for chest pain or ACS within the next 180 days.[113] In addition, the prevalence of chest pain in the absence of obstructive CAD has not declined since it was first reported.[114-117] In those with ACS and no obstructive CAD, there was a 2% risk of death and MI at 30 days post-MI.[118]

An important comparative analysis in 2009 of symptomatic women from the WISE trial and asymptomatic women from the WTH project

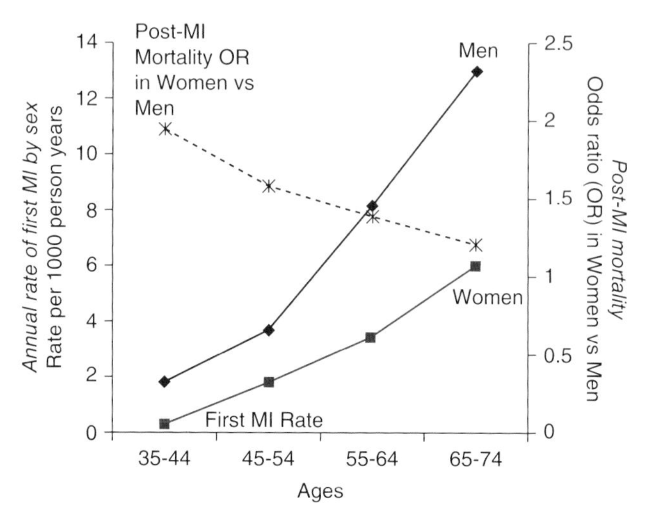

FIGURE 4-20 This graph shows the annual rate of first myocardial infarction (MI) by gender, noting the significantly higher rate across all age groups in men as compared with women.[29]

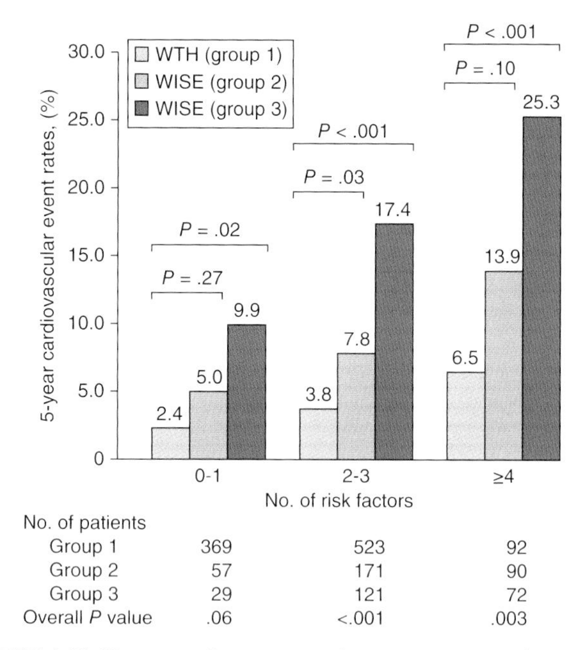

No. of patients	0-1	2-3	≥4
Group 1	369	523	92
Group 2	57	171	90
Group 3	29	121	72
Overall *P* value	.06	<.001	.003

FIGURE 4-21 Five-year primary composite event rate according to risk factor category.[100]

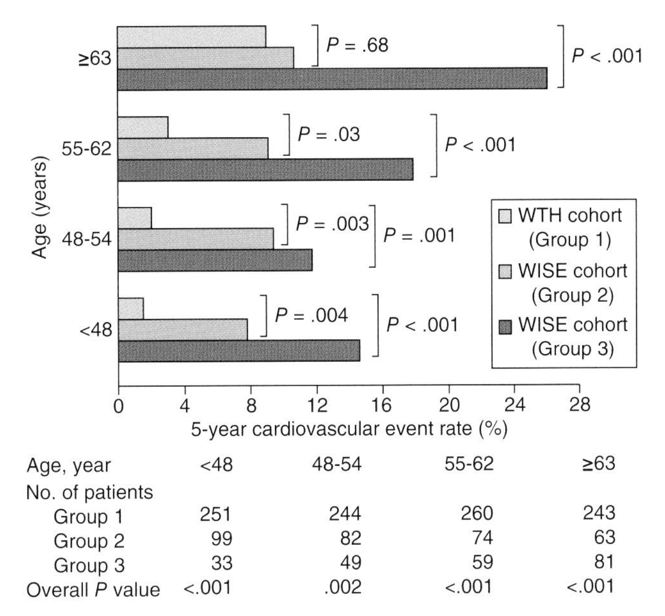

Age, year	<48	48-54	55-62	≥63
No. of patients				
Group 1	251	244	260	243
Group 2	99	82	74	63
Group 3	33	49	59	81
Overall *P* value	<.001	.002	<.001	<.001

FIGURE 4-22 Five-year primary composite event rate according to age.[100]

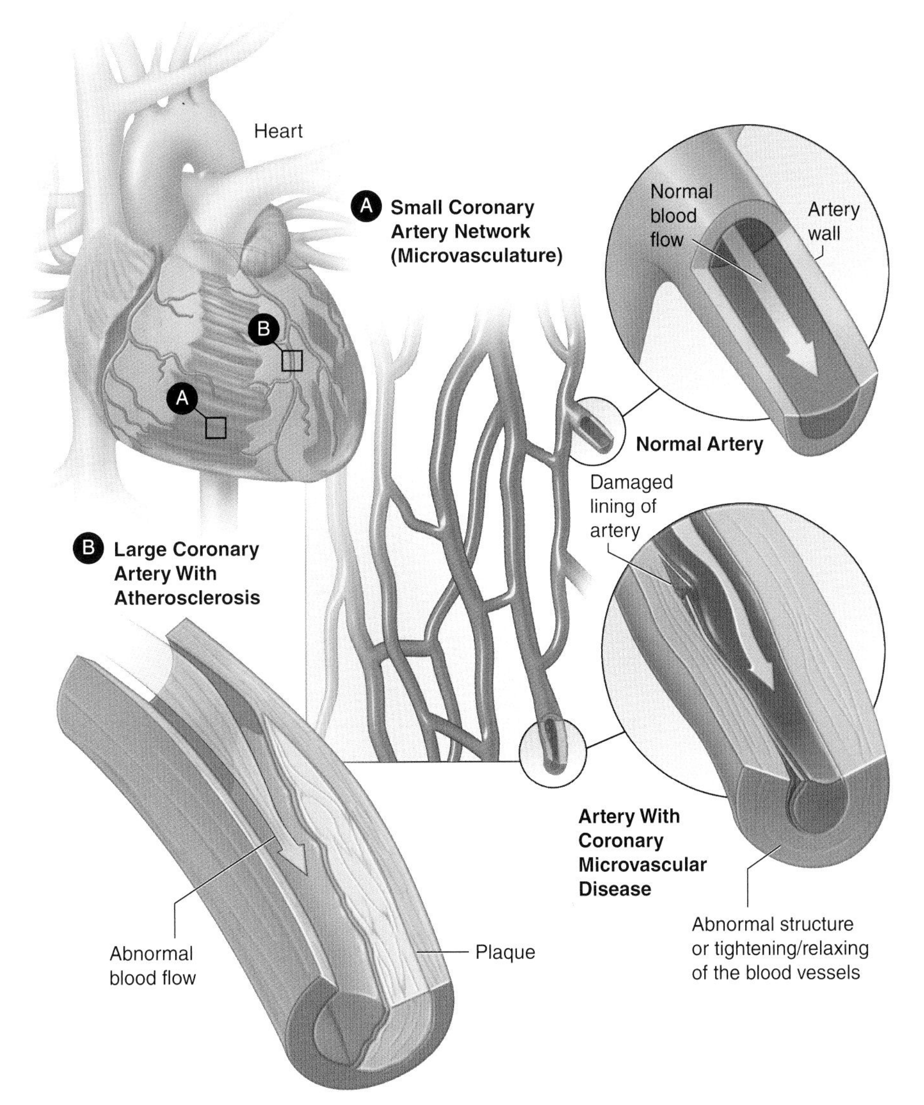

FIGURE 4-23 (A) The small coronary artery network (microvasculature), containing a normal artery and an artery with coronary MVD. (B) A large coronary artery with plaque buildup.
From: http://www.nhlbi.nih.gov/health/health-topics/topics/hdw/. Accessed December 6, 2012.

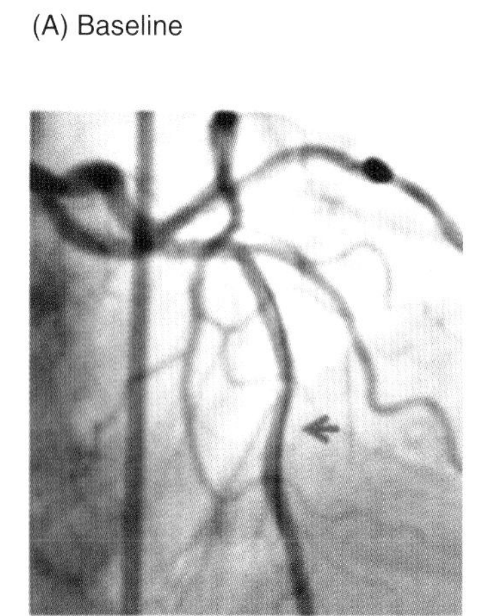

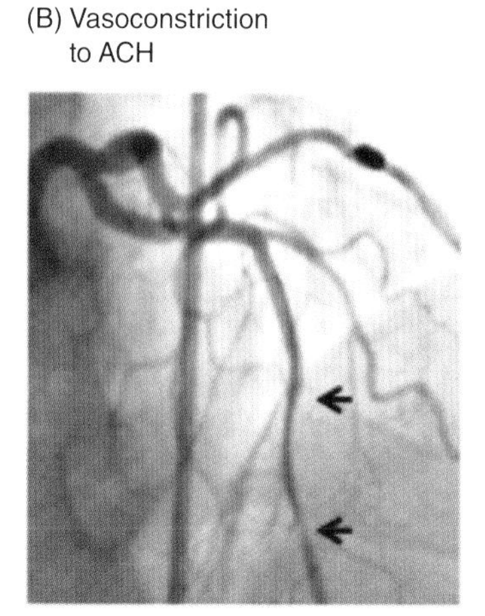

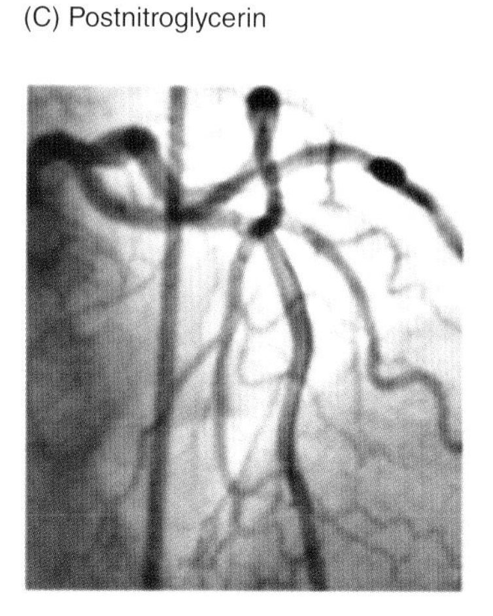

FIGURE 4-24 Coronary angiogram and CRT. (A) The figure shows Doppler flow wire in the left anterior descending artery (red arrow). (B) In response to acetylcholine (ACH) infusion, there is abnormal coronary artery vasoconstriction (black arrows), indicating endothelial dysfunction. (C) This is resolved by intracoronary nitroglycerin. *Abbreviations:* CRT, coronary reactivity testing.[107]

revealed a difference in cardiovascular risk between these 2 populations of women. As seen in Table 4-7, rates of adverse cardiovascular events were highest for the symptomatic women with nonobstructive CAD compared with normal coronary arteries.[100] However, the women with normal coronary arteries had an approximately 3-fold higher risk (16% vs 2.4%) of CVD event rate at 5 years than the asymptomatic cohort of women even after adjusting for cardiovascular risk factors.[100] With an increasing number of risk factors, there was an increased rate of 5-year cardiovascular event in each population of women as shown in Figure 4-21. The symptomatic women had higher event rates compared to the asymptomatic women. And there was a 3-fold increase in event rate in the symptomatic women with ≥4 risk factors versus the asymptomatic women with ≥4 risk factors. Figure 4-22 shows that the relationship between age and cardiovascular events differed by subgroups.[100] Age was an important risk factor in the asymptomatic women from WTH project. This study demonstrates the reason why aggressive medical therapy and risk factor reduction in symptomatic women with normal or nonobstructive CAD is necessary to help reduce their risk for further cardiovascular events.

TREATMENT

Further treatment for nonobstructive CAD has focused on improvement of symptoms or vascular-function response. β-blockers appear to improve symptoms, but calcium channel blockers do not.[119,120] Statins and ACEI improve endothelial dysfunction and may improve symptoms and outcomes.[121-124] In a substudy carried out within WISE, microvascular function improved with ACEI therapy in women with signs and symptoms of ischemia without obstructive CAD and was associated with a reduction in angina.[124] Exercise helps improve symptoms and exercise capacity.[125] Imipramine appears to affect visceral analgesia and improve symptoms.[126] There are concerns regarding the safety of L-arginine, but it may improve endothelial function. Recently, a study of women with angina, myocardial ischemia, and nonobstructive disease revealed that the addition of ranolazine had improved angina symptoms.[127] This was particularly impressive in those with documented microvascular dysfunction.

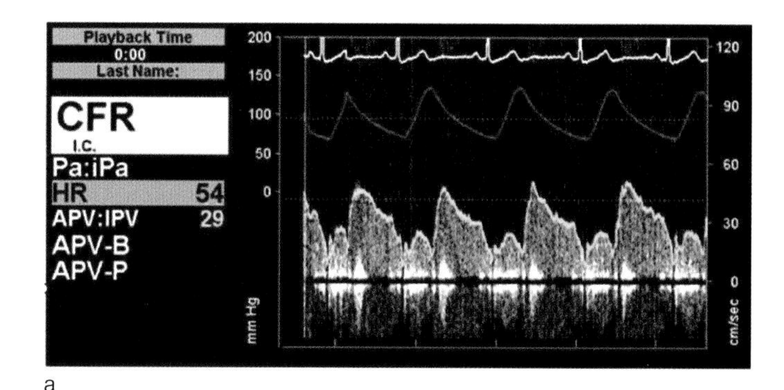

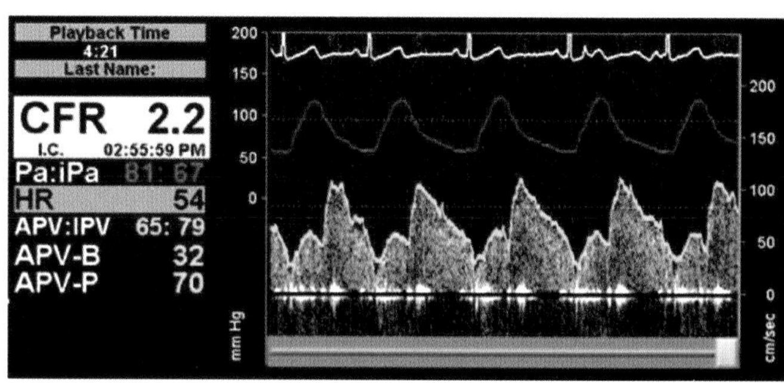

FIGURE 4-25 Intracoronary Doppler blood flow velocity waveforms before intracoronary adenosine (A), and after intracoronary adenosine infusion (B). CFR is the ratio of average peak velocities before and after adenosine.[110]

CONCLUSIONS

Ischemic heart disease has sex-specific differences. Even though the overall prevalence of IHD remains higher in men, women have a higher prevalence of symptoms, ischemia, and mortality relative to men. And despite some improvement in outcomes for women with IHD, the trends show that they still lag behind men. In fact, there are certain populations of women that may be at higher risk. Both novel and traditional risk factors can help identify at-risk women. Better utilization of current diagnostic testing can accurately diagnose myocardial ischemia in symptomatic women and also add prognostic value when evaluating asymptomatic and symptomatic women. There is a suggestion of a "female-pattern disease". This is evidenced by the frequent triad of chest pain, no obstructive CAD, and evidence of myocardial ischemia on stress testing that is more prevalent in women compared to men. Currently, coronary reactivity testing is used to measure MCD and endothelial dysfunction as the primary pathophysiologic mechanisms for ischemia in these women.

Guideline-based therapy is equally effective in both men and women with IHD; however, it is underutilized in women. This underutilization has resulted in continued poorer outcomes after ACS. In the asymptomatic women at risk, there are specific primary

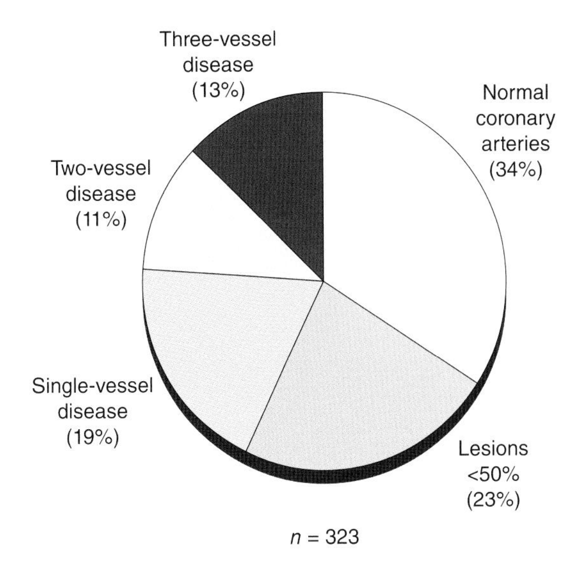

FIGURE 4-26 Detailed angiographic analysis of women with suspected ischemic chest pain and nonobstructive coronary artery disease.
Reproduced with permission from Sharaf BL, Pepine CJ, Kerensky RA, et al. Detailed angiographic analysis of women with suspected ischemic chest pain (pilot phase data from the NHLBI-sponsored Women's Ischemia Syndrome Evaluation [WISE] Study Angiographic Core Laboratory). *Am J Cardiol*. April 2001;87(8):937-941; A933.

TABLE 4-7 Five-year rates of cardiovascular outcomes in asymptomatic women compared with symptomatic women with normal and nonobstructive CAD.[100]

	Asymptomatic Women (WTH) (*n* = 1000)	Symptomatic Women (WISE): Normal Coronary Arteries[a] (*n* = 318)	Symptomatic Women (WISE): Nonobstructive CAD[b] (*n* = 222)	Adjusted *P* Value[c]	Adjusted *P* Value[c,d]
MI, %	0.7	0.9	3.9	0.07	0.31
Hospitalization for CHF, %	0.3	3.3	5.6	< 0.001	0.002
Stroke, %	1.0	2.4	5.2	0.002	0.004
Death due to CV, %	0.6	1.5	4.4	0.11	0.82
All-cause mortality, %	2.1	3.0	8.2	0.04	0.74
Primary composite end point, %[e]	2.4	7.9	16.0	< 0.001	0.002
Secondary composite end point, %[f]	3.9	9.1	19.1	< 0.001	0.008

Abbreviations: CAD, coronary artery disease; CHF, congestive heart failure; CV, cardiovascular causes; MI, myocardial infarction; WISE, Women's Ischemia Syndrome Evaluation; WTH, St James Women Take Heart Project.
[a]Indicates 0% stenosis.
[b]Indicates 1% to 49% stenosis.
[c]Adjusted for age, race, body mass index, systolic blood pressure, diabetes mellitus, education, employment, family history of CAD, smoking history, and the metabolic syndrome.
[d]Compares the WTH cohort with the WISE cohort who had normal coronary arteries.
[e]Consists of MI, hospitalization for heart failure, stroke, or cardiovascular death.
[f]Consists of MI, hospitalization for heart failure, stroke, or death due to any cause.

prevention guidelines that should be followed. Treatment for those asymptomatic women with myocardial ischemia and no obstructive CAD continues to evolve.

REFERENCES

1. Gulati M, Shaw LJ, Bairey Merz CN. Myocardial ischemia in women: lessons from the NHLBI WISE study. *Clin Cardiol.* March 2012;35(3):141-148.
2. Roger VL, Go AS, Lloyd-Jones DM, et al. Heart disease and stroke statistics—2011 update: a report from the American Heart Association. *Circulation.* February 2011;123(4):e18-e209.
3. Shaw LJ, Bairey Merz CN, Pepine CJ, et al. Insights from the NHLBI-sponsored Women's Ischemia Syndrome Evaluation (WISE) study: part I: gender differences in traditional and novel risk factors, symptom evaluation, and gender-optimized diagnostic strategies. *J Am Coll Cardiol.* February 2006; 47(3 Suppl):S4-S20.
4. Bairey Merz N, Bonow RO, Sopko G, et al. Women's Ischemic Syndrome Evaluation: current status and future research directions: report of the National Heart, Lung and Blood Institute workshop: October 2-4, 2002: executive summary. *Circulation.* February 2004;109(6):805-807.
5. Bell DM, Nappi J. Myocardial infarction in women: a critical appraisal of gender differences in outcomes. *Pharmacotherapy.* September 2000;20(9):1034-1044.
6. Ford ES, Capewell S. Coronary heart disease mortality among young adults in the U.S. from 1980 through 2002: concealed leveling of mortality rates. *J Am Coll Cardiol.* November 2007;50(22):2128-2132.
7. Murphy SL. Deaths: final data for 1998. *Natl Vital Stat Rep.* Jul 2000;48(11):1-105.
8. Lampert R, McPherson CA, Clancy JF, et al. Gender differences in ventricular arrhythmia recurrence in patients with coronary artery disease and implantable cardioverter-defibrillators. *J Am Coll Cardiol.* June 2004;43(12):2293-2299.
9. Ni H, Coady S, Rosamond W, et al. Trends from 1987 to 2004 in sudden death due to coronary heart disease: the Atherosclerosis Risk in Communities (ARIC) study. *Am Heart J.* January 2009;157(1):46-52.
10. Pepine CJ. Ischemic heart disease in women: facts and wishful thinking. *J Am Coll Cardiol.* May 2004;43(10):1727-1730.
11. Daly C, Clemens F, Lopez Sendon JL, et al. Gender differences in the management and clinical outcome of stable angina. *Circulation.* January 2006;113(4):490-498.
12. Andreotti F, Marchese N. Women and coronary disease. *Heart.* January 2008;94(1):108-116.
13. Lloyd-Jones DM, Leip EP, Larson MG, et al. Prediction of lifetime risk for cardiovascular disease by risk factor burden at 50 years of age. *Circulation.* February 2006;113(6):791-798.
14. Daviglus ML, Stamler J, Pirzada A, et al. Favorable cardiovascular risk profile in young women and long-term risk of cardiovascular and all-cause mortality. *JAMA.* October 2004;292(13):1588-1592.
15. Mokdad AH, Ford ES, Bowman BA, et al. Prevalence of obesity, diabetes, and obesity-related health risk factors, 2001. *JAMA.* January 2003;289(1):76-79.
16. Lerner DJ, Kannel WB. Patterns of coronary heart disease morbidity and mortality in the sexes: a 26-year follow-up of the Framingham population. *Am Heart J.* February 1986;111(2):383-390.
17. Hokanson JE, Austin MA. Plasma triglyceride level is a risk factor for cardiovascular disease independent of high-density lipoprotein cholesterol level: a meta-analysis of population-based prospective studies. *J Cardiovasc Risk.* April 1996;3(2):213-219.
18. Reuterwall C, Hallqvist J, Ahlbom A, et al. Higher relative, but lower absolute risks of myocardial infarction in women than in men: analysis of some major risk factors in the SHEEP study. The SHEEP Study Group. *J Intern Med.* August 1999;246(2):161-174.
19. Yusuf S, Hawken S, Ounpuu S, et al. Effect of potentially modifiable risk factors associated with myocardial infarction in 52 countries (the INTERHEART study): case-control study. *Lancet.* 2004 September 11-17 2004;364(9438):937-952.
20. Mega JL, Hochman JS, Scirica BM, et al. Clinical features and outcomes of women with unstable ischemic heart disease: observations from metabolic efficiency with ranolazine for less ischemia in non-ST-elevation acute coronary syndromes-thrombolysis in myocardial infarction 36 (MERLIN-TIMI 36). *Circulation.* April 2010;121(16):1809-1817.
21. Ogden CL, Carroll MD, Curtin LR, et al. Prevalence of overweight and obesity in the United States, 1999-2004. *JAMA.* April 2006;295(13):1549-1555.
22. Mosca L, Benjamin EJ, Berra K, et al. Effectiveness-based guidelines for the prevention of cardiovascular disease in women—2011 update: a guideline from the american heart association. *Circulation.* March 2011;123(11):1243-1262.
23. Gami AS, Witt BJ, Howard DE, et al. Metabolic syndrome and risk of incident cardiovascular events and death: a systematic review and meta-analysis of longitudinal studies. *J Am Coll Cardiol.* January 2007;49(4):403-414.
24. Smith SC, Allen J, Blair SN, et al. AHA/ACC guidelines for secondary prevention for patients with coronary and other atherosclerotic vascular disease: 2006 update: endorsed by the National Heart, Lung, and Blood Institute. *Circulation.* May 2006;113(19):2363-2372.
25. Burke AP, Farb A, Malcom GT, et al. Effect of risk factors on the mechanism of acute thrombosis and sudden coronary death in women. *Circulation.* June 1998;97(21):2110-2116.
26. Burke AP, Farb A, Pestaner J, et al. Traditional risk factors and the incidence of sudden coronary death with and without coronary thrombosis in blacks. *Circulation.* January 2002;105(4):419-424.
27. Burke AP, Virmani R, Galis Z, et al. 34th Bethesda Conference: Task force #2—what is the pathologic basis for new atherosclerosis imaging techniques? *J Am Coll Cardiol.* June 2003;41(11):1874-1886.

28. Arbustini E, Dal Bello B, Morbini P, et al. Plaque erosion is a major substrate for coronary thrombosis in acute myocardial infarction. *Heart*. September 1999;82(3):269-272.

29. Bairey Merz CN, Shaw LJ, Reis SE, et al. Insights from the NHLBI-Sponsored Women's Ischemia Syndrome Evaluation (WISE) study: part II: gender differences in presentation, diagnosis, and outcome with regard to gender-based pathophysiology of atherosclerosis and macrovascular and microvascular coronary disease. *J Am Coll Cardiol*. February 2006;47(3 suppl):S21-S29.

30. von Mering GO, Arant CB, Wessel TR, et al. Abnormal coronary vasomotion as a prognostic indicator of cardiovascular events in women: results from the National Heart, Lung, and Blood Institute-Sponsored Women's Ischemia Syndrome Evaluation (WISE). *Circulation*. February 2004;109(6):722-725.

31. Wong TY, Klein R, Sharrett AR, et al. Retinal arteriolar narrowing and risk of diabetes mellitus in middle-aged persons. *JAMA*. May 2002;287(19):2528-2533.

32. Reynolds HR, Srichai MB, Iqbal SN, et al. Mechanisms of myocardial infarction in women without angiographically obstructive coronary artery disease. *Circulation*. September 2011;124(13):1414-1425.

33. Douglas PS, Ginsburg GS. The evaluation of chest pain in women. *N Engl J Med*. May 1996;334(20):1311-1315.

34. Hemingway H, Langenberg C, Damant J, et al. Prevalence of angina in women versus men: a systematic review and meta-analysis of international variations across 31 countries. *Circulation*. March 2008;117(12):1526-1536.

35. Canto JG, Goldberg RJ, Hand MM, et al. Symptom presentation of women with acute coronary syndromes: myth vs reality. *Arch Intern Med*. December 2007;167(22):2405-2413.

36. Milner KA, Funk M, Arnold A, et al. Typical symptoms are predictive of acute coronary syndromes in women. *Am Heart J*. February 2002;143(2):283-288.

37. McSweeney JC, Cody M, O'Sullivan P, et al. Women's early warning symptoms of acute myocardial infarction. *Circulation*. November 2003;108(21):2619-2623.

38. Healy B. The Yentl syndrome. *N Engl J Med*. July 1991;325(4):274-276.

39. Nabel EG, Selker HP, Califf RM, et al. Women's Ischemic Syndrome Evaluation: current status and future research directions: report of the National Heart, Lung and Blood Institute workshop: October 2-4, 2002: section 3: diagnosis and treatment of acute cardiac ischemia: gender issues. *Circulation*. February 2004;109(6):e50-e52.

40. Merz NB, Johnson BD, Kelsey PSF, et al. Diagnostic, prognostic, and cost assessment of coronary artery disease in women. *Am J Manag Care*. Oct 2001;7(10):959-965.

41. Pepine CJ, Balaban RS, Bonow RO, et al. Women's Ischemic Syndrome Evaluation: current status and future research directions: report of the National Heart, Lung and Blood Institute workshop: October 2-4, 2002: section 1: diagnosis of stable ischemia and ischemic heart disease. *Circulation*. February 2004;109(6):e44-e46.

42. Kohli P, Gulati M. Exercise stress testing in women: going back to the basics. *Circulation*. December 2010;122(24):2570-2580.

43. Kwok Y, Kim C, Grady D, et al. Meta-analysis of exercise testing to detect coronary artery disease in women. *Am J Cardiol*. March 1999;83(5):660-666.

44. Alexander KP, Shaw LJ, Shaw LK, et al. Value of exercise treadmill testing in women. *J Am Coll Cardiol*. November 1998;32(6):1657-1664.

45. Shaw LJ, Peterson ED, Shaw LK, et al. Use of a prognostic treadmill score in identifying diagnostic coronary disease subgroups. *Circulation*. October 1998;98(16):1622-1630.

46. Mark DB, Shaw L, Harrell FE, et al. Prognostic value of a treadmill exercise score in outpatients with suspected coronary artery disease. *N Engl J Med*. September 1991;325(12):849-853.

47. Mark DB, Hlatky MA, Harrell FE, et al. Exercise treadmill score for predicting prognosis in coronary artery disease. *Ann Intern Med*. June 1987;106(6):793-800.

48. Kwok JM, Miller TD, Hodge DO, et al. Prognostic value of the Duke treadmill score in the elderly. *J Am Coll Cardiol*. May 2002;39(9):1475-1481.

49. Gulati M, Arnsdorf MF, Shaw LJ, et al. Prognostic value of the Duke treadmill score in asymptomatic women. *Am J Cardiol*. August 2005;96(3):369-375.

50. Gulati M, Black HR, Shaw LJ, et al. The prognostic value of a nomogram for exercise capacity in women. *N Engl J Med*. August 2005;353(5):468-475.

51. Kavanagh T, Mertens DJ, Hamm LF, et al. Peak oxygen intake and cardiac mortality in women referred for cardiac rehabilitation. *J Am Coll Cardiol*. December 2003;42(12):2139-2143.

52. Mieres JH, Shaw LJ, Hendel RC, et al. American Society of Nuclear Cardiology consensus statement: Task Force on Women and Coronary Artery Disease—the role of myocardial perfusion imaging in the clinical evaluation of coronary artery disease in women [correction]. *J Nucl Cardiol*. 2003 January-February 2003;10(1):95-101.

53. Taillefer R, DePuey EG, Udelson JE, et al. Comparative diagnostic accuracy of Tl-201 and Tc-99m sestamibi SPECT imaging (perfusion and ECG-gated SPECT) in detecting coronary artery disease in women. *J Am Coll Cardiol*. January 1997;29(1):69-77.

54. Berman DS, Kang X, Hayes SW, et al. Adenosine myocardial perfusion single-photon emission computed tomography in women compared with men. Impact of diabetes mellitus on incremental prognostic value and effect on patient management. *J Am Coll Cardiol*. April 2003;41(7):1125-1133.

55. Amanullah AM, Berman DS, Hachamovitch R, et al. Identification of severe or extensive coronary artery disease in women by adenosine technetium-99m sestamibi SPECT. *Am J Cardiol*. July 1997;80(2):132-137.

56. Hachamovitch R, Berman DS, Kiat H, et al. Effective risk stratification using exercise myocardial perfusion SPECT in women: gender-related differences in prognostic nuclear testing. *J Am Coll Cardiol.* July 1996;28(1):34-44.

57. Shaw LJ, Iskandrian AE. Prognostic value of gated myocardial perfusion SPECT. *J Nucl Cardiol.* 2004 March-April 2004;11(2):171-185.

58. Mieres JH, Shaw LJ, Arai A, et al. Role of noninvasive testing in the clinical evaluation of women with suspected coronary artery disease: consensus statement from the Cardiac Imaging Committee, Council on Clinical Cardiology, and the Cardiovascular Imaging and Intervention Committee, Council on Cardiovascular Radiology and Intervention, American Heart Association. *Circulation.* February 2005;111(5):682-696.

59. Pilote L, Dasgupta K, Guru V, et al. A comprehensive view of sex-specific issues related to cardiovascular disease. *CMAJ.* March 2007;176(6):S1-S44.

60. Mosca L, Banka CL, Benjamin EJ, et al. Evidence-based guidelines for cardiovascular disease prevention in women: 2007 update. *J Am Coll Cardiol.* March 2007;49(11): 1230-1250.

61. Blomkalns AL, Chen AY, Hochman JS, et al. Gender disparities in the diagnosis and treatment of non-ST-segment elevation acute coronary syndromes: large-scale observations from the CRUSADE (Can Rapid Risk Stratification of Unstable Angina Patients Suppress Adverse Outcomes With Early Implementation of the American College of Cardiology/American Heart Association guidelines) National Quality Improvement Initiative. *J Am Coll Cardiol.* March 2005;45(6):832-837.

62. Alexander KP, Chen AY, Newby LK, et al. Sex differences in major bleeding with glycoprotein IIb/IIIa inhibitors: results from the CRUSADE (Can Rapid Risk Stratification of Unstable Angina Patients Suppress Adverse Outcomes With Early Implementation of the ACC/AHA guidelines) initiative. *Circulation.* September 2006;114(13):1380-1387.

63. Jneid H, Fonarow GC, Cannon CP, et al. Sex differences in medical care and early death after acute myocardial infarction. *Circulation.* December 2008;118(25):2803-2810.

64. Novack V, Cutlip DE, Jotkowitz A, et al. Reduction in sex-based mortality difference with implementation of new cardiology guidelines. *Am J Med.* July 2008;121(7):597-603.e1.

65. Bugiardini R, Yan AT, Yan RT, et al. Factors influencing underutilization of evidence-based therapies in women. *Eur Heart J.* June 2011;32(11):1337-1344.

66. O'Donoghue M, Boden WE, Braunwald E, et al. Early invasive vs conservative treatment strategies in women and men with unstable angina and non-ST-segment elevation myocardial infarction: a meta-analysis. *JAMA.* July 2008;300(1):71-80.

67. Smith SC, Blair SN, Bonow RO, et al. AHA/ACC Scientific Statement: AHA/ACC guidelines for preventing heart attack and death in patients with atherosclerotic cardiovascular disease: 2001 update: a statement for healthcare professionals from the American Heart Association and the American College of Cardiology. *Circulation.* September 2001;104(13): 1577-1579.

68. Vaccarino V, Parsons L, Every NR, et al. Sex-based differences in early mortality after myocardial infarction. National Registry of Myocardial Infarction 2 Participants. *N Engl J Med.* July 1999;341(4):217-225.

69. Nohria A, Vaccarino V, Krumholz HM. Gender differences in mortality after myocardial infarction. Why women fare worse than men. *Cardiol Clin.* February 1998;16(1):45-57.

70. Lagerqvist B, Säfström K, Ståhle E, et al. Is early invasive treatment of unstable coronary artery disease equally effective for both women and men? FRISC II Study Group Investigators. *J Am Coll Cardiol.* July 2001;38(1):41-48.

71. Jacobs AK, Kelsey SF, Brooks MM, et al. Better outcome for women compared with men undergoing coronary revascularization: a report from the bypass angioplasty revascularization investigation (BARI). *Circulation.* September 1998;98(13):1279-1285.

72. Jacobs AK, Johnston JM, Haviland A, et al. Improved outcomes for women undergoing contemporary percutaneous coronary intervention: a report from the National Heart, Lung, and Blood Institute Dynamic registry. *J Am Coll Cardiol.* May 2002;39(10):1608-1614.

73. Mehilli J, Kastrati A, Dirschinger J, et al. Differences in prognostic factors and outcomes between women and men undergoing coronary artery stenting. *JAMA.* October 2000;284(14):1799-1805.

74. Arruda-Olson AM, Juracan EM, Mahoney DW, et al. Prognostic value of exercise echocardiography in 5,798 patients: is there a gender difference? *J Am Coll Cardiol.* February 2002;39(4):625-631.

75. Marwick TH, Shaw LJ, Lauer MS, et al. The noninvasive prediction of cardiac mortality in men and women with known or suspected coronary artery disease. Economics of Noninvasive Diagnosis (END) Study Group. *Am J Med.* February 1999;106(2):172-178.

76. Jacobs AK, Kelsey SF, Yeh W, et al. Documentation of decline in morbidity in women undergoing coronary angioplasty (a report from the 1993-94 NHLBI Percutaneous Transluminal Coronary Angioplasty Registry). National Heart, Lung, and Blood Institute. *Am J Cardiol.* Oct 1997;80(8):979-984.

77. Hochman JS, Tamis JE, Thompson TD, et al. Sex, clinical presentation, and outcome in patients with acute coronary syndromes. Global Use of Strategies to Open Occluded Coronary Arteries in Acute Coronary Syndromes IIb Investigators. *N Engl J Med.* July 1999;341(4):226-232.

78. Hartz RS, Rao AV, Plomondon ME, et al. Effects of race, with or without gender, on operative mortality after coronary artery bypass grafting: a study using The Society of Thoracic Surgeons National Database. *Ann Thorac Surg.* February 2001;71(2): 512-520.

79. Drazner MH, Rame JE, Marino EK, et al. Increased left ventricular mass is a risk factor for the development of a depressed left ventricular ejection fraction within five years:

the Cardiovascular Health Study. *J Am Coll Cardiol.* June 2004;43(12):2207-2215.

80. Ferguson TB, Hammill BG, Peterson ED, et al. A decade of change—risk profiles and outcomes for isolated coronary artery bypass grafting procedures, 1990-1999: a report from the STS National Database Committee and the Duke Clinical Research Institute. Society of Thoracic Surgeons. *Ann Thorac Surg.* February 2002;73(2):480-489; discussion 489-490.
81. Malenka DJ, Wennberg DE, Quinton HA, et al. Gender-related changes in the practice and outcomes of percutaneous coronary interventions in Northern New England from 1994 to 1999. *J Am Coll Cardiol.* December 2002;40(12):2092-2101.
82. Michos ED, Nasir K, Braunstein JB, et al. Framingham risk equation underestimates subclinical atherosclerosis risk in asymptomatic women. *Atherosclerosis.* January 2006;184(1):201-206.
83. Lakoski SG, Greenland P, Wong ND, et al. Coronary artery calcium scores and risk for cardiovascular events in women classified as "low risk" based on Framingham risk score: the multi-ethnic study of atherosclerosis (MESA). *Arch Intern Med.* December 2007;167(22):2437-2442.
84. Pasternak RC, Abrams J, Greenland P, et al. 34th Bethesda Conference: Task force #1—identification of coronary heart disease risk: is there a detection gap? *J Am Coll Cardiol.* June 2003;41(11):1863-1874.
85. Wenger NK. The Reynolds Risk Score: improved accuracy for cardiovascular risk prediction in women? *Nat Clin Pract Cardiovasc Med.* July 2007;4(7):366-367.
86. Wong ND, Pio J, Valencia R, et al. Distribution of C-reactive protein and its relation to risk factors and coronary heart disease risk estimation in the National Health and Nutrition Examination Survey (NHANES) III. *Prev Cardiol.* 2001;4(3):109-114.
87. Bessant R, Hingorani A, Patel L, et al. Risk of coronary heart disease and stroke in a large British cohort of patients with systemic lupus erythematosus. *Rheumatology (Oxford).* July 2004;43(7):924-929.
88. Karim R, Stanczyk FZ, Hodis HN, et al. Associations between markers of inflammation and physiological and pharmacological levels of circulating sex hormones in postmenopausal women. *Menopause.* July 2010;17(4):785-790.
89. Ridker PM, Buring JE, Cook NR, et al. C-reactive protein, the metabolic syndrome, and risk of incident cardiovascular events: an 8-year follow-up of 14 719 initially healthy American women. *Circulation.* January 2003;107(3):391-397.
90. Ridker PM, Rifai N, Cook NR, et al. Non-HDL cholesterol, apolipoproteins A-I and B100, standard lipid measures, lipid ratios, and CRP as risk factors for cardiovascular disease in women. *JAMA.* July 2005;294(3):326-333.
91. Pearson TA, Mensah GA, Alexander RW, et al. Markers of inflammation and cardiovascular disease: application to clinical and public health practice: a statement for healthcare professionals from the Centers for Disease Control and Prevention and the American Heart Association. *Circulation.* January 2003;107(3):499-511.
92. Hlatky MA, Greenland P, Arnett DK, et al. Criteria for evaluation of novel markers of cardiovascular risk: a scientific statement from the American Heart Association. *Circulation.* May 2009;119(17):2408-2416.
93. Bairey Merz CN, Johnson BD, Sharaf BL, et al. Hypoestrogenemia of hypothalamic origin and coronary artery disease in premenopausal women: a report from the NHLBI-sponsored WISE study. *J Am Coll Cardiol.* February 2003;41(3):413-419.
94. Shaw LJ, Bairey Merz CN, Azziz R, et al. Postmenopausal women with a history of irregular menses and elevated androgen measurements at high risk for worsening cardiovascular event-free survival: results from the National Institutes of Health—National Heart, Lung, and Blood Institute sponsored Women's Ischemia Syndrome Evaluation. *J Clin Endocrinol Metab.* April 2008;93(4):1276-1284.
95. Bellamy L, Casas JP, Hingorani AD, et al. Pre-eclampsia and risk of cardiovascular disease and cancer in later life: systematic review and meta-analysis. *BMJ.* November 2007;335(7627):974.
96. Ratner RE, Christophi CA, Metzger BE, et al. Prevention of diabetes in women with a history of gestational diabetes: effects of metformin and lifestyle interventions. *J Clin Endocrinol Metab.* December 2008;93(12):4774-4779.
97. Jones LW, Haykowsky MJ, Swartz JJ, et al. Early breast cancer therapy and cardiovascular injury. *J Am Coll Cardiol.* October 2007;50(15):1435-1441.
98. Shaw LJ, Shaw RE, Merz CN, et al. Impact of ethnicity and gender differences on angiographic coronary artery disease prevalence and in-hospital mortality in the American College of Cardiology-National Cardiovascular Data Registry. *Circulation.* April 2008;117(14):1787-1801.
99. Hochman JS, McCabe CH, Stone PH, et al. Outcome and profile of women and men presenting with acute coronary syndromes: a report from TIMI IIIB. TIMI Investigators. Thrombolysis in Myocardial Infarction. *J Am Coll Cardiol.* July 1997;30(1):141-148.
100. Gulati M, Cooper-DeHoff RM, McClure C, et al. Adverse cardiovascular outcomes in women with nonobstructive coronary artery disease: a report from the Women's Ischemia Syndrome Evaluation Study and the St James Women Take Heart Project. *Arch Intern Med.* May 2009;169(9):843-850.
101. Pohost GM, Biederman RW, Doyle M. Cardiovascular magnetic resonance imaging and spectroscopy in the new millennium. *Curr Probl Cardiol.* August 2000;25(8):525-620.
102. Panting JR, Gatehouse PD, Yang GZ, et al. Abnormal subendocardial perfusion in cardiac syndrome X detected by cardiovascular magnetic resonance imaging. *N Engl J Med.* June 2002;346(25):1948-1953.
103. Buchthal SD, den Hollander JA, Merz CN, et al. Abnormal myocardial phosphorus-31 nuclear magnetic resonance spectroscopy in women with chest pain but normal coronary angiograms. *N Engl J Med.* March 2000;342(12):829-835.

104. Johnson BD, Shaw LJ, Buchthal SD, et al. Prognosis in women with myocardial ischemia in the absence of obstructive coronary disease: results from the National Institutes of Health-National Heart, Lung, and Blood Institute-Sponsored Women's Ischemia Syndrome Evaluation (WISE). *Circulation*. June 2004;109(24):2993-2999.

105. Pilz G, Klos M, Ali E, et al. Angiographic correlations of patients with small vessel disease diagnosed by adenosine-stress cardiac magnetic resonance imaging. *J Cardiovasc Magn Reson*. 2008;10:8.

106. Phan A, Shufelt C, Merz CN. Persistent chest pain and no obstructive coronary artery disease. *JAMA*. April 2009;301(14):1468-1474.

107. Wei J, Mehta PK, Johnson BD, et al. Safety of coronary reactivity testing in women with no obstructive coronary artery disease: results from the NHLBI-sponsored WISE (Women's Ischemia Syndrome Evaluation) study. *JACC Cardiovasc Interv*. June 2012;5(6):646-653.

108. Prinzmetal M, Kennamer R, Merliss R, et al. Angina pectoris. I. A variant form of angina pectoris; preliminary report. *Am J Med*. September 1959;27:375-388.

109. Sun H, Mohri M, Shimokawa H, et al. Coronary microvascular spasm causes myocardial ischemia in patients with vasospastic angina. *J Am Coll Cardiol*. March 2002;39(5):847-851.

110. Kothawade K, Bairey Merz CN. Microvascular coronary dysfunction in women: pathophysiology, diagnosis, and management. *Curr Probl Cardiol*. August 2011;36(8): 291-318.

111. Bugiardini R, Bairey Merz CN. Angina with "normal" coronary arteries: a changing philosophy. *JAMA*. January 2005;293(4):477-484.

112. Lanza GA, Crea F. Primary coronary microvascular dysfunction: clinical presentation, pathophysiology, and management. *Circulation*. June 2010;121(21):2317-2325.

113. Humphries KH, Pu A, Gao M, et al. Angina with "normal" coronary arteries: sex differences in outcomes. *Am Heart J*. February 2008;155(2):375-381.

114. Kemp HG, Elliott WC, Gorlin R. The anginal syndrome with normal coronary arteriography. *Trans Assoc Am Physicians*. 1967;80:59-70.

115. Likoff W, Segal BL, Kasparian H. Paradox of normal selective coronary arteriograms in patients considered to have unmistakable coronary heart disease. *N Engl J Med*. May 1967;276(19):1063-1066.

116. Sullivan AK, Holdright DR, Wright CA, et al. Chest pain in women: clinical, investigative, and prognostic features. *BMJ*. April 1994;308(6933):883-886.

117. Kennedy JW, Killip T, Fisher LD, et al. The clinical spectrum of coronary artery disease and its surgical and medical management, 1974-1979. The Coronary Artery Surgery study. *Circulation*. November 1982;66(5 pt 2):III16-III23.

118. Diver DJ, Bier JD, Ferreira PE, et al. Clinical and arteriographic characterization of patients with unstable angina without critical coronary arterial narrowing (from the TIMI-IIIA Trial). *Am J Cardiol*. September 1994;74(6):531-537.

119. Sütsch G, Oechslin E, Mayer I, et al. Effect of diltiazem on coronary flow reserve in patients with microvascular angina. *Int J Cardiol*. November 1995;52(2):135-143.

120. Lanza GA, Colonna G, Pasceri V, et al. Atenolol versus amlodipine versus isosorbide-5-mononitrate on anginal symptoms in syndrome X. *Am J Cardiol*. October 1999;84(7):854-856, A858.

121. Pizzi C, Manfrini O, Fontana F, et al. Angiotensin-converting enzyme inhibitors and 3-hydroxy-3-methylglutaryl coenzyme A reductase in cardiac syndrome X: role of superoxide dismutase activity. *Circulation*. January 2004;109(1):53-58.

122. Kayikcioglu M, Payzin S, Yavuzgil O, et al. Benefits of statin treatment in cardiac syndrome-X1. *Eur Heart J*. November 2003;24(22):1999-2005.

123. Chen JW, Hsu NW, Wu TC, et al. Long-term angiotensin-converting enzyme inhibition reduces plasma asymmetric dimethylarginine and improves endothelial nitric oxide bioavailability and coronary microvascular function in patients with syndrome X. *Am J Cardiol*. November 2002;90(9): 974-982.

124. Pauly DF, Johnson BD, Anderson RD, et al. In women with symptoms of cardiac ischemia, nonobstructive coronary arteries, and microvascular dysfunction, angiotensin-converting enzyme inhibition is associated with improved microvascular function: a double-blind randomized study from the National Heart, Lung and Blood Institute Women's Ischemia Syndrome Evaluation (WISE). *Am Heart J*. October 2011;162(4): 678-684.

125. Eriksson BE, Tyni-Lennè R, Svedenhag J, et al. Physical training in syndrome X: physical training counteracts deconditioning and pain in syndrome X. *J Am Coll Cardiol*. November 2000;36(5):1619-1625.

126. Cannon RO, Quyyumi AA, Mincemoyer R, et al. Imipramine in patients with chest pain despite normal coronary angiograms. *N Engl J Med*. May 1994;330(20):1411-1417.

127. Mehta PK, Goykhman P, Thomson LE, et al. Ranolazine improves angina in women with evidence of myocardial ischemia but no obstructive coronary artery disease. *JACC Cardiovasc Imaging*. May 2011;4(5):514-522.

5 CARDIAC SURGERY IN WOMEN

Jennifer M. Worth, MD
Juan Crestanello, MD

NATURAL HISTORY

According to the American Heart Association, more than 42 million women are affected with some form of cardiovascular disease that is responsible for 2,935,000 hospitalizations and 419,730 deaths every year (Roger).[1] This is about 1 death per minute among women, which makes cardiovascular disease the leading cause of death in US women nationally (Roger).[1] Heart disease causes more deaths in women than cancer, lung disease, and Alzheimer disease combined (Roger).[1] Coronary artery disease, valvular heart disease, congestive heart failure, and aortic aneurysms account for the majority of cardiovascular disease and related deaths in women (Roger).[1] Cardiac surgery is an effective treatment for many patients afflicted with these disorders.

CORONARY ARTERY BYPASS GRAFTING

Approximately 500,000 patients undergo coronary artery bypass grafting (CABG) surgery in the United States annually; however, only 25% of these surgeries are performed in women (Roger).[1]

Coronary artery disease usually manifests differently in women than in men. Symptoms in women are usually subtle, leading to delays in diagnosis and presentation at more advanced stages (Blankstein).[2] For example, after a myocardial infarction women present more often with heart failure and cardiogenic shock symptoms, and they more frequently require support with intra-aortic balloon pumps or with inotropic drugs (Blankstein).[2] In addition, women have a higher prevalence of diabetes and other risk factors associated with adverse outcomes after CABG such as renal failure, stage III or IV heart failure, and valvular heart disease (Blankstein).[2]

CABG surgery is not only performed less often in women but is also performed differently. The left internal mammary artery (LIMA) bypass to the left anterior descending coronary artery is used less often than in men (Blankstein).[2] This is particularly relevant since LIMA bypass (Figure 5-1) has been associated with the best long-term primary patency rate and with improved long-term survival (Edwards).[3] Women have smaller coronary arteries, leading to a lower number of bypass grafts performed per patient and to incomplete revascularization. Incomplete revascularization has been associated with adverse long-term outcomes (Edwards).[3] Early outcomes after CABG are also less favorable in women. Women have an increased incidence of perioperative morbidity and mortality compared to men. The 30-day mortality in women can be about twice that of men (4.2% vs 2.2%) (Blankstein).[2]

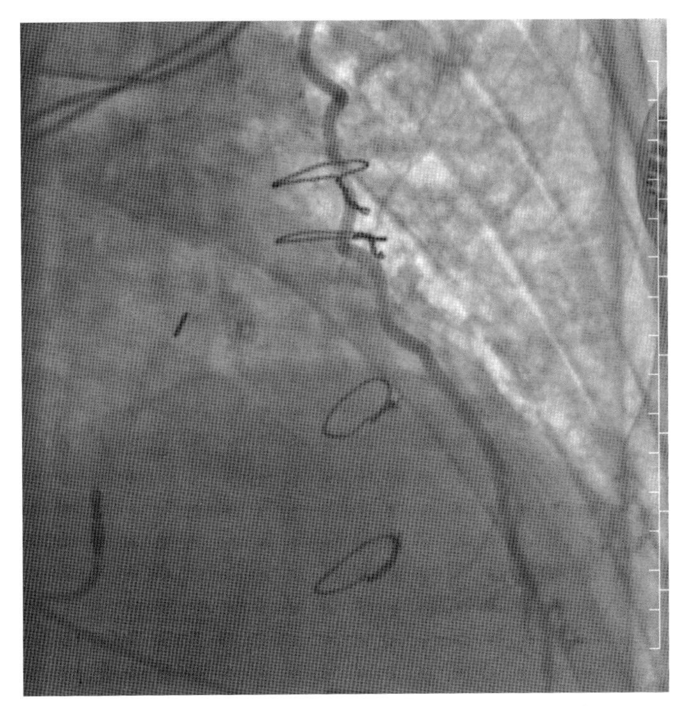

FIGURE 5-1 Angiogram of left internal mammary artery to left anterior descending coronary artery. This bypass is performed less frequently in women than in men despite demonstrated improvement in survival.

MITRAL VALVE SURGERY

Mitral valve disease is the most common valvular lesion in the United States (Roger).[1] According to the Framingham study, the prevalence of moderate or severe mitral regurgitation is 15.5% in adult men and

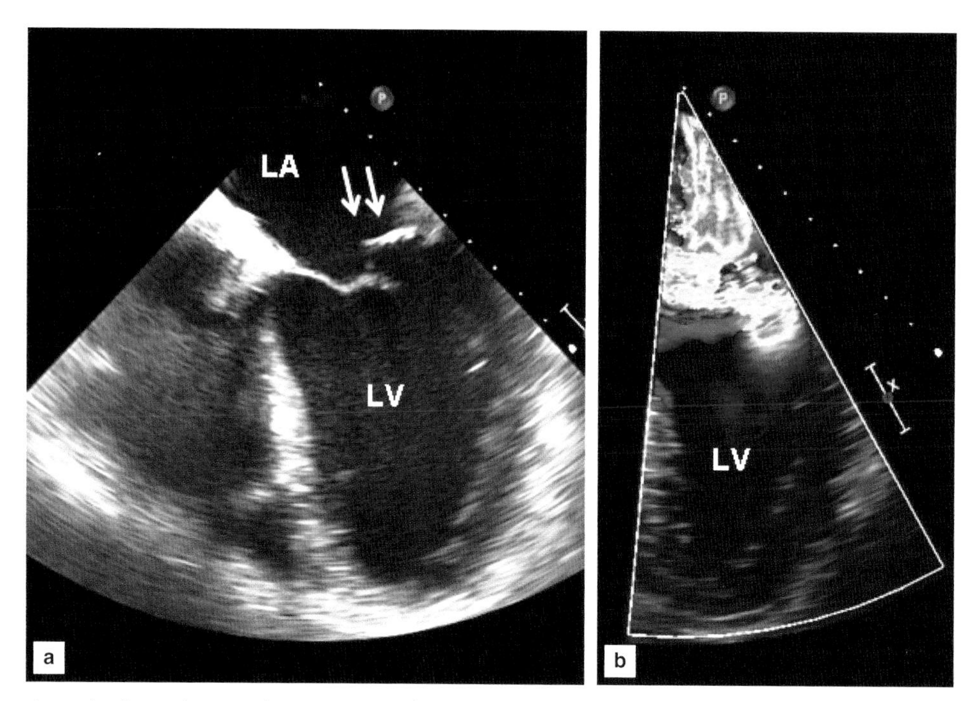

FIGURE 5-2 Transesophageal echocardiogram demonstrating a flail segment of the posterior leaflet of the mitral valve (A, arrows) resulting in severe mitral regurgitation (B). LA, left atrium; LV, left ventricle.

4.2% in women (Singh)[4] (Figure 5-2). Isolated mitral stenosis is more common in women (Roger).[1] Mitral stenosis occurs secondary to rheumatic heart disease and its prevalence has significantly decreased in the developed world (Roger).[1]

Mitral valve disease may present with heart failure symptoms, atrial fibrillation, chest pain, and hemoptysis.

The treatment for the majority of patients with degenerative severe mitral valve regurgitation is mitral valve repair. Mitral valve repair is safe, effective, and durable. It reestablishes valve competency and improves the patient's life expectancy. Restoration of the competency of the mitral valve is achieved by resection of the flail leaflet segment or by insertion of artificial chordae tendineae. The repair is reinforced by the insertion of an annuloplasty ring (Figure 5-3). This procedure can be performed in a minimally invasive manner through a right mini-thoracotomy or mini-sternotomy. Mitral valve replacement is rarely required. Operative mortality after mitral valve repair is increased for younger women compared to younger men and is believed to be related to hormonal effects (Song).[5] Percutaneous mitral valvuloplasty has become the preferred treatment for mitral stenosis (Figure 5-4).

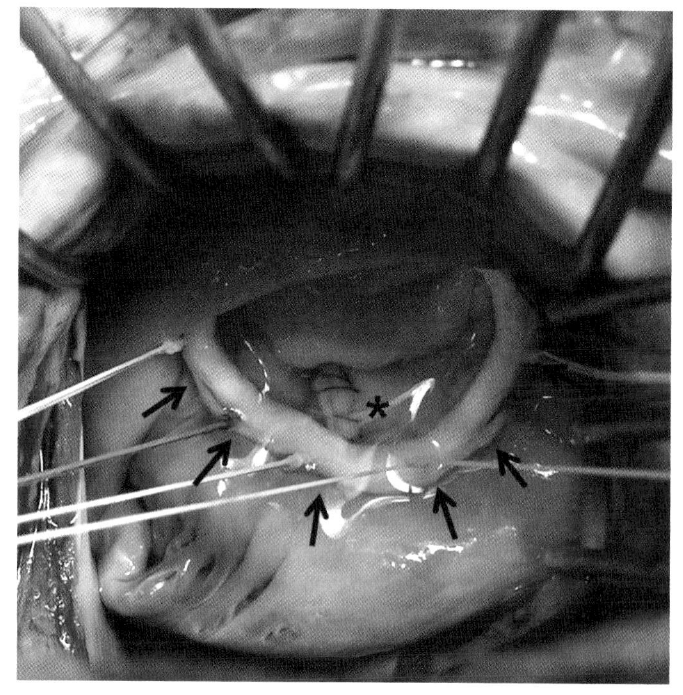

FIGURE 5-3 Mitral valve repair of the patient shown in Figure 5-2. The valve was repaired by excising the flail segment of the posterior leaflet (*) and inserting an annuloplasty band (arrows).

The incidence of functional mitral regurgitation is rising secondary to the increase of ischemic and nonischemic cardiomyopathy. In functional mitral regurgitation, the mitral valve leaflets are normal. Leaflet coaptation is impeded secondary to leaflet tethering by the remodeled ventricle. Mitral valve repair with a restrictive, undersized annuloplasty ring restores competency. Recurrence rates are high and patient survival is limited due to the underlying cardiomyopathy.

AORTIC VALVE SURGERY

Aortic stenosis is a disease of the elderly (Figure 5-5). Two percent of adults over the age of 65 have severe aortic stenosis. It is less common in women (Roger).[1] Symptoms of aortic stenosis include heart

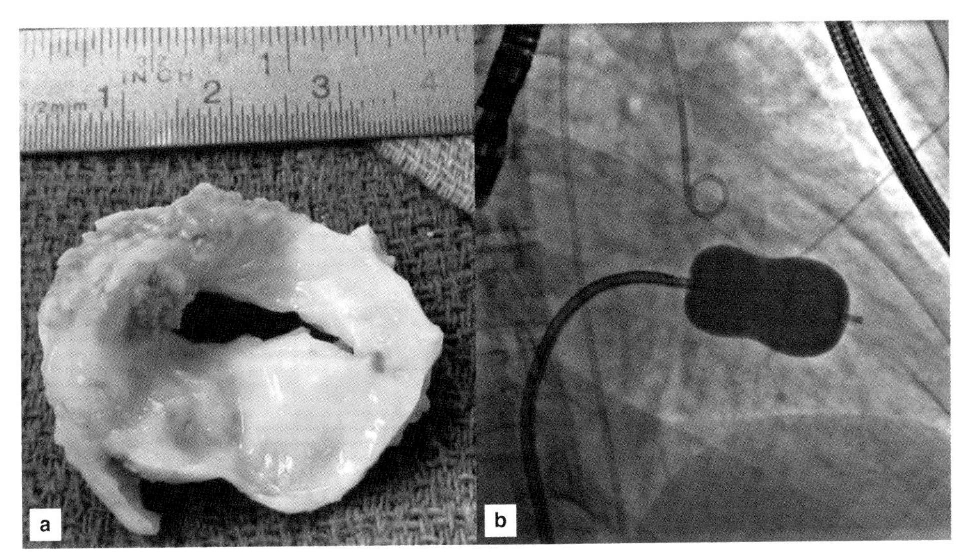

FIGURE 5-4 (A) Surgical specimen of a patient with severe mitral stenosis showing thickened mitral valve leaflets, leaflet calcification, and fusion of commissures. (B) Mitral balloon valvuloplasty is the preferred treatment for severe mitral stenosis.

failure, fatigue, dizziness, syncope, and angina. Once aortic stenosis becomes symptomatic, the prognosis is poor. More than 50% of patients are dead within a year (Leon).[6]

Surgical aortic valve replacement (AVR) is the standard treatment for severe symptomatic aortic stenosis. AVR can be done through a full sternotomy or through a minimally invasive approach. AVR is associated with low mortality. Thirty day and one-year survival is similar in both genders (Stamou).[7]

Replacement can be done with a mechanical or a biological prosthesis. Mechanical valves require life-long anticoagulation. Biological prostheses are associated with structural deterioration over time and need for reoperation.

Transcatheter aortic valve replacement (TAVR) has become an alternative to AVR for high-risk and inoperable patients (Figure 5-6). TAVR is associated with similar periprocedural mortality, higher stroke rates, but faster recovery than surgical AVR. Women appear to have significantly better survival than men after TAVR despite increased rates of bleeding, vascular complications, and stroke (Smith Humphries).[8,9]

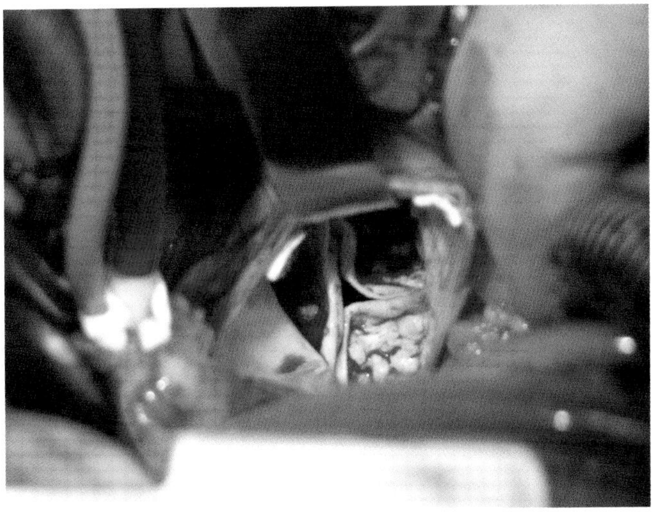

FIGURE 5-5 Aortic valve with severe degenerative stenosis showing extensive calcification and thickening of leaflets with decreased leaflet mobility.

HEART FAILURE

More than 5 million Americans are affected by congestive heart failure (Roger).[1] For patients with end-stage heart failure, medical management is not effective. For those patients, mechanical circulatory support or heart transplantation is the only treatment that improves survival and quality of life.

Less than 4000 heart transplants are performed every year in the world (Stehlik).[10] Their epidemiological impact in heart failure is minimal. Only 23% of heart transplant recipients are females. This underrepresentation of women in transplant recipients is likely due to a size mismatch between donor and recipient body habitus. Transplant outcomes in females are similar to males. There is a slightly higher incidence of rejection seen in women; however, this does not seem to influence long-term outcomes for the graft as long-term survival rates are similar across genders (Stehlik).[10]

Mechanical circulatory support can be used as a bridge to recovery, bridge to transplantation, or as a destination therapy. Intracorporeal or paracorporeal devices are used for support of the left ventricle, the right ventricle, or both (Figure 5-7). Women are also underrepresented as ventricular assist device (VAD) recipients. Only 22% of the VAD recipients are women. Female gender has been identified as a risk factor associated with increased mortality in VAD patients (Kirklin).[11]

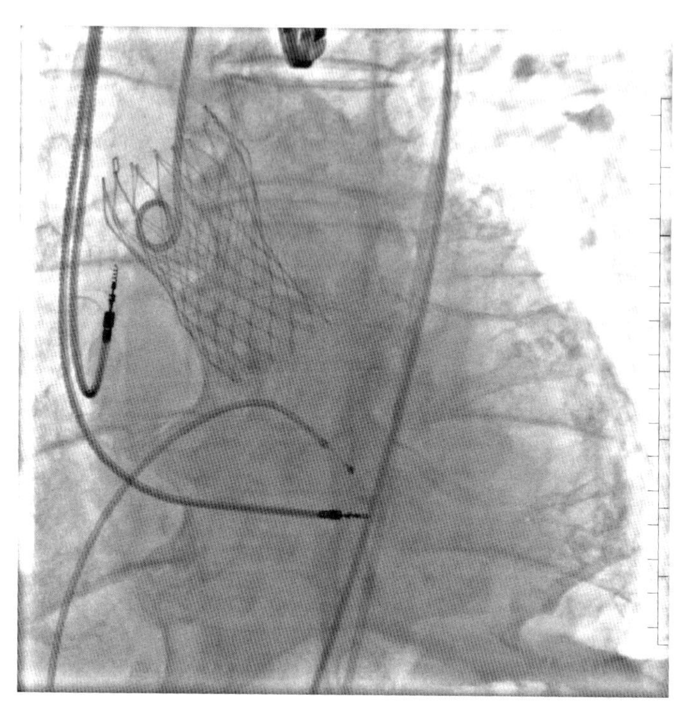

FIGURE 5-6 Transcatheter aortic valve (Medtronic CoreValve) deployed in the aortic root.

THORACIC AORTIC ANEURYSMS AND AORTIC DISSECTIONS

Aortic aneurysm refers to the dilatation of the aorta beyond the normal aortic diameter. The normal aortic diameter is influenced by age, sex, body size, and location of measurements. Thoracic aortic aneurysms are less common in females. Patients with thoracic aortic aneurysm are at increased risk for aortic rupture or dissection (Figure 5-8). Aortic aneurysms should be operated on when the risk of the surgery is less than the risk of rupture or dissection. This is influenced by the size of the aneurysm and the presence of connective tissue disorders and other risk factors for rupture.

Aortic dissection refers to disruption of the media and intima layer of the aorta with the creation of a false lumen with flow of blood within the aortic media. Patients with dissections may present with chest pain, hyper or hypotension, end-organ ischemia, cardiac tamponade, aortic insufficiency, heart failure, or shock. A type A dissection involves the ascending aorta. If not operated on, it is usually lethal. A type B dissection does not involve the ascending aorta. Type B dissections are usually treated medically. Aortic dissection, as aortic aneurysms, is less common in women. Women with aortic dissection are usually older than men. They are usually diagnosed late and are more likely to present with end organ ischemia, changes in mental status, or congestive heart failure. They have a significantly higher hospital mortality compared to men (Grubb).[12]

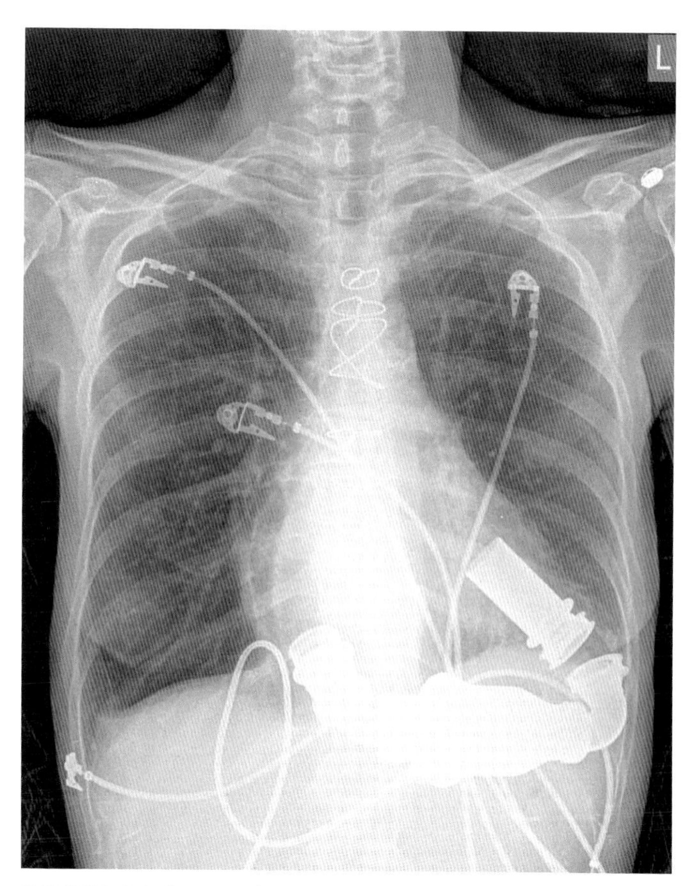

FIGURE 5-7 Left ventricular assist device, Thoratec HeartMate II.

REFERENCES

1. Roger VL, et al. Heart disease and stroke statistics-2012 update: a report from the American Heart Association. *Circulation*. 2012;125(22):e1002.

2. Blankstein R, et al. Female gender is an independent predictor of operative mortality after coronary artery bypass graft surgery: contemporary analysis of 31 midwestern hospitals. *Circulation*. 2005;112(9):I323-I327.

3. Edwards FH, et al. Gender-specific practice guidelines for coronary artery bypass surgery: perioperative management. *Ann Thorac Surg*. 2005;79(6):2189-2194.

4. Singh JP, et al. Prevalence and clinical determinants of mitral, tricuspid and aortic regurgitation (The Framingham Heart Study). *Am J Cardiol*. 1999;83(6):897-902.

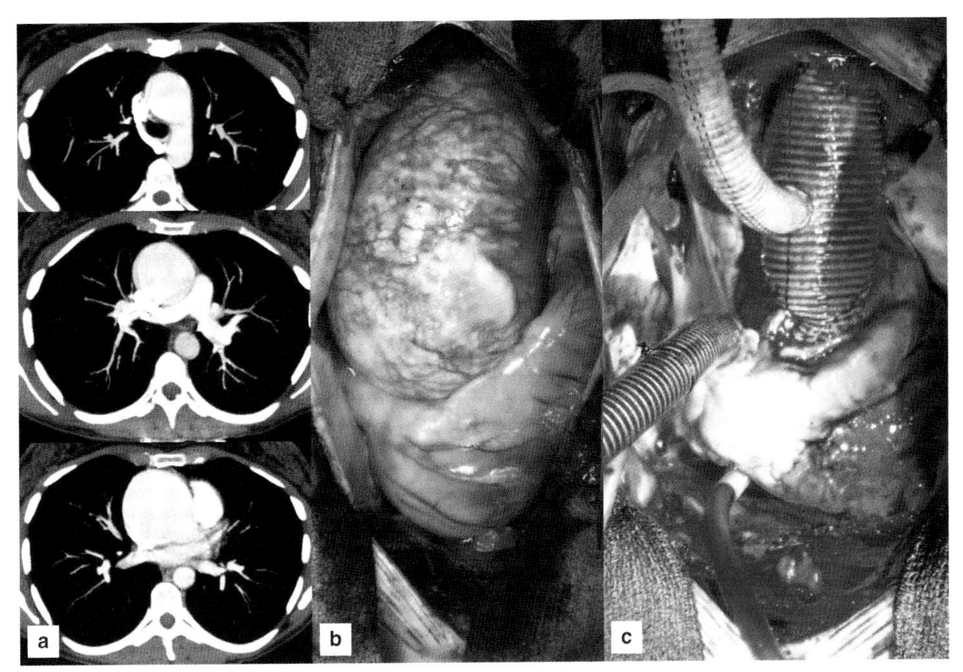

FIGURE 5-8 Ascending aortic aneurysm. (A) Computed tomography–demonstrated ascending aortic aneurysm extending from the sinotubular junction to the aortic arch. (B) Intraoperative picture of the ascending aortic aneurysm. (C) Replacement of the ascending aorta and proximal arch with a Dacron graft.

5. Song HK, et al. Gender differences in mortality after mitral valve operation: evidence for higher mortality in perimenopausal women. *Ann Thorac Surg*. 2008;85(6):2040-2025.

6. Leon MB, et al. Transcatheter aortic-valve implantation for aortic stenosis in patients who cannot undergo surgery. *N Engl J Med*. 2010;363(17):1597-607.

7. Stamou SC, et al. Effects of gender and ethnicity on outcomes after aortic valve replacement. *J Thorac Cardiovasc Surg*. 2012;144(2):486-492.

8. Smith CR, et al. Transcatheter versus surgical aortic-valve replacement in high-risk patients. *N Engl J Med*. 2011;364(23):2187-98.

9. Humphries KH, et al. Sex differences in mortality after transcatheter aortic valve replacement for severe aortic stenosis. *J Am Coll Cardiol*. 2012;60(10):882-886.

10. Stehlik J, et al. The registry of the International Society for Heart and Lung Transplantation: twenty-eighth adult heart transplant report-2011. *J Heart Lung Transplant*. 2011;30(10):1078-1094.

11. Kirklin JK, et al. The fourth INTERMACS annual report: 4,000 implants and counting. *J Heart Lung Transplant*. 2012;31(2):117-126.

12. Grubb KJ, Kron IL. Sex and gender in thoracic aortic aneurysms and dissection. *Semin Thoracic Surg*. 2011;23(2):124-125.

6 SCREENING PROCEDURES AND TESTS FOR THE DIAGNOSIS OF CAD IN WOMEN

Gina Mentzer, MD
Jennifer Dickerson, MD

CLINICAL CASE PRESENTATION

A 53-year-old woman with a history of hypertension (HTN), diabetes mellitus Type 2 (Type 2 DM), and tobacco abuse presents to urgent care for symptoms of nausea, chest tightness, and bilateral shoulder pain. The discomfort started 4 hours ago and was not relieved with aspirin or antacid. She had recently been going to a chiropractor for pain in her neck and shoulders, which had been persisting over the past week, but felt this pain was more intense. Her blood pressure was elevated to 165/84 mm Hg and pulse to 93 beats per minute (bpm). Physical examination was unremarkable for cardiac findings with a normal S_1 and S_2, no rubs, murmurs or gallops, no pulmonary abnormalities, and no signs of heart failure. Further evaluation demonstrated no arrhythmias or acute ischemic changes on a normal-appearing electrocardiogram (ECG). Biomarkers for ischemia were negative.

CLINICAL FEATURES OF ISCHEMIC HEART DISEASE

- Angina pectoris is a common presentation of ischemic heart disease (IHD). Based on data from the CASS trial in women who had typical angina, 62% had coronary artery disease (CAD), and even those with atypical features, 40% had CAD.[1-3]
- During an acute ischemic event, many women do not experience typical angina, but have atypical symptoms. This may cause a delay in presentation, evaluation, and therapy. Lack of symptoms with an acute coronary syndrome (ACS) can occur in both men as well as women. But pooled data from large cohort studies have shown this to be more common in women, 37% versus 27%.[4] Myocardial infarction (MI) without chest pain has been more common in younger women, under the age of 55 years. And this group has a higher associated mortality than men within the same age group.[5]
- Other symptoms common in women presenting with ACS include upper abdominal discomfort, dyspnea, and fatigue as well as middle or upper back pain, nausea, indigestion, and loss of appetite.[4]

EPIDEMIOLOGY OF ISCHEMIC HEART DISEASE

- Heart disease accounts for more deaths in women than cancer. Looking at data from the Centers for Disease Control from 2008, IHD accounts for 24.5% of deaths among women of all races[6] (see Table 6-1).

TABLE 6-1 Data regarding all-cause mortality for all ages and races of women from 2008.

Cause	%
Heart disease	24.5%
Cancer	21.7%
Stroke	6.5%
Chronic lower respiratory disease	5.9%
Alzheimer's disease	4.6%

Adapted from data provided by the Centers for Disease Control, 2008. www.cdc.gov/women/lcod/.

- Women are 5.5 times more likely to die from heart disease than breast cancer. Lifetime risk of developing IHD after 40 years of age is 32% for women.[7]
- Nearly 250,000 women die annually in the United States from IHD. The mortality rate for women is higher than men at initial presentation of MI (52% vs 42%) and within 1 year following an MI (23% vs 18%).[8-10]
- Women, on average, present with IHD 10 years later than men, and occurrence of a clinical event such as MI and sudden death lags behind men by 20 years. However, by the time they reach the eighth decade, both men and women have similar rates of mortality and morbidity. However, mortality and morbidity is higher at the extremes of ages, that is, 35 to 44 years and 75 to 84 years.[1,9,11,12]
- IHD is an under-recognized and untreated cause of death among women, with only 8% to 20% aware that cardiovascular disease is the major cause of death for women.[9]

PATHOPHYSIOLOGY AND ETIOLOGY OF ISCHEMIC HEART DISEASE

- Epicardial coronary IHD is an inflammatory vascular process that involves lipid deposition, smooth muscle cell migration, and proliferation with calcification. Without risk factor modification, it evolves over time with progression that may lead to plaque rupture and thrombosis, causing significant disease burden and can even result in an acute myocardial event.
- Risk factors in women include advanced age, smoking tobacco, African American ethnicity, family history of IHD, central obesity, metabolic syndrome, DM, HTN or history of preeclampsia, history of autoimmune disease, premature menopause, and poor exercise capacity.[13] (The strongest risk factors for women are DM, smoking, and HTN.)
- Of the women suffering from typical or atypical chest pain who undergo coronary angiography, 50% have nonobstructive CAD and 50% of those continue with angina. In ACS/STEMI (ST-segment elevation myocardial infarction), approximately 10% to 25% of women as compared to 6% to 10% of men have nonobstructive CAD, which is 60,000 to 150,000 women a year in the United States.[14] The CASS trial showed 50% of women referred with angina pectoris had minimal or no atherosclerotic epicardial artery obstruction compared to 17% of men.[3]
- Microvascular coronary disease and abnormal coronary vasoreactivity are also causes of ischemia that is mediated by endothelial dysfunction and physiological stimuli such as exercise, mental stress, and acetylcholine.[1,15]
- Women have smaller coronary arteries as indexed by body surface area. This can lead to increased risk of vascular complications with percutaneous coronary procedures as well as decreased graft patency with surgical revascularization.[16-18]
- In those >40 years old after an initial ACS, women have higher mortality rates than men at 1 year (23% vs 18%, respectively) and within 5 years (43% vs 33%, respectively). Women also have higher rates or recurrent and fatal cardiovascular events as well as heart failure (HF), that is, 40% of initial cardiovascular events are fatal in women.[19,20]

NONINVASIVE DIAGNOSTIC TESTING AND FUNCTIONAL ASSESSMENT

PRETEST ASSESSMENT AND RISK STRATIFICATION

- When a woman presents with chest pain, a process for evaluation begins with a comprehensive history and physical. Assessment is needed to determine her pretest probability for IHD. This will aid in clinical decision-making and test selection.
- Evaluation begins with consideration of the pretest probability of IHD for symptomatic patients and with calculation of a 10-year cardiovascular event-absolute risk score for asymptomatic patients. Risk factors such as those previously mentioned can be assessed using risk calculators such as the National Cholesterol Education Program Adult Treatment Panel III (NCEP-ATP III), ACC/AHA Practice Guidelines on Exercise testing or the Framingham Heart Study equation to categorize individuals into low, intermediate, and high risk.[8,21-23] The lower prevalence and incidence of disease in the female population can cause the risk assessment to have a lower specificity and lower positive predictive value (PPV); therefore, evaluation should also be done on an individual basis with reference to this calculation.
- In symptomatic patients, age and assessment of anginal chest pain are used to determine the pretest probability of IHD as very low <5%, low <10%, intermediate 10% to 90%, and high >90%.[21]
- Framingham risk categorizes absolute CHD risk over 10 years in asymptomatic women to low as 0 to 10%, moderate >10% to <20%, and high >20%.[8] In addition, NCEP-ATP III categorizes those with ≥2 risk factors with a 10-year risk <10% as moderate risk and those with a 10-year risk of 10% to 20% to moderately high risk.[23]

REST TESTING

- Resting ECG: On initial evaluation, the resting ECG is a powerful negative predictive value (NPV) if it is normal. Abnormalities such as Q-waves, ST-segment changes, T-wave inversions, LV hypertrophy, arrhythmias, or bundle branch block patterns may indicate potential disease and need for further cardiac evaluation.[3]
- Coronary artery calcium (CAC) scoring is a noncontrast coronary imaging modality reserved for asymptomatic individuals. This is utilized for additional risk stratification beyond traditional Framingham assessment. CAC is standard cinefluoroscopy, which is used in screening for IHD and identifies those at risk using either electron beam tomography (EBT) or a noncontrast multidetector computed tomography (MDCT) scan. It is used in low-risk and a few select intermediate-risk patients. Patients must be able to hold still with arms above their shoulders. It also uses radiation that although small, poses future risks for cancer. This modality helps to identify individuals at increased risk of cardiovascular disease beyond the traditional Framingham risks. The ACC/AHA recommends this test for selected asymptomatic, intermediate-risk women for coronary artery disease detection and risk factor modification.[20] The Multi-Ethnic Study of Atherosclerosis (MESA) is a longitudinal epidemiological study that included over 3000 women with a mean

follow-up of 3.75 years.[24] In the MESA study, 90% of women were classified as low risk based on Framingham assessment. Any calcium score >0 was associated with increased risk of CAD and was predictive of increased cardiovascular events. CAC scores are typically expressed as Agatston score that is a weighted unit of calcium density to represent calcium burden of coronary vessels.[25,26] Figure 6-1 is a noncontrast MDCT scan providing a calcium score. While the overall cardiovascular event rate in the MESA study was low, women with CAC score ≥300 with an absolute rate of a cardiovascular event of 8.6% over a 3.75-year period.[20,24]

- Coronary computed tomographic angiography (CTA) is a contrast-enhanced imaging using an MDCT scanner. Imaging technology is constantly evolving. The current published trials typically use 64 multidetector row equipment, with a spatial resolution of 0.6 to 1.0 mm. This provides a sensitivity of 85% to 87% range and specificity of 96%. This modality provides anatomic assessment for IHD typically in combination with CAC. With this study, the most optimal imaging is accomplished using β-blockers or calcium channel blockers to a goal heart rate of 60. In addition, intravenous contrast is used to visualize the coronary arteries. In the obese population, there is concern for decreased signal to noise, resulting in a decreased sensitivity of the imaging examination. Patients with decreased renal function are excluded due to the use of contrast and further renal compromise. Caution is utilized in testing young women due to the heightened lifetime cancer risk with radiation exposure (12.7 milli-Sievert [mSV] for women); however, with advancements in protocols and techniques, the dose of ionizing radiation has continued to decrease. Because this examination is an anatomic assessment, the physiologic data acquired with exercise testing is not obtained and this can limit the clinical usefulness in risk stratification. However, overall with a high NPV in the range of 99%, there is a wide range of clinical applications for this test. Trials have demonstrated comparable diagnostic accuracy between both men and women. With anatomical assessment of the entire vessel lumen and wall, the appearance may show positive remodeling. The phenomenon of positive remodeling is more common in women and may be missed with traditional invasive coronary angiography.[27-29] This is identified in Figure 6-2.

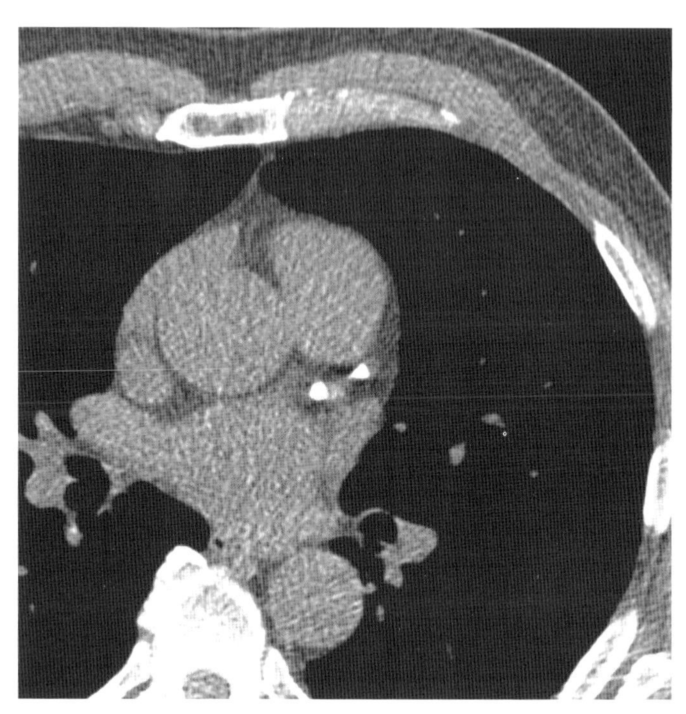

FIGURE 6-1 Noncontrast MDCT scan showing dense calcium in the left anterior descending coronary artery.

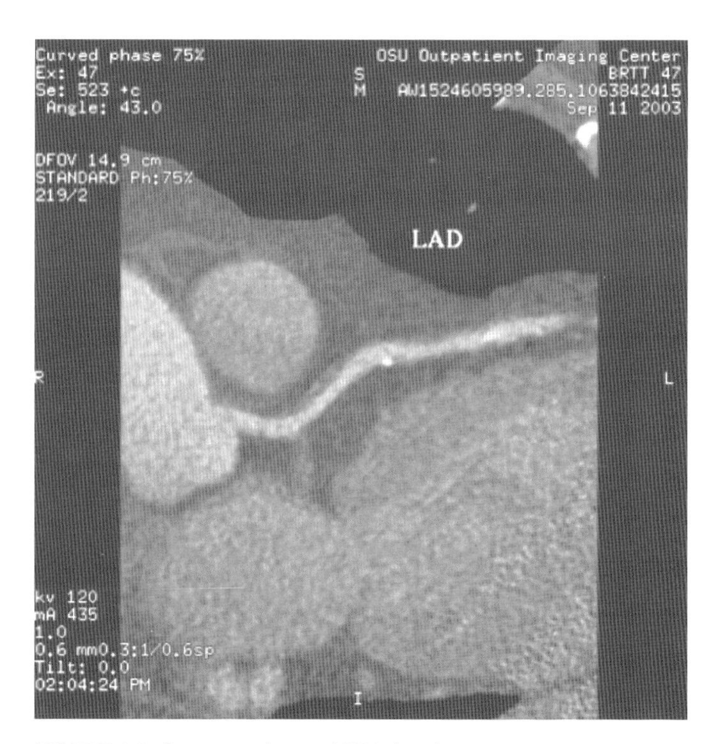

FIGURE 6-2 Contrast-enhanced CTA that demonstrates positive remodeling in the left anterior descending coronary artery in a woman. This oftentimes is missed on coronary angiography.

STRESS TESTING

- Diagnostic cardiac stress testing is performed in symptomatic women to identify those patients with CAD that may be flow limiting. This can be assessed with traditional exercise in the form of treadmill stress or supine bike stress. For patients unable to exercise, pharmacologic stress is accomplished with either an ionotropic agent, such as dobutamine, or a vasodilator agent, such as adenosine or regadenoson. Dobutamine increases myocardial contractility and increased chronotropy. Vasodilator agents work to increase a maximal hyperemic response with increasing myocardial blood flow 3.5 to 4 times normal. The area with hemodynamically significant obstruction has an attenuated response that is manifested as perfusion heterogeneity with imaging.
- Exercise stress ECG according to the ACC/AHA guidelines is recommended as the initial test for symptomatic woman at intermediate risk for CAD with a normal resting ECG and capable of maximal exercise on a treadmill.[20] This has a sensitivity of 60% to 70% and specificity of 70% to 75%. Due to the high NPV, this test

is also appropriate in low and low-to-intermediate risk (pretest likelihoods <20%) when the patient has a normal baseline ECG. (ACC class I intermediate, class IIb low risk.)

- Criticisms of this modality exist as it has a lower detection for CAD in women than in men for many reasons. There is a bias toward patient selection for this test and a lower prevalence of obstructive CAD in women. This reduces the sensitivity and specificity for ST-segment depression in women as compared to men.[30,31] Furthermore, women must be able to achieve adequate heart rates, which is challenging for women as this condition is based on algorithms and exercise programs previously designed by male-dominated trials (ideally ≥85% maximal predicted HR on the Bruce protocol).
- In addition to ST deviation, functional information is obtained with the exercise test. The Duke Treadmill score (DTS) takes into account not only ST deviation, but also duration of exercise and symptoms, which have shown to more accurately predict IHD in women.[32] Additional parameters such as functional capacity and heart rate recovery have improved the diagnostic functionality of this test. Those patients unable to achieve target heart rates, defined as ≥85% age-predicted maximum heart rate or <5-metabolic equivalents (METS), are at higher risk for all-cause mortality as well as MI and IHD.[31,33,34]
- Exercise stress ECG adds very little to clinical assessment in low-risk pretest patient and high-risk pretest patient management. For intermediate pretest-risk patients, a low-risk stress ECG will assist in prognosis, but does not clarify the presence of disease or etiology of symptoms; therefore, an imaging test is more helpful.

Imaging With Stress

The addition of cardiovascular imaging to exercise stress testing provides more clinical information and adds value to the diagnostic study in women with suspected IHD. It has also been shown to be cost-effective as it is more specific than exercise ECG alone. According to the AHA/ACC guidelines, imaging added to stress testing should be done in symptomatic women with intermediate and high pretest probabilities for CAD (≥40%) with an abnormal ECG.[20] A variety of different modalities can be combined with both exercise as well as pharmacologic stress. Those modalities include multi-gated acquisition scanning (MUGA), single-photon emission computed tomography (SPECT), echocardiography, or magnetic resonance.

MUGA

Stress MUGA is typically performed with a supine bike exercise protocol. Imaging interpretation is limited to stress-induced wall motion abnormalities as well as assessment of overall left ventricular function augmentation with stress. Gender-related differences in ventricular response to exercise limit the diagnostic and prognostic value of exercise ventriculography in women. This is not a useful diagnostic stress modality for IHD as 1 in 3 women with normal hearts and normal coronary arteries fail to augment left ventricular ejection fraction (LVEF) with exercise. Women increase stroke volume during exercise by increasing left ventricular end-diastolic volume (LVEDV) with little or no change in LVEF. With quality interpretation and experience, wall motion abnormalities can be helpful and improve sensitivity and specificity; however, other modalities are now preferred.

SPECT

The 2 most common radioactive isotopes include 2 technetium 99m agents (Tc-99 sestamibi and Tc-99m tetrofosmin), as well as thallium 201, a potassium analog that is actively transported into the myocyte. (Thallium [Tl] sensitivity 75%, specificity 90% and technetium [Tc] sestamibi sensitivity 87%-87% and specificity 73%-75%). The spatial resolution for SPECT imaging is in the order of 10 mm with Tc-99. SPECT imaging is the most commonly performed stress-imaging test in the United States and provides information on perfusion defects, global and regional function as well as LV volume. As demonstrated in Figure 6-3, with SPECT scanning the patient lies supine in the scanner with her hands over her head. Artifact can be introduced with excessive movement or with excessive soft tissue, such as breast tissue. Although radionuclide-based exercise testing has a higher sensitivity and specificity compared to exercise stress testing, breast attenuation and smaller ventricles, both of which are predominantly found in female patients, can cause false-positive results. Imaging technology and the recognition of artifacts have improved this modality to a sensitivity and specificity that is found in men; however, more strict criteria for interpretation have increased the false-negative and nondiagnostic results. In women, a normal study portends an annual IHD event rate of 0.6% while moderate-to-severe perfusion abnormalities yield a 5% annual IHD mortality.[35,36]

Echocardiography Stress Imaging

Stress echocardiography has a high sensitivity and specificity in women. In addition, the echocardiographic imaging provides incremental prognostic data beyond that of the exercise component alone. Stress echocardiography has a sensitivity of 80% to 85% and specificity 80% to 86%. Stress echocardiography can provide information on ventricular systolic and diastolic function, rest and post-stress wall motion, valvular disease, and extent of infarction/ischemia as well as viability. Wall motion abnormalities are the most specific, while LVEF augmentation can have similar issues seen with MUGA imaging. Sensitivity is diminished with intermediate stenosis and single-vessel obstructive CAD, but the high NPV makes it useful in the evaluation of disease in younger women.[20] Exercise forms used with echocardiography can be obtained with the treadmill or supine bike, but technical concerns for optimal window imaging remain a challenge. As in Figure 6-4, immediately after exercise the patient quickly returns to the scanning table in a left lateral decubitus position for optimal imaging.[37]

- In patients unable to exercise, echocardiographic imaging can be combined with pharmacologic stress, most typically using dobutamine. The use of pharmacologic stress testing coupled with echocardiography has been shown to be safe, highly feasible, and effective in risk stratification. It has sensitivity in the range of 75% to 93% and specificity from 79% to 92%.[20] Diagnostic accuracy is similar in men and women. The prognosis of a normal dobutamine stress echo (DSE) is more favorable in women versus men.[38] When wall motion abnormalities are present, they are easily identified as demonstrated in Figure 6-5.[39]
- Cardiac magnetic resonance imaging (CMR) with magnetic perfusion imaging (MPI) is an advanced imaging technique that is

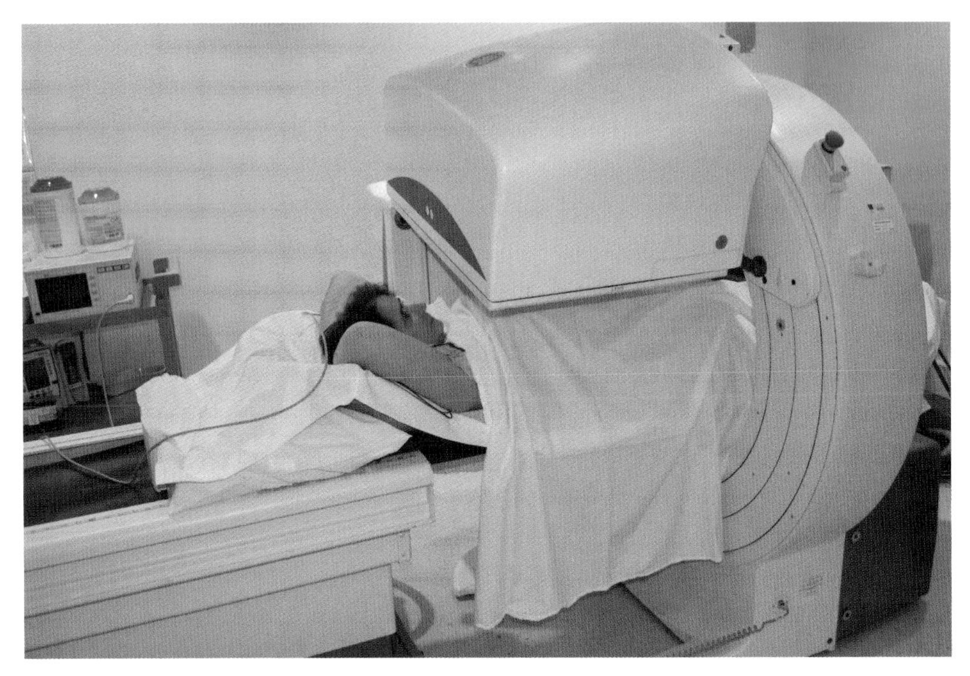

FIGURE 6-3 SPECT scanner imaging of a patient at the Wexner Medical Center, The Ohio State University, which lasts approximately 15 minutes. The patient lies supine in the scanner with her hands over her head.

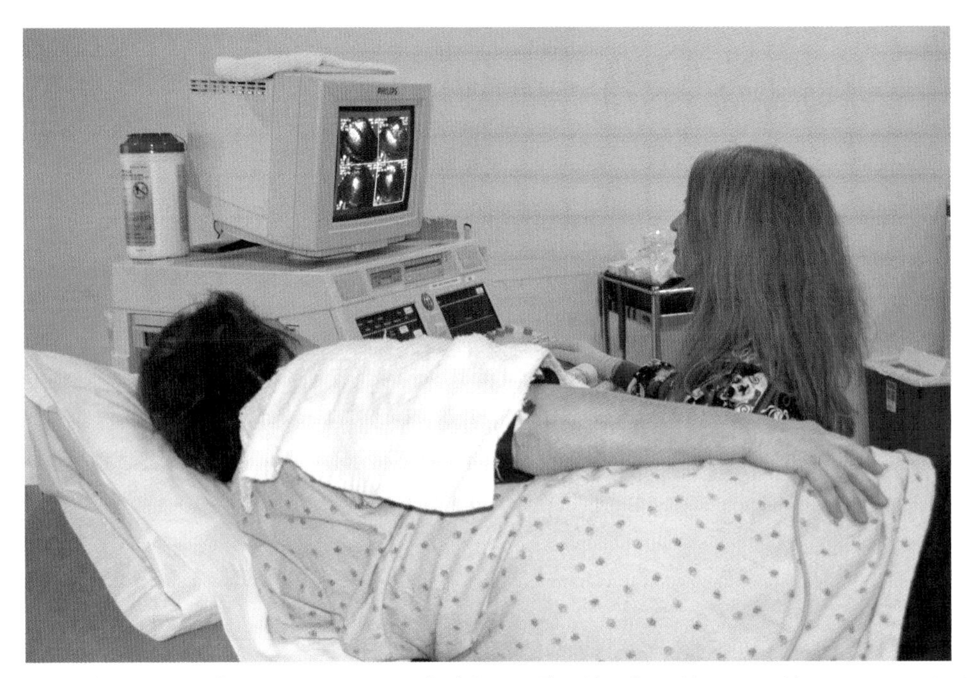

FIGURE 6-4 Stress echocardiographic imaging of patient at Wexner Medical Center, The Ohio State University. After stress exercise is completed, the patient quickly returns to the scanning table in a left lateral decubitus position for optimal imaging. During pharmacological stress echocardiography testing, the patient remains in this position for the entire time of testing.

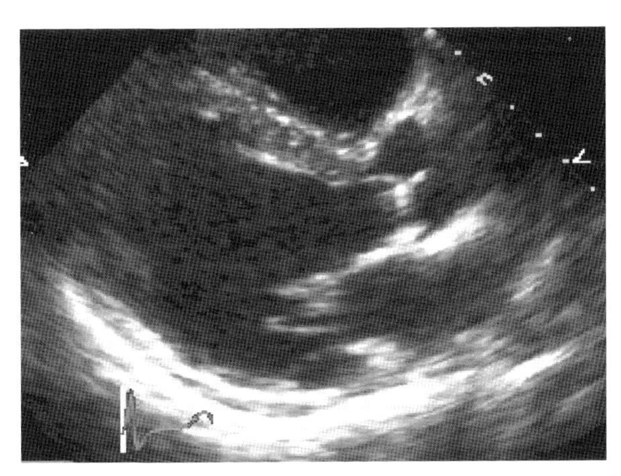

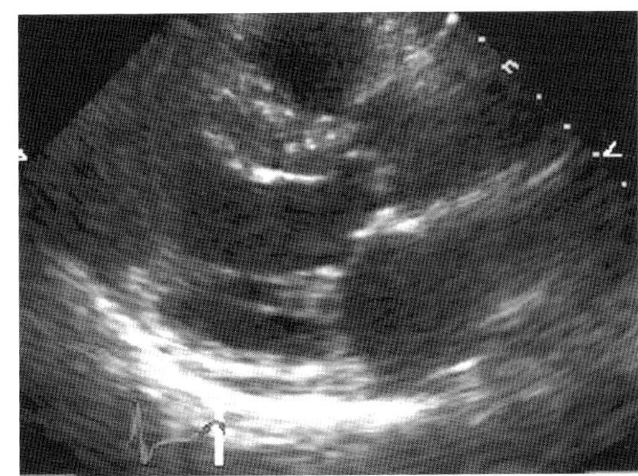

FIGURE 6-5 An echocardiogram in a parasternal long axis projection at both an end-diastolic frame (A) and end-systolic frame (B) to identify a wall motion abnormality of the posterior wall.

emerging as a powerful tool for ischemic evaluation in women, especially given an inherent spatial resolution of 3 mm. The use of CMR for cardiovascular stress can assess biventricular function, myocardial ischemia (both due to epicardial disease as well as microvascular disease) in addition myocardial viability/scar. Traditional CMR stress testing involves the use of a vasodilator agent or dobutamine. With the use of adenosine or regadenoson, gadolinium is used as the MRI contrast to assess for regional perfusion abnormalities. Late-gadolinium hyperenhancement is then present in regions of scar. Perfusion defects may be in patterns of coronary distributions or in diffuse, subendocardial perfusion defects. This subendocardial pattern as imaged by CMR may correlate to abnormal coronary vasoreactivity. This is seen most typically in patients with chest pain due to microvascular dysfunction and correlates with invasive testing. In women who present with recurrent angina, despite having nonobstructive CAD with traditional coronary angiography, microvascular dysfunction is high on the differential.[40] To introduce a state-of-the-art advancement with CMR stress testing, an MRI-compatible treadmill was designed by Raman and colleagues at Wexner Medical Center, The Ohio State University. Figure 6-6 shows the proximity of the treadmill to the table of the MRI scanner. A multicenter clinical trial is currently under way to validate this method of stress testing. With utilization of these technologies, there forms a powerful bond of functional assessment with exercise stress and high spatial resolution with CMR imaging.[41] More traditionally, CMR can be safely used with dobutamine and regadenoson stress; however, studies for sensitivity and specificity for IHD in women are still being done. Figure 6-7 identifies a stres-induced perfusion abnormality in the septum of the left ventricle. Figure 6-8 is an image of delayed myocardial hyperenhancement, where the areas of scar are bright as noted in the inferior wall.

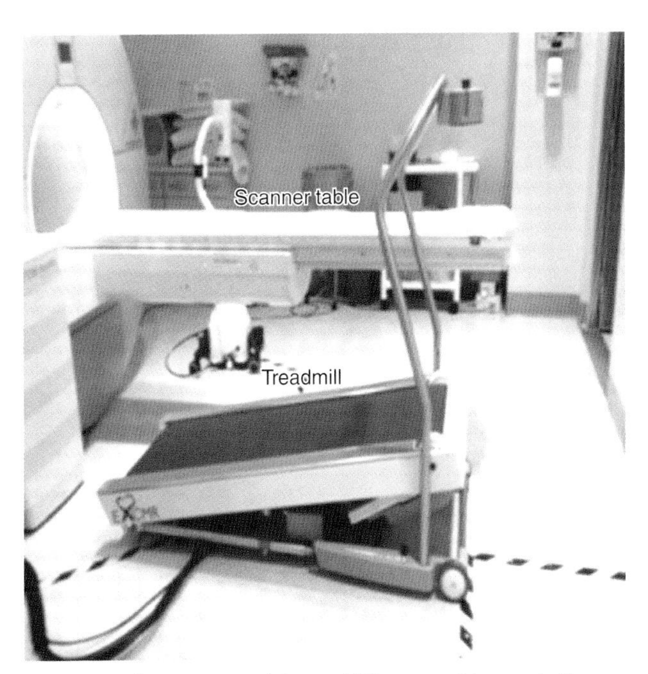

FIGURE 6-6 This is a state-of-the-art MRI-compatible treadmill designed by Raman and colleagues at Wexner Medical Center, The Ohio State University.

- Positron emission tomography (PET) stress imaging has a reported sensitivity and specificity of 95% with an inherent spatial resolution of 5 to 8 mm.[42,43] Clinically, this modality remains underutilized due to high expense, technological requirements, and expertise for interpretation. Overall, it has great promise for improved stress imaging for ischemia and viability that leads to better outcomes and cost-effectiveness in women once it becomes more clinically friendly and attains lower doses of radiation with testing. It has the capability to quantify absolute values of regional and global myocardial blood flow to assess microvascular disease and an improved evaluation in the obese woman. This is also an emerging advanced imaging technology that is undergoing evaluation at Wexner Medical Center, The Ohio State University.

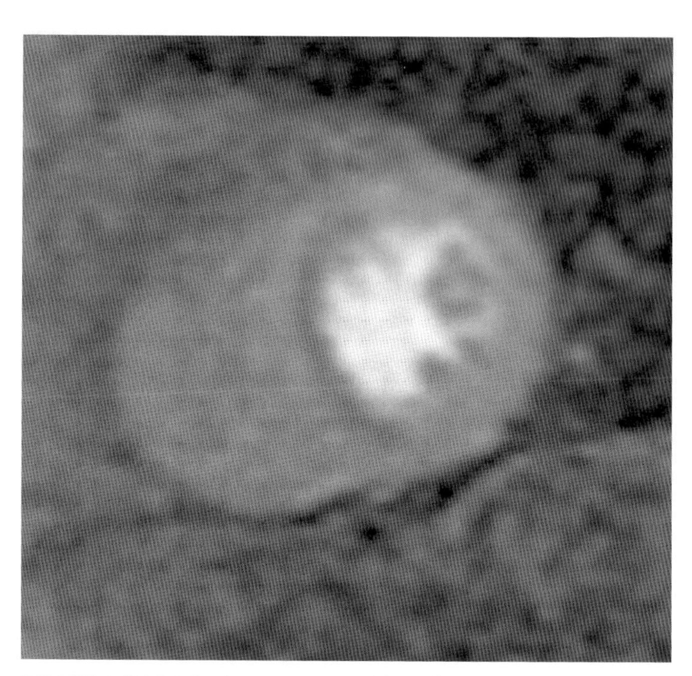

FIGURE 6-7 Middle short-axis view of the left ventricle with a myocardial perfusion abnormality of the septum identified poststress with gadolinium injection.

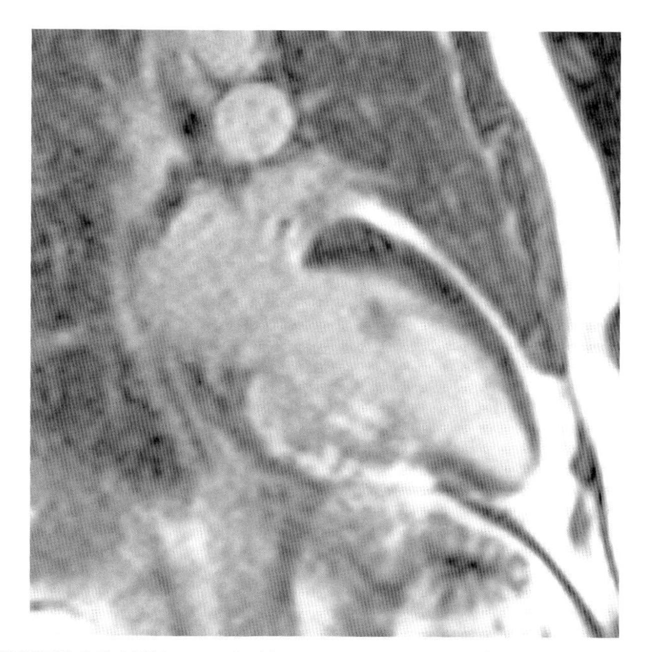

FIGURE 6-8 MRI in a vertical long-axis projection with dense scar in the inferior wall with late gadolinium imaging.

CLINICAL CONSIDERATIONS FOR DIAGNOSTIC REST/STRESS MODALITY

Symptomatic Women

- Patients with a low likelihood for IHD and a probability of <5% undergo assessment and are given reassurance and observed. For an individual where the probability is >5% and symptoms are disabling, a new exercise program is considered. Besides, if the patient is in a high-risk occupation, she should undergo a resting ECG. If she has an interpretable ECG then exercise stress test should also be considered. Should the posttest probability be elevated due to stress-induced abnormalities, consider a radionuclide stress or cardiac catheterization in select patients.
- Intermediate and intermediate-to-high probability for IHD with absence of ongoing ischemia. Perform a resting ECG. If the resting ECG is interpretable and the patient is able to exercise, an exercise treadmill test should be done. Furthermore, imaging such as nuclear or echocardiography can be considered as a component of the exercise stress test in those with an intermediate-risk Duke Treadmill score (DTS) or exercise ECG abnormalities.
  1. Stress testing with cardiac imaging is recommended if the patient has any of the following: DM, abnormal rest ECG, or questionable exercise tolerance.[20]
  2. Pharmacologic stress testing is preferred with patients with left bundle branch blocks (LBBB) and those who are unable to exercise.

In patients with evidence of ongoing cardiac ischemia or a high-risk pretest probability, an invasive strategy should be considered. An algorithm, shown in Figure 6-9, has been suggested by Kohli and colleagues for stress testing evaluation in women with IHD symptoms.[20,31]

Asymptomatic Women

In the low-risk, asymptomatic female population, there is no clinical indication for screening with stress or stress imaging testing. There is a lack of cost-benefit ratio to support this testing as well as undue risk, a high rate of false positives due to the low prevalence of disease, and prior demonstration of inaccurate testing. Clinical risk assessment is recommended as a part of the routine evaluation with risk factor modification and reassurance. In special, asymptomatic populations such as those with diabetes, strong family history or other high-risk individuals, there is a IIb recommendation from the ACC/AHA guideline committee for exercise ECG stress testing.[44]

PROGNOSTIC IMPLICATIONS OF NONINVASIVE TESTING

- The DTS accurately predicts IHD mortality in women and the St. James Women Take Heart Study demonstrated a 9% reduction in the risk of death for every unit increase in the DTS as well as

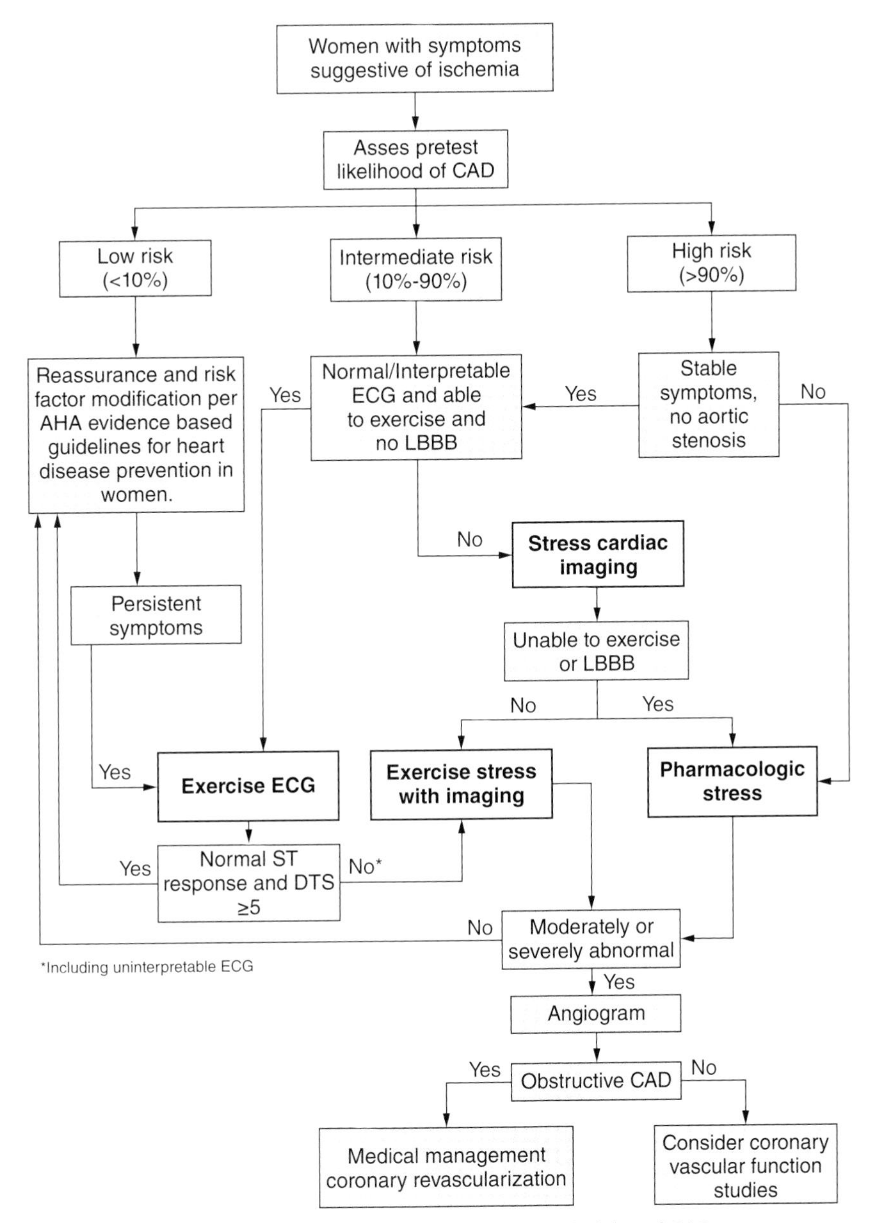

FIGURE 6-9 Algorithm for stress testing in a symptomatic woman based on pretest probability of CAD.
Reproduced with permission from Kohli and Gulati, Algorithm for stress testing in a symptomatic woman based on pre-test probability of CAD. *Circulation* 2010.

a 17% reduction in mortality for every metabolic equivalent (MET) increase in exercise capacity.[32,33,35]

- Women with IHD and nonobstructive CAD have a 2% risk of death and MI at 30 days of follow-up. In fact, 30% of women with chest pain and normal coronaries by catheterization develop obstructive CAD within the 10-year follow-up.[14] The 5-year CV event rates are 16% for those with mild CAD, 7.9% with no coronary stenosis, and 2.4% with asymptomatic women.[34]

CLINICAL CASE SUMMARY

After further discussion on the diagnostic testing modalities, the patient presented underwent an exercise stress cardiac SPECT study. She exercised for 6 minutes on a Bruce protocol. With stress, she

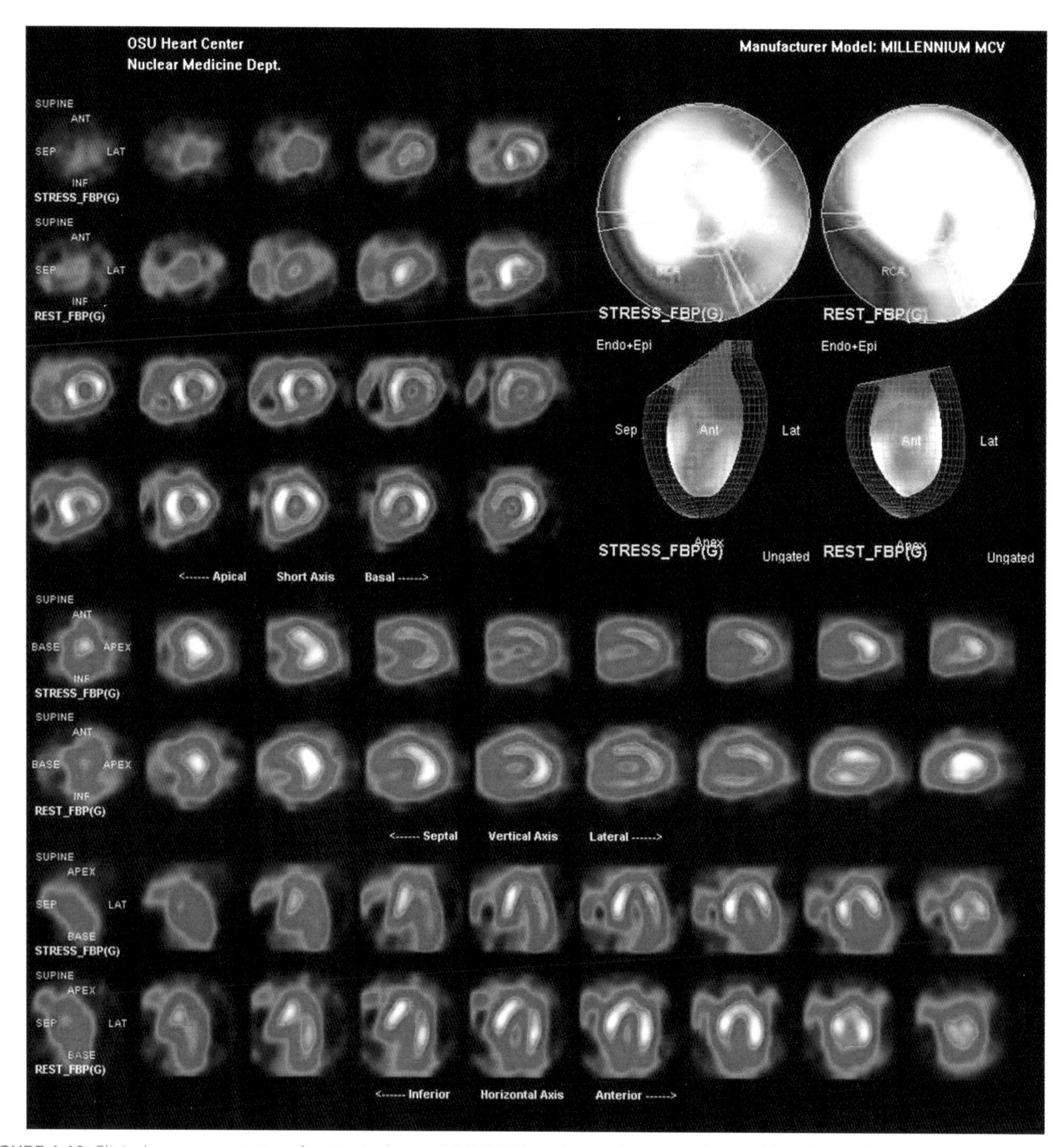

FIGURE 6-10 Clinical case presentation of patient's abnormal SPECT. There is a moderate-sized reversible inferior defect visualized that corresponds to the RCA territory.

developed 2-mm ST depression and within 4 minutes had reproduction of her angina chest discomfort. With the cessation of exercise, the ST depression resolved as well as her angina chest pain. The DTS was moderate-risk [6 minutes − (5 × 2) − (4 × 1) = −8] with a probability of significant CAD upto 58% and a 5-year mortality of 27%. SPECT demonstrated ischemia in the inferior and inferolateral segments as seen in Figure 6-10 and LV function of 40%. Based on the pretest probability, DTS, and abnormal perfusion imaging by SPECT, her posttest probability of having significant CAD was high and she was referred for a cardiac catheterization for further anatomic

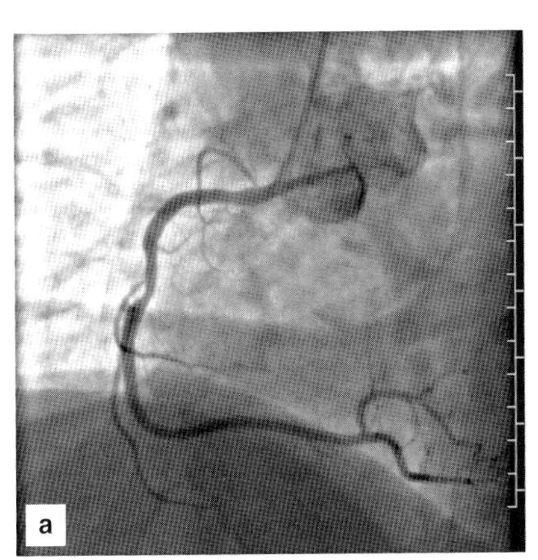

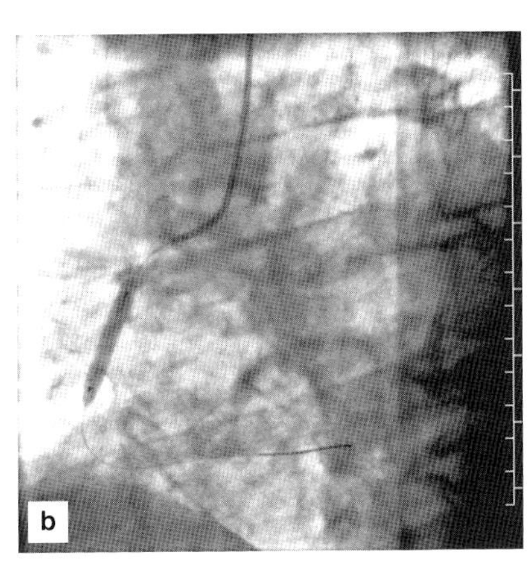

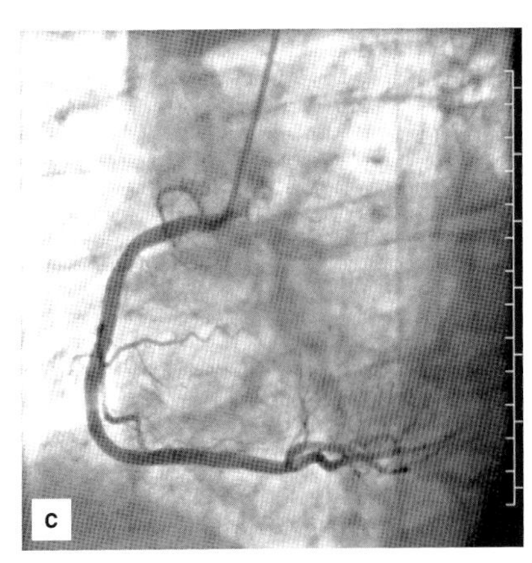

FIGURE 6-11 Clinical case presentation of patient's invasive coronary angiogram demonstrating a high-grade, mid-RCA lesion. Additional images show stent placement during percutaneous intervention (PCI) and post-PCI coronary flow.

evaluation. A high-grade, mid–right coronary artery (RCA) stenosis was identified that correlated to the deficit found through stress testing, Figure 6-11. With symptomatic, high-grade IHD, revascularization was successfully performed with a drug-eluting stent with complete resolution of symptoms. Medically, she was treated with aspirin, clopidogrel, β-blocker, ace inhibitor, and statin therapy and follows routinely with our outpatient cardiology clinic.

REFERENCES

1. Wenger NW, Collins P, eds. *Women & Heart Disease*. 2nd ed. Boca Raton, FL: Taylor & Francis Group; 2005.
2. Weiner DA, Ryan TJ, McCabe CH, et al. Exercise stress testing. Correlations among history of angina, ST-segment response and prevalence of coronary-artery disease in the coronary artery surgery study (CASS). *N Engl J Med*. 1979;301(5):230-235.
3. Chaitman BR, Bourassa MG, Davis K, et al. Angiographic prevalence of high-risk coronary artery disease in patient subsets (CASS). *Circulation*. 1981;64(2):360-367.
4. Canto JG, Goldberg RJ, Hand MM, et al. Symptom presentation of women with acute coronary syndromes: myth vs reality. *Arch Intern Med*. 2007;167(22):2405-2413.
5. Canto JG, Rogers WJ, Goldberg RJ, et al. Association of age and sex with myocardial infarction symptom presentation and in-hospital mortality. *JAMA*. 2012;307(8):813-822.
6. Center for Disease Control and Prevention. Leading causes of death in females. The Center for Disease Control and Prevention. www.cdc.gov/women/lcod/. 2008. Updated 2008. Accessed January 2013.
7. Roger VL, Go AS, Lloyd-Jones DM, et al. Heart disease and stroke statistics—2011 update: a report from the American Heart Association. *Circulation*. 2011;123(4):e18-e209.
8. Kannel WB, Sorlie P, McNamara PM. Prognosis after initial myocardial infarction: the Framingham study. *Am J Cardiol*. 1979;44(1):53-59.

9. Lloyd-Jones D, Adams RJ, Brown TM, et al. Executive summary: heart disease and stroke statistics—2010 update: a report from the American Heart Association. *Circulation*. 2010;121(7):948-954.

10. Vaccarino V, Parsons L, Every NR, et al. Sex-based differences in early mortality after myocardial infarction. National Registry of Myocardial Infarction 2 Participants. *N Engl J Med*. 1999;341(4):217-225.

11. Yusuf S, Hawken S, Ounpuu S, et al. Effect of potentially modifiable risk factors associated with myocardial infarction in 52 countries (the INTERHEART study): case-control study. *Lancet*. 2004;364(9438):937-952.

12. Thom T, Haase N, Rosamond W, et al. Heart disease and stroke statistics—2006 update: a report from the American Heart Association Statistics Committee and Stroke Statistics Subcommittee. *Circulation*. 2006;113(6):e85-e151.

13. Mosca L, Benjamin EJ, Berra K, et al. Effectiveness-based guidelines for the prevention of cardiovascular disease in women—2011 update: a guideline from the American Heart Association. *Circulation*. 2011;123(11):1243-1262.

14. Shaw LJ, Bugiardini R, Merz CN. Women and ischemic heart disease: evolving knowledge. *J Am Coll Cardiol*. 2009;54(17):1561-1575.

15. Gulati M, Shaw LJ, Bairey Merz CN. Myocardial ischemia in women: lessons from the NHLBI WISE study. *Clin Cardiol*. 2012;35(3):141-148.

16. Dickerson JA, Nagaraja HN, Raman SV. Gender-related differences in coronary artery dimensions: a volumetric analysis. *Clin Cardiol*. 2010;33(2):E44-E49.

17. Berger JS, Brown DL. Gender-age interaction in early mortality following primary angioplasty for acute myocardial infarction. *Am J Cardiol*. 2006;98(9):1140-1143.

18. Kim C, Redberg RF, Pavlic T, et al. A systematic review of gender differences in mortality after coronary artery bypass graft surgery and percutaneous coronary interventions. *Clin Cardiol*. 2007;30(10):491-495.

19. Lloyd-Jones D, Adams RJ, Brown TM, et al. Executive summary: heart disease and stroke statistics—2010 update: a report from the American Heart Association. *Circulation*. 2010;121(7):948-954.

20. Mieres JH, Shaw LJ, Arai A, et al. Role of noninvasive testing in the clinical evaluation of women with suspected coronary artery disease: consensus statement from the Cardiac Imaging Committee, Council on Clinical Cardiology, and the Cardiovascular Imaging and Intervention Committee, Council on Cardiovascular Radiology and Intervention, American Heart Association. *Circulation*. 2005;111(5):682-696.

21. Gibbons RJ, Balady GJ, Bricker JT, et al. ACC/AHA 2002 guideline update for exercise testing: summary article: a report of the American College of Cardiology/American Heart Association Task Force on Practice Guidelines (committee to update the 1997 exercise testing guidelines). *Circulation*. 2002;106(14):1883-1892.

22. Stone NJ, Bilek S, Rosenbaum S. Recent National Cholesterol Education Program Adult Treatment Panel III update: adjustments and options. *Am J Cardiol*. 2005;96(4A):53E-59E.

23. National Cholesterol Education Program (NCEP) Expert Panel on Detection, Evaluation, and Treatment of High Blood Cholesterol in Adults (Adult Treatment Panel III). Third report of the National Cholesterol Education Program (NCEP) expert panel on detection, evaluation, and treatment of high blood cholesterol in adults (Adult Treatment panel III) final report. *Circulation*. 2002;106(25):3143-3421.

24. Lakoski SG, Greenland P, Wong ND, et al. Coronary artery calcium scores and risk for cardiovascular events in women classified as "low risk" based on Framingham risk score: the Multi-Ethnic Study of Atherosclerosis (MESA). *Arch Intern Med*. 2007;167(22):2437-2442.

25. Detrano R, Guerci AD, Carr JJ, et al. Coronary calcium as a predictor of coronary events in four racial or ethnic groups. *N Engl J Med*. 2008;358(13):1336-1345.

26. Budoff MJ, Nasir K, McClelland RL, et al. Coronary calcium predicts events better with absolute calcium scores than age-sex-race/ethnicity percentiles: MESA (Multi-Ethnic Study of Atherosclerosis). *J Am Coll Cardiol*. 2009;53(4):345-352.

27. Budoff MJ, Dowe D, Jollis JG, et al. Diagnostic performance of 64-multidetector row coronary computed tomographic angiography for evaluation of coronary artery stenosis in individuals without known coronary artery disease: results from the prospective multicenter ACCURACY (Assessment by Coronary Computed Tomographic Angiography of Individuals Undergoing Invasive Coronary Angiography) trial. *J Am Coll Cardiol*. 2008;52(21):1724-1732.

28. Tsang JC, Min JK, Lin FY, et al. Sex comparison of diagnostic accuracy of 64-multidetector row coronary computed tomographic angiography: results from the multicenter ACCURACY trial. *J Cardiovasc Comput Tomogr*. 2012;6(4):246-251.

29. Kornowski R, Lansky AJ, Mintz GS, et al. Comparison of men versus women in cross-sectional area luminal narrowing, quantity of plaque, presence of calcium in plaque, and lumen location in coronary arteries by intravascular ultrasound in patients with stable angina pectoris. *Am J Cardiol*. 1997;79(12):1601-1605.

30. Kwok Y, Kim C, Grady D, et al. Meta-analysis of exercise testing to detect coronary artery disease in women. *Am J Cardiol*. 1999;83(5):660-666.

31. Kohli P, Gulati M. Exercise stress testing in women: going back to the basics. *Circulation*. 2010;122(24):2570-2580.

32. Shaw LJ, Peterson ED, Shaw LK, et al. Use of a prognostic treadmill score in identifying diagnostic coronary disease subgroups. *Circulation*. 1998;98(16):1622-1630.

33. Gulati M, Black HR, Shaw LJ, et al. The prognostic value of a nomogram for exercise capacity in women. *N Engl J Med*. 2005;353(5):468-475.

34. Gulati M, Shaw LJ, Thisted RA, et al. Heart rate response to exercise stress testing in asymptomatic women: the St. James Women Take Heart Project. *Circulation*. 2010;122(2):130-137.

35. Shaw LJ, Bugiardini R, Merz CN. Women and ischemic heart disease: evolving knowledge. *J Am Coll Cardiol*. 2009;54(17):1561-1575.

36. Berman DS, Kang X, Hayes SW, et al. Adenosine myocardial perfusion single-photon emission computed tomography in women compared with men. Impact of diabetes mellitus on incremental prognostic value and effect on patient management. *J Am Coll Cardiol*. 2003;41(7):1125-1133.

37. Heupler S, Mehta R, Lobo A, et al. Prognostic implications of exercise echocardiography in women with known or suspected coronary artery disease. *J Am Coll Cardiol*. 1997;30(2):414-420.

38. Cortigiani L, Dodi C, Paolini EA, et al. Prognostic value of pharmacological stress echocardiography in women with chest pain and unknown coronary artery disease. *J Am Coll Cardiol*. 1998;32(7):1975-1981.

39. Biagini E, Elhendy A, Bax JJ, et al. Seven-year follow-up after dobutamine stress echocardiography: impact of gender on prognosis. *J Am Coll Cardiol*. 2005;45(1):93-97.

40. Panting JR, Gatehouse PD, Yang GZ, et al. Abnormal subendocardial perfusion in cardiac syndrome X detected by cardiovascular magnetic resonance imaging. *N Engl J Med*. 2002;346(25):1948-1953.

41. Raman SV, Dickerson JA, Jekic M, et al. Real-time cine and myocardial perfusion with treadmill exercise stress cardiovascular magnetic resonance in patients referred for stress SPECT. *J Cardiovasc Magn Reson*. 2010;12:41.

42. Patterson RE, Eisner RL, Horowitz SF. Comparison of cost-effectiveness and utility of exercise ECG, single photon emission computed tomography, positron emission tomography, and coronary angiography for diagnosis of coronary artery disease. *Circulation*. 1995;91(1):54-65.

43. Bateman TM, Heller GV, McGhie AI, et al. Diagnostic accuracy of rest/stress ECG-gated Rb-82 myocardial perfusion PET: comparison with ECG-gated Tc-99m sestamibi SPECT. *J Nucl Cardiol*. 2006;13(1):24-33.

44. Greenland P, Alpert JS, Beller GA, et al. 2010 ACCF/AHA guideline for assessment of cardiovascular risk in asymptomatic adults: a report of the American College of Cardiology Foundation/American Heart Association Task Force on Practice Guidelines. *J Am Coll Cardiol*. 2010;56(25):e50-e103.

7 CARDIAC REHABILITATION IN WOMEN

Rita Szymanski, RN, BSN
Kameswari Maganti, MD

INTRODUCTION

Although death rates from cardiovascular disease (CVD) have declined in recent years, CVD continues to be the leading cause of death for women in the United States. In the years between 1997 and 2007, the overall death rate from CVD declined 26.3%; however, the rate of death has been increasing by an average of 1.3% annually between 1997 and 2002, which is statistically significant.[1]

Cardiac rehabilitation (CR) involves exercise training, education, counseling regarding risk reduction and lifestyle modification, and, frequently, behavior interventions in patients with cardiac events or chronic cardiac disease. For many women who experience a cardiac event, a structured CR is their first opportunity to become physically active. CR is an important component of multidisciplinary approach for management of the patients with various presentations of coronary heart disease. CR improves functional capacity, recovery, and psychological well-being. It is a class I recommendation endorsed by American Heart Association and American College of Cardiology in treatment of patients with CVD. Moreover, it is a cost-effective intervention following an acute coronary event and chronic heart failure (CHF)[2-4] as it improves prognosis by reducing recurrent hospitalization and health-care expenditures, while prolonging life.

In addition to a structured exercise program, components of a CR program often include medical history and physical examination; nutrition counseling; weight, blood pressure, and lipid management; diabetes education; psychosocial evaluation and treatment; and tobacco cessation programs.[5] The benefits of participation in CR program include improved exercise capacity, improvement in lipid profile, reduction of obesity, prevention or reduction of Type 2 diabetes mellitus, improvement in depression and anxiety, and improvement in overall quality of life.[6]

Despite the role of cardiac rehabilitation having been extensively documented, endorsed, and promoted by a number of health-care organizations for the comprehensive secondary prevention of cardiovascular events, it continues to remain vastly underutilized; much more so in women. They are less likely to be referred for rehabilitation program, and even when referred, are less likely to attend.[7] The Evidence-Based Guidelines for Cardiovascular Disease Prevention in Women strongly endorse cardiac rehabilitation after a coronary event.[8] Barriers to participation for women include the lack of financial resources, transportation difficulties, and lack of social and emotional support.

HISTORICAL PERSPECTIVE

Following the clinical description of myocardial infarction by Herrick in 1912, prolonged bed rest up to 2 months was advocated for fear of infarct expansion, aneurysm formation, congestive heart failure, cardiac rupture, and sudden death. Strenuous activities were restricted for prolonged periods, and sometimes indefinitely. Resumption of normal life style was rare.[9]

By late 1940s, Levine and Lown advocated the use of chair therapy as an alternative to prolonged bed rest.[10] It was erroneously believed that the dependent lower extremities resulted in reduced venous return, thereby decreasing the stroke work and cardiac output.[11] Early ambulation was defined as 3 to 5 minutes of walking, twice daily, 4 weeks after infarction by Newman et al.[12] This was then tried at 14 days after an acute event.[13] In 1961, Cain et al recommended the efficacy and safety of early graded activity.[14]

Clinicians began to realize that early ambulation following an acute event helped decrease the incidence of pulmonary embolism and deconditioning. Early ambulation was increasingly advocated at earlier intervals, and finally evolved into what we currently define as phase I cardiac rehabilitation. Wenger et al refined the technique and promoted its wide clinical use.[15]

Goals of Cardiac Rehabilitation[16-18]

Short-Term Goals of CR	Long-Term Goals of CR
Reconditioning sufficient to resume customary activities; increasing exercise tolerance	Identification and treatment of risk factors
Limiting psychological effects of heart disease	Stabilizing or even reversing the athero-sclerotic process
Reduction in mortality, recurrent myocardial infarction, and requirement for myocardial revascularization procedures	Reduction in mortality, recurrent myocardial infarction, and requirement for myocardial revascularization procedures
Improvement in symptoms	Enhancing psychological status of patients

INDICATIONS AND CONTRAINDICATIONS

Medicare-Approved Indications

- Recent myocardial infarction
- Stable angina
- Coronary angioplasty

- Coronary bypass surgery
- Heart valve surgery
- Heart transplantation or heart/lung transplantation

There are many studies demonstrating the benefit of cardiac rehabilitation in patients with advanced heart failure, and asymptomatic patients at high risk for coronary heart disease, though they are not Medicare-approved indications yet.

Contraindications for Cardiac Rehabilitation

- Severe residual angina
- Decompensated heart failure
- Uncontrolled arrhythmias
- Severe ischemia, LV dysfunction, or arrhythmia during exercise testing
- Poorly controlled hypertension
- Hypertensive or any hypotensive systolic blood pressure response to exercise
- Unstable concomitant medical problems (eg, poorly controlled or "brittle" diabetes, diabetes prone to hypoglycemia, ongoing febrile illness, active transplant rejection)
- Active pericarditis
- Severe orthopedic problems

REFERRAL TO CARDIAC REHABILITATION

Risk stratification is typically performed following a cardiac event utilizing a stress test prior to referring a patient to a cardiac rehabilitation program. Either a submaximal stress test or a symptom-limited stress test is utilized. The exercise prescription and surveillance are based on results of exercise testing. These are individualized.

Phases of CR

- **Phase I (in-hospital phase):** The purpose is to provide education and to prevent deconditioning. It prepares patients to return to normal daily activities. In CCU, assisted range of motion should be performed within the first 24 to 48 hours. Low-risk patients are made to sit on a chair and perform self-care activities. On being transferred to the step-down unit, patients should be encouraged to ambulate as tolerated. Walking is resumed with target heart rate of <20 beats above the resting heart rate. This can be started with 5 to 10 minutes of walking each day, with exercise time being gradually increased to 30 minutes daily.
- **Phase II (supervised exercise):** The purpose of this phase to progressively improve functional capacity, lower risk factors, and prepare patients for return to work. It includes exercises which are performed following dismissal from hospital. It typically lasts 1 week to 3 months following an event. During phase II CR, the BP, heart rate, telemetry, dyspnea scale, Borg scale, and angina scale are all monitored (Figure 7-1).
- **Phase III (late outpatient maintenance phase):** The purpose of this phase is continued patient education, risk factor modification, and improved functional status. This phase is unsupervised and should ideally last lifetime (Figure 7-2).

CORE COMPONENTS OF CR

Cardiac rehabilitation/secondary prevention (SP) programs are expected to deliver patient-centered care services provided by a multidisciplinary team of health-care providers. Communication between these disciplines is critical.

The American Association of Cardiovascular and Pulmonary Rehabilitation (AACVPR) has defined core components to assure the provision of high-quality care within evidence-based guidelines. Initially introduced as performance measures in 2007, these components were established with the support of the American Heart Association and The American College of Cardiology.[19]

Initially, all patients starting a CR program should have a comprehensive clinical examination, including assessment of risk stratification for adverse events. Assessment continues to guide an individual's treatment plan including determination of a risk factor profile, interventions, goal setting, and on-going evaluation (Figure 7-3). While planning and implementing CR for women, one needs to consider that women are more likely to be older; have clustering of comorbidities such as hypertension, diabetes, hypercholesterolemia, obesity, heart failure, as well as lower exercise and functional capacity compared to male patients; and may therefore carry a higher cardiac risk as a CR population. Beyond the impact of the cardiac disease, older women in particular are more likely to experience activity limitations and other exercise-limiting comorbid conditions such as arthritis, osteoporosis, and urinary incontinence. At recruitment to CR, women typically score lower in health-related quality of life and they are more likely to be diagnosed with depressive disorders and higher scores of anxiety.

Essential care components include the following steps:

- Tobacco cessation as an ultimate goal utilizing behavioral interventions, pharmaceuticals, referral to a tobacco cessation program, and on-going support as needed.
- Hypertension management utilizing frequent and repeated blood pressure measurements; assessment of medication compliance, sodium intake, patient's understanding of the complexity of factors affecting blood pressure; and empowering patients to become active partners in blood pressure control through education and self-monitoring. Collaboration with the patient's physician is important.
- Individual assessment of optimal lipid control. This also includes collaboration with the patient's physician as well as a dietician. Education should include target lipid goals and the importance of treatment compliance and lifestyle modifications.
- Assessment of current physical activity levels, with return to or establishment of safely meeting the goal of 30 to 60 minutes of activity most days of the week. On-going evaluation of ECG-monitored exercise training sessions and hemodynamic response allows safe progression of exercise prescription. Behavioral counseling is part of the education related to this goal.
- Each participant should be evaluated for body weight and composition to guide in a collaborative effort for weight management. Besides, nutritional and dietary habits should be assessed as a baseline for nutritional counseling as well as behavioral intervention.

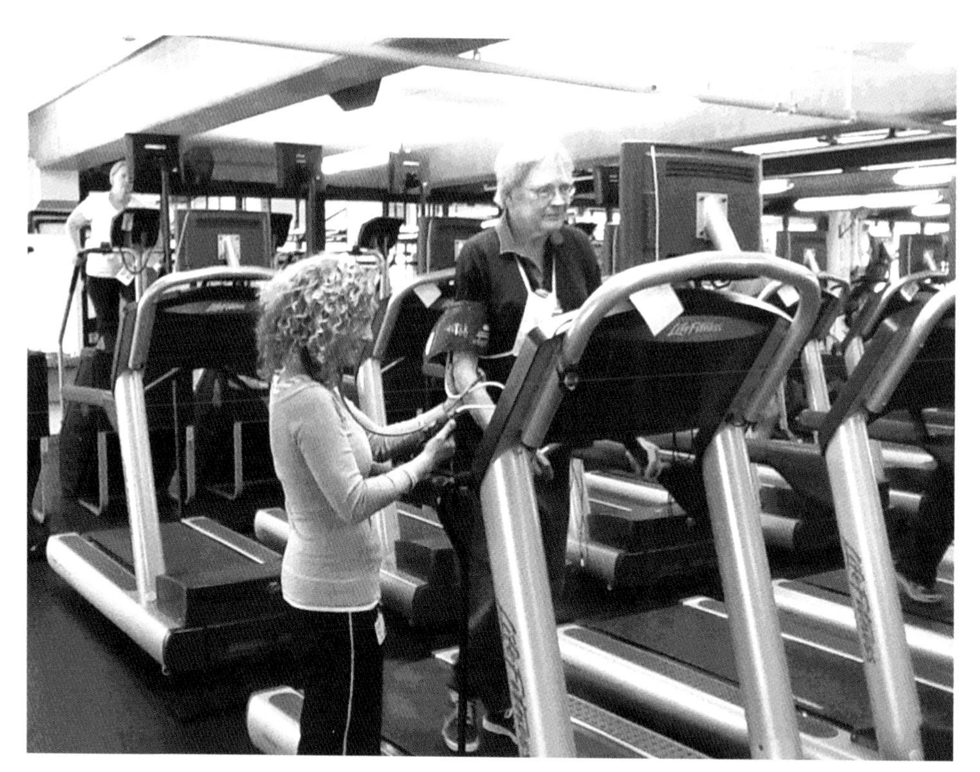

FIGURE 7-1 Hemodynamic monitoring during phase 2 CR.

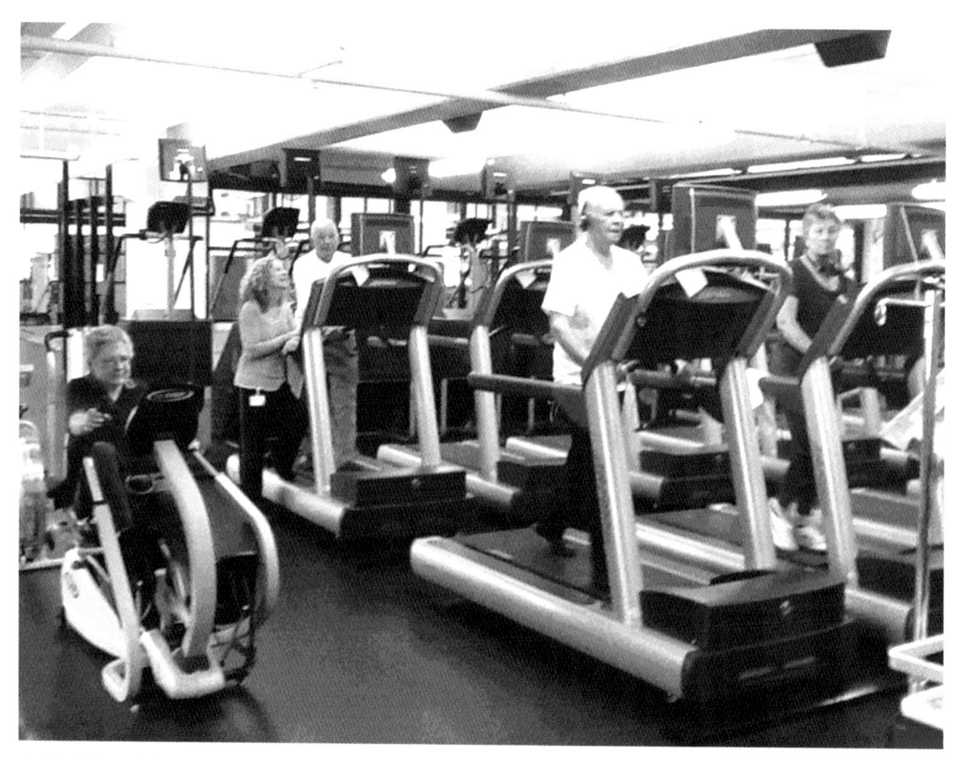

FIGURE 7-2 Phase: 3 CR.

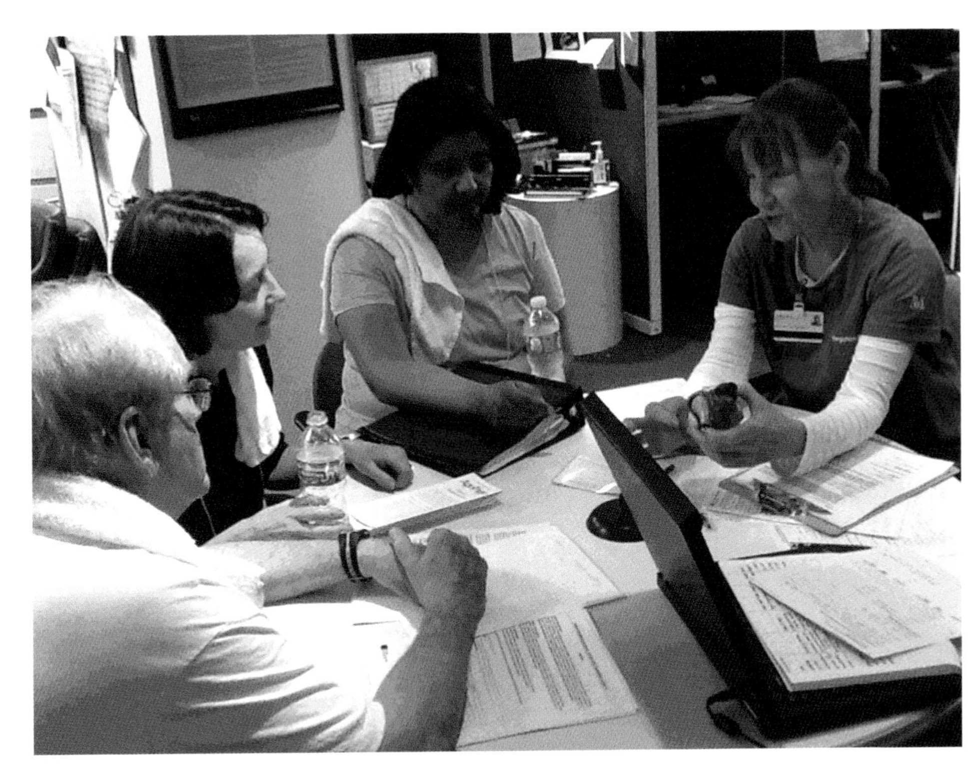

FIGURE 7-3 Assessment and counseling during phase 2 CR.

- A diagnosis of diabetes mellitus directs us to focus on assessment and management of blood glucose levels. Monitoring of blood glucose levels around physical activities allows for opportunity to educate patients regarding self-management techniques. Collaboration with the patient's physician and other practitioners is often necessary to achieve optimal diabetes management.

Screening for depression should be an integral part of the initial assessment for CR/SP program participants. Because of its high prevalence in cardiac patients and its identification as an independent risk factor for cardiac mortality after an acute myocardial infarction or unstable angina, cannot be ignored. The opportunity to bridge cardiac care and mental health through communication with physicians and appropriate referral promotes psychosocial well being, which is critical to optimizing patient outcomes.[20]

Most recently, an update published in 2010 describes core competencies for health-care professionals working in CR/SP programs that address the necessary knowledge and skill sets in order to meet the requirements of the core components.[21]

EXERCISE PRESCRIPTION

The recommended time between an event and the start of an exercise program is typically 6 weeks following a coronary artery bypass surgery, 4 weeks after an acute myocardial infarction, and 3 weeks after a percutaneous coronary intervention. Exercise prescription is individualized and is typically based on the results of a submaximal or a symptom-limited stress test for prognostic, diagnostic, and therapeutic purposes. Exercise testing carries a predictive value for mortality. In addition to mortality, the stress test will stratify the patient's risk for cardiac events during exercise participation.[22,23]

Both aerobic and strength training aspects are recommended. Isotonic, rhythmic, and aerobic exercise using large muscle groups such as walking, jogging, swimming, and cycling is preferred. Strength training at least twice a week is recommended after participating in endurance training for several weeks. The calorie expenditure and a positive influence on risk factors is less with strength training than with endurance training; however, the resultant increased muscle mass correlates with the increased strength and functional mobility. High-intensity isometric exercises should be avoided because of the resultant increase in afterload.

Strength training should be avoided in patients with congestive heart failure, uncontrolled arrhythmias, systolic blood pressure >160 mm Hg, diastolic blood pressure >100 mm Hg, severe valvular disease, or unstable angina.[24]

The components of exercise prescription typically include the following:

- **Mode:** Recommend the type that requires the use of large muscle groups and aerobic exercises. Low-impact activities are typically recommended due to lesser risk of physical injury. The mode or modes of exercise chosen should be enjoyable and simple to carry out to maximize compliance.
- **Frequency:** Typically performed 3 to 5 times a week, to achieve a significant improvement in functional capacity.
- **Content and duration:**
  - i. Warm-up: Usually lasts 5 to 10 minutes. These include stretching, flexibility movements, and aerobic activity that gradually increases the heart rate into the target range. This gradual increment in oxygen demand minimizes the risk of exercise-related cardiovascular complications.
  - ii. Conditioning or training phase: This usually lasts a minimum of 20 minutes, and preferably lasts 30 to 45 minutes of continuous or discontinuous aerobic activity.
  - iii. Cool-down: Usually lasts 5 to 10 minutes. This involves low-intensity exercise and permits a gradual recovery from the conditioning phase. Omission of cool-down can result in a transient decrease in venous return, reducing coronary blood flow while heart rate and myocardial oxygen consumption remain high.
- **Intensity:** This ranges from 40% to 85% of functional capacity (VO_{2max}), which corresponds to 55% to 90% of maximal heart rate. Categorized using the percent HR_{max} as light (<60%), moderate (60%-79%), and heavy (80%).
- **Supervision:** Low-risk patients may initially benefit from medically supervised ECG-monitored exercise (6-12 sessions), which help to reassure the patient about the safety of the program. Self-monitored, home-based exercise programs also have been shown to be effective and safe in these patients and result in better rates of adherence when compared to group-based programs.

It is recommended that patients at moderate or high risk complete their phase II cardiac rehabilitation in a medically supervised program, with ECG monitoring and personnel and equipment suitable for advanced cardiac life support. This level of medical supervision should be continued for 8 to 12 weeks until the safety of the prescribed exercise regimen has been established.

BENEFITS OF CR

CR program is designed to provide disease management that complements and supports the goals and treatment plan of an individual's health-care providers. There is a vast evidence to indicate that CR is a useful and effective therapy that maximizes an individual's health and clinical outcomes. Meta-analyses of randomized controlled trials of CR have demonstrated 15% to 28% reductions in all-cause mortality.[25-28]

The largest study to date of CR in elderly has been published by Suaya et al comprising >600,000 Medicare beneficiaries aged 65 and over, who were hospitalized for coronary conditions or cardiac revascularization procedures. Notably, this study redemonstrated a low utilization of CR (12%). Participants in cardiac rehabilitation were more likely to be white, male, younger, and of higher socioeconomic class. At 1-year and 5-year follow-up, there were statistically significant RR reductions of 58% and 34%, respectively, in favor of cardiac rehabilitation. The benefits were seen in all groups, including those with chronic heart failure who gained greater benefit than those without heart failure, and those following revascularization procedures. Importantly, there was a "dose-dependent" response—those who attended more sessions experienced a greater mortality reduction than those who attended fewer sessions. Mortality reductions were increased in older age groups (>75 years of age) and women gained greater benefit than men across all age groups[29] (Figure 7-4).

All curves begin 1 month after discharge. Observed and adjusted differences in cumulative mortality rates between cardiac rehabilitation (CR) users and nonusers at each time point shown were significant ($p = 0.0001$). Adjusted cumulative mortality rates for CR use from instrumental variables were lower at each time point than rates from single probit ($p = 0.001$ for 12 months, $p = 0.01$ for 24 and 48 months, and $p = 0.05$ for 36 and 60 months). Adjusted differences in annual mortality rates between CR use and non-CR use from instrumental variables were 6.0% in year 1, 2.4% in year 2, 2.9% in year 3, 1.5% in year 4, and 1.5% in year 5 (all at $p < 0.001$).

A recent meta analysis[30] had confirmed that CR not only decreases cardiovascular mortality and all-cause mortality, but also a statistically significant reduction in reinfarction when used as a secondary prevention postmyocardial infarction (Figure 7-5).

In addition to improvements in mortality and morbidity, CR has been shown to reduce symptoms such as angina, shortness of breath, and fatigue. Depression and rehospitalization rates are lower. Adherence to heart-healthy diet, prescribed medications, and regular exercise training, which positively affects all modifiable cardiac risk factors, is higher in patients who attend CR programs.[31]

Participants in CR programs have demonstrated improved quality of life, increased knowledge of disease processes and prevention strategies, leading to improved adherence to healthy lifestyle choices thereby reducing lifestyle-related risks.

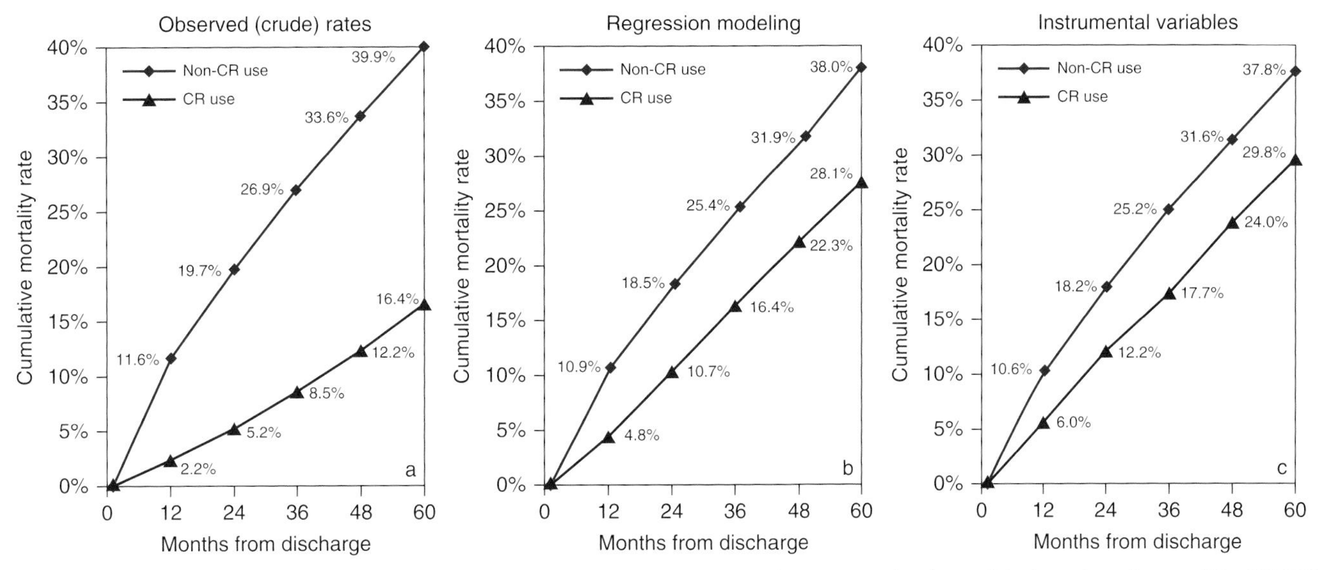

FIGURE 7-4 Crude and adjusted cumulative mortality rates for CR use and nonuse in the entire study cohort of Medicare beneficiaries (N = 601,099).[29]

RISKS OF CR

In 2007, the American Heart Association estimated the risk of any major adverse cardiac event during cardiac rehabilitation, including myocardial infarction, cardiac arrest, or death, as one event in 60,000 to 80,000 hours of supervised exercise.[32] Patients at risk of experiencing an ischemic event during cardiac rehabilitation include those with postoperative angina, left ventricular ejection fraction <35%, New York Heart Association grade III or IV congestive heart failure, ventricular tachycardia, or fibrillation in the postoperative period. Besides, if the patient experiences a drop in systolic blood pressure of 10 points or more with exercise, excessive ventricular ectopy with exercise, and myocardial ischemia with exercise, he/she can be said to be at risk.

Overall, there is a 30% incidence of ventricular tachycardia with up to 1 urgent complication in 138 patient-hours of exercise; however, there were only 1.3 fatalities per 1 million patient-hours. The rate of arrhythmias is similar in men and women. Incorporating a warm-up and a cool-down period for each exercise session decreases the frequency of arrhythmias by promoting coronary perfusion. The initiation of cardiac rehabilitation should occur 6 weeks after the implantation of an automatic implantable cardioverter defibrillator (AICD) to prevent the dislodgement of the device leads.[33]

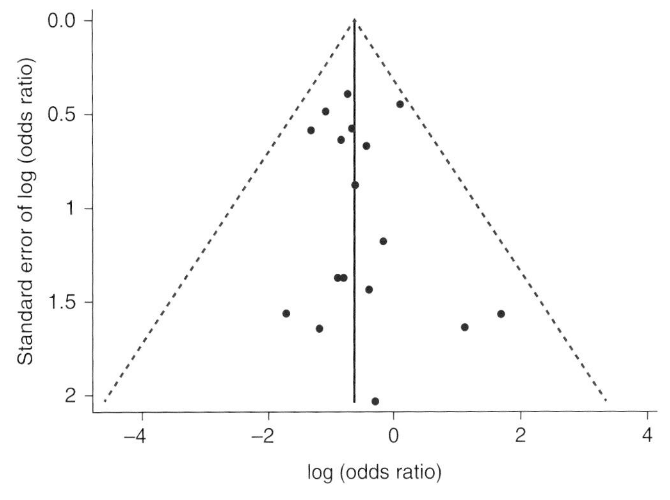

FIGURE 7-5 Funnel plot for meta-analysis examining the effect of exercise-based CR on the risk of reinfarction. Dashed lines represent pseudo 95% CIs.[30]

SPECIAL POPULATIONS

ELDERLY

Elderly patients are more likely to encounter complications of myocardial infarction and myocardial revascularization procedures due to clustering of risk factors, and may have greater rehabilitation needs. More than half of cardiac rehabilitation candidates are older than 65 years. Older patients rarely quit cardiac rehabilitation and achieve excellent outcomes with a low risk of adverse events. Even so, older individuals are less likely to be referred to and participate in cardiac rehabilitation.[34,35]

MINORITIES

According to the American Heart Association 2011 Heart Disease and Stroke Statistics Update, the prevalence of cardiovascular disease for black men (44.8%) and women (47.3%) far exceeds those for their white counterparts (37.4% and 33.8%, respectively).[36]

Even after controlling factors such as socioeconomic status, health insurance, and clinical causes, racial and ethnic inequalities in health status and care exist. Minority Americans lag behind on nearly every health indicator.[37] National standards in assuring cultural competence in health care have been proposed by the US Department of Health and Human Services, Office of Minority Health with the intention to help eliminate such discrepancies.

HEART FAILURE

Clinically stable class II and class III heart failure patients without complex arrhythmias should exercise in the absence of particular contraindications to exercise. Exercise training in stable heart failure patients was associated with significant reductions in all-cause mortality or hospitalization and cardiovascular mortality or hospitalization because of heart failure[38] and significant improvement in health status compared with usual care. These results have persisted over a 2.5-year follow-up.[39]

CARDIAC TRANSPLANT

Cardiac transplant recipients experience exercise intolerance of 40% to 50% below that of age-matched controls. This is thought to be secondary to myocardial sympathetic denervation; residual skeletal muscle abnormalities developed before transplantation and decreased strength.[40] The denervated myocardium and increased plasma norepinephrine seen in these patients causes elevated resting heart rate (often >90 bpm), elevated systolic and diastolic blood pressures, an attenuated increase in heart rate during submaximal work, a lower peak heart rate and peak stroke volume, and a delayed slowing of heart rate in recovery. Exercise intensity relies more on the perceived exertion (the Borg scale) than on specific heart rate, and the exercise prescription involves gradual increase in activity.

PERIPHERAL ARTERY DISEASE

At least one-third of patients with known coronary artery disease have coexistent peripheral artery disease (PAD) and more than half of the patients with known PAD have coexistent coronary artery disease.[41] Functional capacity in patients with PAD is often <50% of the predicted value because of claudication and exercise limitation. Patients are made to exercise till they reach their claudication threshold within 3 to 5 minutes. This is followed by a brief period of rest to permit the symptoms to resolve, and exercise is resumed once again. The exercise-rest-exercise cycle is repeated several times during a 30- to 60-minute period to stimulate collateral formation.

Arm ergometry is a safe and effective method for improving cardiovascular fitness and efficiency of arm work in a patient with dysvascular amputation.[42]

STROKE

One-third of patients with known coronary artery disease have coexistent ischemic cerebrovascular accident, and more than half of the patients with known ischemic cerebrovascular accident have coexistent coronary artery disease. One should reduce walking speed in stroke patients so that they are safe and comfortable. Leg and arm ergometers have been adapted for use by hemiparetic persons.[41] The rehabilitation program needs to be individualized based on the degree of mobility dysfunction and the nature of cognitive impairment.[43]

NEW APPROACHES TO CR

Different approaches have been tried to improve efficiencies and maximize outcomes in cardiac rehabilitation. Traditional cardiac rehabilitation sessions burn 700 to 800 cal/wk. High calorie expenditure (HCE) exercise has been designed to burn 3000 to 3500 cal/wk. HCE exercise has resulted in more favorable cardiac risk profile, with a significant decrease in triglycerides, insulin resistance, blood pressure, and plasminogen activator inhibitor-1, and a significant increase in high-density lipoprotein cholesterol. HCE exercise also leads to doubling of the weight loss as compared with traditional cardiac rehabilitation, and the benefits could be reaped even a year later.[44]

High-intensity interval training (HIIT) is another form of aerobic training with alternating short episodes of high- and low-intensity exercises. Numerous contemporary studies suggest that HIIT is safe and more effective for improving maximal aerobic capacity, endurance, and endothelial function.[45,46]

UNDERUTILIZATION OF CR

Despite evidence showing significant benefit, CR remains underutilized. Nearly 12.5 million Americans are eligible for secondary prevention programs; yet there is a great disparity between those individuals and the number of participants completing a phase II program. Of the eligible patients, only 14% to 35% participate in CR programs after an acute myocardial infarction and approximately 31% of patients do so after coronary artery bypass graft surgery. Participation is lowest in women, minorities, socioeconomically disadvantaged patients, and the elderly.[47]

A small prospective study[48] demonstrated that the predictors of cardiac rehabilitation participation included younger age, male sex, lack of diabetes, ST-elevation MI, receipt of reperfusion therapy, having a cardiologist as primary provider in the hospital, lack of prior MI, no prior cardiac rehabilitation attendance, and receiving a referral to cardiac rehabilitation while in the hospital. Psychosocial predictors of cardiac rehabilitation participation include placing a high importance and feeling a need for rehabilitation, better perceived health before MI, the ability to drive, and higher education level. As with prior studies, older age, female sex, lack of physician referral, not feeling that rehabilitation is necessary, an inability to drive, and lower education level have all been shown to decrease participation (Figure 7-6).

When examining the barriers to participation in a CR program among women with CAD, barriers were identified at provider level, system level, and individual level. Lack of a physician referral[49-52] as well as disparities in referral of women to CR by ethnicity and

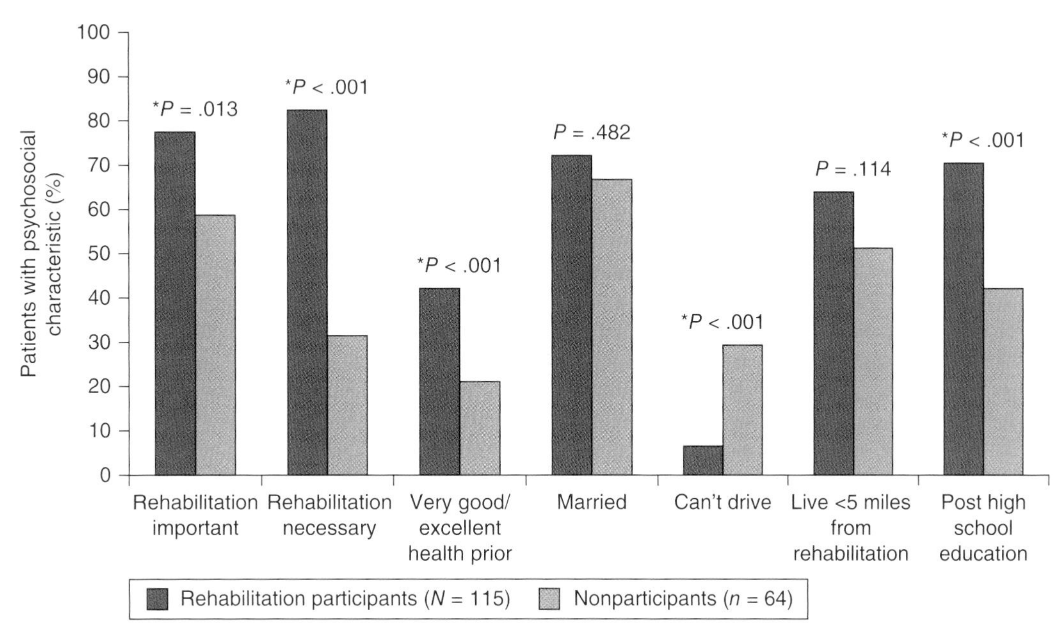

FIGURE 7-6 Difference in psychosocial characteristics between CR participants vs non participants.[48]

socioeconomic status were noted.[49] Despite being given a referral, physician involvement and encouragement seem to be key to assure participation of women in CR.[53] Pertaining to system-level factors, lack of insurance coverage or financial concerns[50] and transportation problems appears to hinder the participation in CR.[54-57]

Individual level factors including poor perceived health, comorbid conditions,[53-55,58] and perceptions about CR were identified as barriers to CR. Among female nonparticipants, comorbid conditions were rated as significant barriers when compared with male counterparts.[59] Lack of awareness and misperceptions of CR programs and its benefits may be another important factor in the decision to participate for women who are eligible for CR.[60]

Farley et al[61] reported that women identified personal preferences for lack of participation in CR, which included not wanting to dwell on or be reminded of cardiac problems, wanting to deal with the problems by themselves, and feeling uncomfortable in groups. Additionally, women also identified lack of perceived need for CR as a reason for not attending the same in a qualitative study.[62]

CONCLUSION

Cardiac rehabilitation is an effective intervention with a large and increasing evidence base. It is estimated that one 5-year death would be averted for every 12 patients receiving cardiac rehabilitation[29]—a statistic not easily rivaled by most modern drug therapies.[63] Although cardiac rehabilitation has been an established intervention for decades, there is exciting new research in a variety of areas, including exploring the benefit of cardiac rehabilitation in new patient populations, finding ways to improve cardiac rehabilitation referral and participation, and developing variations in exercise regimens. Cardiac rehabilitation is beneficial in some of the most pervasive diseases in modern society.[64] Maximizing the benefit from this intervention through further research has the potential to significantly reduce the individual and societal burden from these diseases.

REFERENCES

1. Roger VL, Go AS, Lloyd-Jones DM, et al. Heart disease and stroke statistics—2012 update: a report from the American Heart Association. *Circulation*. 2012 January 3;125(1):e2-e220.
2. Antman EM, Anbe ST, Armstrong PW, et al. ACC/AHA guidelines for the management of patients with ST-elevation myocardial infarction: executive summary: a report of the American College of Cardiology/American Heart Association Task Force on Practice Guidelines. *J Am Coll Cardiol*. 2004;44: 671-719.
3. Braunwald E, Antman EM, Beasley JW, et al. ACC/AHA 2002 guideline update for the management of patients with unstable angina and non–ST-segment elevation myocardial infarction: summary article: a report of the American College of Cardiology/American Heart Association Task Force on Practice Guidelines. *J Am Coll Cardiol*. 2002;40:1366-1374.
4. Gibbons RJ, Abrams J, Chatterjee K, et al. ACC/AHA 2002 guideline update for the management of patients with chronic stable angina: summary article: a report of the American College of Cardiology/American Heart Association Task Force on Practice Guidelines. *Circulation*. 2003;107:149-158.
5. Balady GJ, Williams M, Ades PA, et al. Core components of Cardiac Rehabilitation/Secondary Prevention Programs: 2007 update. A scientific statement from the American Heart Association Exercise, Cardiac Rehabilitation, and Prevention Committee, the Council on Clinical Cardiology; the Councils on Cardiovascular Nursing, Epidemiology and Prevention, and Nutrition, Physical Activity, and Metabolism; and the American Association of Cardiovascular and Pulmonary Rehabilitation. *Circulation*. 2007;115:2675-2682.
6. Lavie CJ, Thomas RJ, Squires RW, et al. Exercise training and cardiac rehabilitation in primary and secondary prevention of coronary heart disease. *Mayo Clin Proc*. 2009;84(4):373-383.
7. Wenger NK. Current status of cardiac rehabilitation. *J Am Coll Cardiol*. 2008;51:1619-1631.
8. Mosca L, Banka CL, Benjamin EJ, et al., for the Expert Panel/Writing Group. Evidence-based guidelines for cardiovascular disease prevention in women: 2007 update. *Circulation*. 2007;115:1481-1501.
9. Forelicher V. Cardiac rehabilitation. In: Parmley W, Chatterjee K. eds. *Cardiology*. Philadelphia, PA: JB Lippincott; 1988:1-17.
10. Levine SA. Some harmful effects of recumbency in the treatment of heart disease. *JAMA*. 1944;126:80-84.
11. Levine S, Lown B. "Armchair" treatment of acute coronary thrombosis. *JAMA*. 1952;148:1356-1369.
12. Newman L, Andrews M, Koblish M. Physical medicine and rehabilitation in acute myocardial infarction. *Arch Intern Med*. 1952;82:552-561.
13. Brummer P, Linko E, Kasanen A. Myocardial infarction treated by early ambulation. *Am Hear J*. 1956;52:269-272.
14. Cain HD, Fraser WG, Stivelman R. Graded activity program for safe return to self-care after myocardial infarction. *JAMA*. 1961;177:111-115.
15. Wenger N, Gilbert C, Skorapa M. Cardiac conditioning after myocardial infarction. An early intervention program. *J Cardiac Rehabil*. 1971;2:17-22.
16. Oldridge NB, Guyatt GH, Fischer ME, Rimm AA. Cardiac rehabilitation after myocardial infarction. Combined experience of randomized clinical trials. *JAMA*. 1988;260:945-950.
17. Taylor RS, Brown A, Ebrahim S, et al. Exercise-based rehabilitation for patients with coronary heart disease: systematic review and meta-analysis of randomized controlled trials. *Am J Med*. 2004;116:682-692.
18. Clark AM, Hartling L, Vandermeer B, McAlister FA. Meta-analysis: secondary prevention programs for patients with coronary artery disease. *Ann Intern Med*. 2005;143:659-672.
19. Thomas RJ, King M, Lui K, et al. AACVPR/ACC/AHA 2007 performance measures on cardiac rehabilitation for referral to and delivery of cardiac rehabilitation/secondary prevention services endorsed by the American College of Chest Physicians, American College of Sports Medicine, American Physical Therapy Association, Canadian Association of Cardiac Rehabilitation, European Association for Cardiovascular Prevention and Rehabilitation, Inter-American Heart Foundation, National Association of Clinical Nurse Specialists, Preventive Cardiovascular Nurses Association, and the Society of Thoracic Surgeons. *J Am Coll Cardiol*. 2007 October 2;50(14):1400-1433.
20. Herridge ML, Stimler CE, Southard DR, King ML; AACVPR Task Force. Depression screening in cardiac rehabilitation: AACVPR Task Force Report. *J Cardiopulm Rehabil*. 2005 January-February;25(1):11-13.
21. Thomas RJ, King M, Lui K, et al. AACVPR/ACCF/AHA 2010 Update: performance measures on cardiac rehabilitation for referral to cardiac rehabilitation/secondary prevention services endorsed by the American College of Chest Physicians, the American College of Sports Medicine, the American Physical Therapy Association, the Canadian Association of Cardiac Rehabilitation, the Clinical Exercise Physiology Association, the European Association for Cardiovascular Prevention and Rehabilitation, the Inter-American Heart Foundation, the National Association of Clinical Nurse Specialists, the Preventive Cardiovascular Nurses Association, and the Society of Thoracic Surgeons. *J Am Coll Cardiol*. 2010 September 28;56(14):1159-1167.
22. Kavanagh T, Mertens DJ, Hamm LF, et al. Prediction of long-term prognosis in 12169 men referred for cardiac rehabilitation. *Circulation*. 2002;106:666-671.
23. Myers J, Prakash M, Froelicher V, et al. Exercise capacity and mortality among men referred for exercise testing. *N Engl J Med*. 2002;346:793-801.
24. Dingwall H, Ferrier K, Semple J. Exercise prescription in cardiac rehabilitation. In: Thow MK, ed. *Exercise Leadership in Cardiac Rehabilitation: An Evidence Based Approach*. West Sussex, England: Whurr Publishers Limited; 2006:102-118.
25. Oldridge N, Guyatt G, Fischer M. Cardiac rehabilitation after myocardial infarction. Combined experience of randomized clinical trials. *JAMA*. 1988;260:945-950.

26. O'Connor G, Buring J, Yusuf S, et al. An overview of randomized trials of rehabilitation with exercise after myocardial infarction. *Circulation*. 1989;80:234-244.

27. Taylor R, Brown A, Ebrahim S, et al. Exercise-based rehabilitation for patients with coronary heart disease: systematic review and meta-analysis of randomized controlled trials. *Am J Med*. 2004;116:682-692.

28. Clark A, Hartling L, Vandermeer B, et al. Meta-analysis: secondary prevention programs for patients with coronary artery disease. *Ann Intern Med*. 2005;143:659-672.

29. Suaya J, Stason W, Ades P, et al. Cardiac rehabilitation survival in older coronary patients. *J Amer Coll Cardiol*. 2009;54;25-33.

30. Lawler PR, Filion KB, Eisenberg MJ. Efficacy of exercise-based cardiac rehabilitation post-myocardial infarction: a systematic review and meta-analysis of randomized controlled trials. *Am Heart J*. 2011 October;162(4):571-584.

31. Herridge ML, Stimler CE, Sousthard DR, et al. Depression screening in cardiac rehabilitation. AACVPR Task Force Report. *J Cardiopulm Rehabil*. 2005;25:11-13.

32. Thompson PD, Franklin BA, Balady GJ, et al. Exercise and acute cardiovascular events placing the risks into perspective. A scientific statement from the American Heart Association Council on Nutrition, Physical Activity, and Metabolism and the Council on Clinical Cardiology. *Circulation*. 2007;115:2358-2368.

33. Sears SF, Kovacs AH, Conti JB, et al. Expanding the scope of practice for cardiac rehabilitation: managing patients with implantable cardioverter defibrillators. *J Cardiopulm Rehabil*. 2004;24:209-215.

34. Strahle A, Mattsson E, Ryden L, et al. Improved physical fitness and quality of life following training of elderly patients after acute coronary events. A 1 year follow-up randomized controlled study. *Eur Heart J*. 1999;20:1475-1484.

35. Balady GJ, Jette D, Scheer J, et al. Changes in exercise capacity following cardiac rehabilitation in patients stratified according to age and gender. Results of the Massachusetts Association of Cardiovascular and Pulmonary Rehabilitation Multicenter Database. *J Cardiopulm Rehabil*. 1996;16:38-46.

36. Roger VL, Go AS, Lloyd-Jones DM, et al. Heart disease and stroke statistics 2011 update: a report from the American Heart Association. *Circulation*. 2011;123:e18-e209.

37. Ren XS, Amick BC, Williams DR. Racial/ethnic disparities in health: the interplay between discrimination and socioeconomic status. *Ethn Dis*. 1999;9:151-165.

38. O'Connor CM, Whellan DJ, Lee KL, et al. Efficacy and safety of exercise training in patients with chronic heart failure: HF-ACTION randomized controlled trial. *JAMA*. 2009;310:1439-1450.

39. Flynn KE, Pina IL, Whellan DJ, et al. Effects of exercise training on health status in patients with chronic heart failure: findings from the HF-ACTION randomized controlled trial. *JAMA*. 2009:301:1451-1459.

40. Schairer JR, Keteyian SJ. Exercise in patients with cardiovascular disease. In: Kraus WE, Keteyian SJ, eds. *Cardiac Rehabilitation*. Totowa, NJ: Humana Press; 2007:169-183.

41. Aronow WS, Ahn C. Prevalence of coexistence of coronary artery disease, peripheral arterial disease, and atherothrombotic brain infarction in men and women > or = 62 years of age. *Am J Cardiol*. 1994;74:64-65.

42. Davidoff GN, Lampman RM, Westbury L, et al. Exercise testing and training of persons with dysvascular amputation: safety and efficacy of arm ergometry. *Arch Phys Med Rehabil*. 1992;73:334-338.

43. Gitter A, Halar EM. Cardiac rehabilitation of the patient with stroke. *Phys Med Rehabil Clin North Am*. 1995;6:297-310.

44. Ades PA, Savage PD, Toth MJ, et al. High-calorie-expenditure exercise: a new approach to cardiac rehabilitation for overweight coronary patients. *Circulation*. 2009;119:2671-2678.

45. Rognmo O, Hetland E, Helgerud J, et al. High intensity aerobic interval exercise is superior to moderate intensity exercise for increasing aerobic capacity in patients with coronary artery disease. *Eur J Cardiovasc Prev Rehabil*. 2004;11:216-222.

46. Guiraud T, Juneau M, Nigam A, et al. Optimization of high intensity interval exercise in coronary heart disease. *Eur J Appl Physiol*. 2010;108:733-740.

47. Suaya JA, Shepard DS, Normand ST, et al. Use of cardiac rehabilitation by Medicare beneficiaries after myocardial infarction or coronary bypass surgery. *Circulation*. 2007;116:1653-1662.

48. Dunlay SM, Witt BJ, Allison TG, et al. Barriers to participation in cardiac rehabilitation. *Am Heart J*. 2009;158(5):852-859.

49. Mochari HY, Lee JWR, Klingfield P, et al. Ethnic differences in barriers to cardiac rehabilitation among women hospitalized with coronary heart disease. *Circulation*. 2002;106(19): Abstract 3514.

50. Missik E. Women and cardiac rehabilitation: accessibility issues and policy recommendations. *Rehabil Nurs*. 2001;26(4):141-147.

51. Heid HG, Schmelzer M. Influences on women's participation in cardiac rehabilitation. *Rehabil Nurs*. 2004;29(4):116-121.

52. Allen JK, Scott LB, Stewart KJ, Young DR. Disparities in women's referral to and enrollment in outpatient cardiac rehabilitation. *J Gen Intern Med*. 2004;19(7):747-753.

53. Sanderson B, Shewchuk R, Bittner V. Cardiac rehabilitation and women: what keeps them away? *J Cardiopulm Rehabil Prev*. 2010;30(1):12-21.

54. Halm M, Penque S, Doll N, Beahrs M. Women and cardiac rehabilitation: referral and compliance patterns. *J Cardiovasc Nurs*. 1999;13(3):83-92.

55. Brown TM, Hernandez AF, Bittner V, et al. Predictors of cardiac rehabilitation referral in coronary artery disease patients: findings from the American Heart Association's Get With the Guidelines Program. *J Am Coll Cardiol*. 2009;54(6):515-521.

56. Marcuccio E, Loving N, Bennett SK, Hayes SN. A survey of attitudes and experiences of women with heart disease. *Womens Health Issues*. 2003;13(1):23-31.

57. Gallagher R, McKinley S, Dracup K. Predictors of women's attendance at cardiac rehabilitation programs. *Prog Cardiovasc Nurs*. 2003;18(3):121-126.

58. Grace SL, Gravely-Witte S, Kayaniyil S, Brual J, Suskin N, Stewart DE. A multisite examination of sex differences in cardiac rehabilitation barriers by participation status. *J Womens Health (Larchmt)*. 2009;18(2):209-216.

59. Lieberman L, Meana M, Stewart D. Cardiac rehabilitation: gender differences in factors influencing participation. *J Womens Health*. 1998;7(6):717-723.

60. Caulin-Glaser T, Blum M, Schmeizl R, Prigerson HG, Zaret B, Mazure CM. Gender differences in referral to cardiac rehabilitation programs after revascularization. *J Cardiopulm Rehabil*. 2001;21(1):24-30.

61. Farley RL, Wade TD, Birchmore L. Factors influencing attendance at cardiac rehabilitation among coronary heart disease patients. *Eur J Cardiovasc Nurs*. 2003;2(3):205-212.

62. McSweeney JC, Crane PB. An act of courage: women's decision-making processes regarding outpatient cardiac rehabilitation attendance. *Rehabil Nurs*. 2001;26(4):132.

63. Freemantle N, Cleland J, Young P, et al. Beta blockade after myocardial infarction: systematic review and meta regression analysis. *BMJ*. 1999; 318:1730-1737.

64. Lloyd-Jones D, Adams RJ, Brown TM, et al. Executive summary: heart disease and stroke statistics—2010 update: a report from the American Heart Association. *Circulation*. 2010 February 23;121(7):948-954.

8 HEART FAILURE IN WOMEN

Adam Pleister, MD
Ayesha Hasan MD, FACC

CASE PRESENTATION

A 31-year-old woman was admitted in a state of cardiogenic shock 6 months after she was diagnosed with nonischemic cardiomyopathy. Nearly 9 to 12 months ago, she had started experiencing fatigue and dyspnea while climbing stairs and was diagnosed with left ventricular systolic dysfunction a few months later. She had ejection fraction of 15% and dilated left ventricle of 6.8 cm and was started on medicines and evidence-based treatment. More recently, she developed intolerance toward her current carvedilol dose that had to be reduced as it caused hypotension and nausea. Currently, the patient was admitted with blood pressure of 88/62 mm Hg, heart rate of 105 beats per minute, S_3 gallop on examination, elevated jugular venous distention to 6 cm above the clavicle, cool extremities, brain natriuretic peptide of 953 pg/mL, serum sodium of 134 mmol/L, and total bilirubin of 4 mg/dL. The physician started her on an inotrope upon admission. After diuresis, her right heart catheterization revealed elevated filling pressures (right atrial pressure of 15 mm Hg, wedge pressure of 36 mm Hg), pulmonary hypertension (mean pulmonary artery pressure of 49 mm Hg), and low cardiac index <1.8 on dobutamine 5 µg/kg/min. Echo now revealed progression of left ventricular dilation to 7.2 cm, moderate mitral regurgitation, and moderate right ventricular dysfunction in addition to left-sided failure. Due to advanced stage of the disease and clinical decline in patient's condition, she was worked up for cardiac transplantation and listed with blood type O. Meanwhile, she continued to decline requiring 2 inotropes, and a repeat hemodynamic evaluation showed a high pulmonary vascular resistance of 4.5 Wood units. Her chances of receiving a cardiac transplant were also limited by both her blood type (type O) and worsening pulmonary hypertension. Besides, she could not tolerate attempts to wean her off the inotrope or pressor support, and continued to become more tachycardic. So a decision was made to implant ventricular assist device that would act as a bridge to cardiac transplantation by extending the life of the patient.

INTRODUCTION

Heart failure is a complex clinical syndrome with increasing prevalence and incidence in developed and developing nations. Among adults in the United States, heart failure is now the leading etiology for inpatient admissions. Women represent half of these hospital admissions and heart failure accounts for approximately one-third of all deaths from cardiovascular disease in women.[1-3] Although women bear a significant burden of heart failure mortality and morbidity, they are historically very poorly represented in clinical trials: prior to 2002, only one-fifth of patients enrolled in randomized controlled trials were women.[4] Therefore a paucity of evidence exists regarding gender-specific differences in the diagnosis, treatment, and prognosis of heart failure.

GENETIC EXPRESSION

Recent analysis revealed differential autosomal gene expression in men versus women with heart failure.[5-7] Women overexpressed genes related to adrenergic and angiotensin signaling, cyclic nucleotide metabolism, and glucose transport (*GATAD1*, *PDE6B*, and *SCLA12*, respectively). Those genes upregulated in men with heart failure were associated with potassium channel/arrhythmia regulation, cellular homeostasis, and immune system regulation (*KCNK1*, *PLEKHA8*, and *CD24*, respectively). These initial genetic studies may provide an early foundation to explain the gender differences noted in etiology (eg, ischemic vs nonischemic secondary to hypertensive heart disease), presentation (eg, with age differences), clinical course, and response to treatment in heart failure—or personalized medicine based on sex-related heart failure management.

EPIDEMIOLOGY

The prevalence of heart failure increases in both men and women as the population ages. However, the initial diagnosis of heart failure occurs later in women, and more women than men have heart failure after the age of 80.[8] The most recent population data from the last decade reveal an incidence of 550,000 cases per year and approximately equal numbers of men and women with heart failure, overall affecting 3.1 million males and 2.6 million females.[2] Women and men are admitted for inpatient care for acute exacerbations of heart failure at an almost equal rate, but women appear to have improved overall survival compared to men. One exception to the survival advantage in women versus men appears to lie in the specific subpopulation of patients with depressed left ventricular systolic function in the setting of coronary heart disease and ischemic cardiomyopathy; the Beta-Blocker Evaluation of Survival Trial (BEST) study suggested that survival is better for women with a nonischemic etiology versus those with ischemic etiology.[9-10] In addition, in both the acute and chronic settings, women present more often with heart failure with preserved ejection fraction (HFPEF, defined as ejection fraction ≥50%) and often in the setting of multiple chronic medical conditions such as obesity, diabetes mellitus, sleep apnea, and hypertension.[11-12] This increased incidence of HFPEF in women compared to men may at least partially account for the survival advantage in women due to the higher systolic ejection fraction and prevalence of nonischemic disease in HFPEF.[13]

PRESENTATION

Despite apparent overall survival advantages, women with heart failure present more often with symptoms of heart failure, poorer functional class, more significant physical examination findings consistent with heart failure (eg, jugular venous distension or S_3), and increased diuretic requirements when compared to men.[14] As per the ADHERE (Acute Decompensated Heart Failure National Registry) database, women were more hypertensive than men upon admission for acute heart failure exacerbations (systolic BP of 148 mm Hg vs 139.4 mm Hg, $p < 0.0001$); despite a lower creatinine, women had a lower glomerular filtration rate of 51.3 mL/min/1.73 m^2 vs 55.7 mL/min/1.73 m^2 in men ($p < 0.0001$).[15] Gender differences in this registry support data that women are less likely to have an ischemic etiology and associated risk factors but are more likely to have hypertension. Population data also suggest that women with heart failure have poorer quality-of-life scores and a greater incidence of depression.[16]

Comorbid medical conditions upon presentation with heart failure also differ between women and men. While men are more likely to have chronic obstructive pulmonary disease, coronary heart disease (CAD), and peripheral vascular disease, women most often present in the setting of thyroid disease, valvular heart disease, and systemic hypertension[15,17] (Tables 8-1 and 8-2).

Diabetes mellitus and systemic hypertension have long been known risk factors for the development of heart failure in women, even in the absence of coronary heart disease.[2]

In terms of racial diversity associated with risk factors for heart disease, ethnicity has been underrepresented in clinical trials, similar to underrepresentation of women in general. Limited studies have focused on ethnic differences among women; more recently, as part of the Women's Health Initiative, incident rates of heart failure hospitalization among different racial/ethnic groups were studied in postmenopausal women without self-reported heart failure, who were followed for an average of 7.8 years.[18] Findings showed the highest incidence among black women (380 in 100,000 person-years) and lowest risk among Hispanic and Asian/Pacific Islander women (193 and 103 in 100,000 person-years, respectively). The effects of low income and diabetes mellitus, but not hypertension, explained the higher risk in black women; lower risk in Hispanic and Asian/Pacific Islander women persisted despite adjustment for socioeconomic status, age, and traditional risk factors. Such data emphasize the need for further evaluation of the effect of racial differences on the mechanism of heart failure among women.

TABLE 8-1 Gender-related differences in comorbidities in in-patient heart failure registry data from the ADHERE database[15] and EHFS[17]

Women are more likely to have • Thyroid disease
Women are less likely than men to have • COPD • PVD • Renal failure • Smokers
Conflicting data: Diabetes & Anemia based on heart failure registry data

ADHERE found no gender difference in the prevalence of diabetes mellitus but more men presented with anemia; whereas EHFS noted more women presented with diabetes mellitus and anemia when admitted with acute exacerbations of heart failure.

Abbreviations: ADHERE, Acute Decompensated Heart Failure National Registry; EHFS, European Heart Failure Survey.

ETIOLOGY

Comorbid conditions are also associated with heart failure in women. Systemic hypertension is a significant risk factor and causative agent of heart failure in women.[13,15] In particular, increased blood pressure is noted after menopause due to changes in arterial structure and function that increase stiffness of the vessels with age and hormonal changes. Hypertension has a higher prevalence in the elderly population, black patients, and women.[19]

Diabetes mellitus and obesity are also known etiologies of heart failure, which result in a significant burden on women with heart failure.[20,21] In fact, glycemic control has been linked to the incidence of heart failure. Each 1% increase in hemoglobin A_{1C} has been associated with an 8% increased risk of heart failure after adjustment for gender and other risk factors (race, education level, smoking, use of medical therapy) in a study of over 40,000 patients without a prior history of heart failure.[20] A hemoglobin A_{1C} of >10% relative to a hemoglobin A_{1C} of <7% was associated with a 1.56-fold greater risk of heart failure. The risk of developing heart failure is increased by a factor of 4 to 5 times in diabetic women compared to nondiabetic women and twice that of diabetic men.[7]

Additionally, the endothelial dysfunction of diabetes has known pathological effects that can lead to the development of heart failure. Increased interstitial connective tissue and myocardial hypertrophy are caused by angiotensin II and endothelin, both derived from the endothelium, and could contribute to the higher left ventricular mass in those patients with both diabetes mellitus and systemic hypertension, compared to patients with hypertension alone. The significant correlation in women between heart failure and diabetes is also especially relevant given the higher occurrence of heart failure with preserved ejection fraction in women, where diabetes has been a more common risk factor for women compared to men.[14]

Obesity also plays a significant role in metabolic syndrome and comorbidities such as hypertension, type II diabetes mellitus, and sleep-disordered breathing; obesity alone is an independent etiology for the development of heart failure.[21,22] Detrimental effects of fatty acids on the myocardium as well as toxic proteins released by adipose tissue contribute to structural alterations. Although this appears to be an equal risk factor for both women and men, the emerging obesity epidemic in developed nations warrants significant attention. More recent studies have mentioned the "obesity paradox" of heart failure, but this phenomenon refers to a protective effect of obesity in chronic, more advanced heart failure compared to the poorer prognosis associated with a leaner body mass in these patients, regardless of gender.[23]

Valvular heart disease is a well-known source of heart failure, and a significant number of women have valvular heart disease with approximately two-thirds of women discharged from the hospital in 1987 with mitral or aortic valve disease and more than half of valve replacements occurring in women.[24] Mitral stenosis tends to have a higher predominance in women than men. Although rheumatic mitral stenosis, caused by rheumatic fever during childhood, has decreased recently in developed countries, this condition continues to be a significant burden in developing and underdeveloped countries. In developed countries, aortic stenosis in older populations is more common, due to calcific and degenerative processes. Valvular disease presents more commonly as a comorbid condition in women with heart failure compared to men with heart failure.

Pregnancy carries a potential risk based on the type of valvular heart disease. Mitral stenosis has the greatest risk of maternal cardiac complications whereas regurgitant lesions, asymptomatic aortic stenosis, and hypertrophic cardiomyopathy with mild-to-moderate left ventricular outflow obstruction are usually fairly well tolerated.[25] Pregnancy is not recommended in Marfan syndrome with a dilated aortic root >4 cm, and a normal dimension aortic root in this population still carries a risk of dissection beyond that of a woman without connective tissue disease.

TABLE 8-2 Gender differences in characteristics, management, and outcomes for patients hospitalized with heart failure[15]

	Women vs Men
Women are More Likely to Have	
Diastolic heart failure or HFPEF	51% vs 28%
Higher ejection fraction upon admission	42% vs 32.9%
Older age on presentation for admission	74.5 vs 70.1 years
Hypertension as risk factor	76% vs 70%
More hypertensive on admission (mean SBP)	148 vs 139 mm Hg
Nonischemic etiology of heart failure	
Men are More Likely to Have	
Coronary artery disease	51% vs 64%
Ischemic etiology of heart failure	19% vs 32%
Utilization of Therapy and Outcomes	
Similar intravenous diuretic use	
Less vasoactive drug use in women	
Less procedure-oriented therapy in women	
Similar but underutilized oral evidence-based therapy in both	
Similar mean length of stay	
Similar adjusted in-hospital mortality	

N = 105,388.
Abbreviations: ADHERE: acute decompensated heart failure national registry; HFPEF: heart failure with preserved ejection fraction.
Data from the ADHERE registry.

Coronary artery disease is the most common form of cardiovascular disease and a leading cause of death among men and women.[26] Along with hypertension, ischemic heart disease accounts for the largest number of newly diagnosed cases of heart failure annually. Gender differences have been found among risk factors. Women have a higher prevalence of hypertension after age 55, more hypertriglyceridemia, greater mortality risk from diabetes, and higher total cholesterol after age 50. Women diagnosed with acute coronary syndrome are more likely to have noncritical CAD with the hypothesis that endothelial and microvascular dysfunctions play a role in symptoms and outcomes in these patients without obstructive disease. The WISE study (Women's Ischemia Syndrome Evaluation) showed abnormal coronary flow reserve after intracoronary adenosine infusion in women and was associated with adverse cardiovascular outcomes.[27] Estrogen seems to have a protective effect on the reaction to acute coronary ischemia in women by reducing apoptosis and, therefore, infarct expansion and remodeling after an acute myocardial infarction (MI).[26] Women have a greater risk of developing heart failure post-MI, yet appear to have a long-term survival advantage compared to men in many studies, although this remains controversial since not all studies agree on this issue. Underrepresentation of women in clinical trials limits conclusions regarding gender differences. Figure 8-1 compares cardiac magnetic resonance imaging (MRI) in ischemic versus nonischemic etiology of heart failure.

Stress cardiomyopathy, or takotsubo cardiomyopathy, is a nonischemic cause of heart failure that occurs more often in women and, in particular, postmenopausal women[28] (Figure 8-2). Severe left ventricular dysfunction, most often at the apex, is noted in the setting of preceding emotional, physical, or medical stress (eg, loss of a loved one, trauma, or significant infection); left ventricular function usually normalizes in most patients after a few weeks. Elevated biomarkers, such as brain natriuretic peptide (BNP) and troponin, as well as ST elevation on electrocardiogram are often noted, similar to a presentation of acute coronary syndrome and/or acute decompensated heart failure. The coronary angiogram, however, will reveal normal coronary arteries with no significant obstruction. The pathology of this condition is still not well understood, although an acute catecholamine release and possibly a localized acute inflammatory response are thought to play a role. The diagnosis of stress cardiomyopathy is one of exclusion and depends on multiple findings, including history, demographics, biomarker levels, electrocardiogram, echocardiogram or MRI, and cardiac catheterization results. Treatment includes standard heart failure therapies in addition to supportive care.

Women appear to be more susceptible to certain toxins known to damage the myocardium and result in cardiomyopathy. In particular, the cardiotoxic effect of chemotherapeutic agents is more often observed in women compared to men.[29] It does not appear, however, that there is a difference in the duration of cardiotoxicity and resultant heart failure between genders. Cardiotoxicity may occur, at times acutely, within a few weeks of treatment or within a year to many years later. Risk factors also include type of drug, cumulative dose, schedule, coexisting cardiac disease, age >65 years, previous mediastinal radiation, and simultaneous use of other cardiotoxic drugs. For example, combination therapy of anthracyclines with trastuzumab, a monoclonal antibody against the human epidermal growth factor receptor-2 (HER2), enhances survival at the expense of augmented

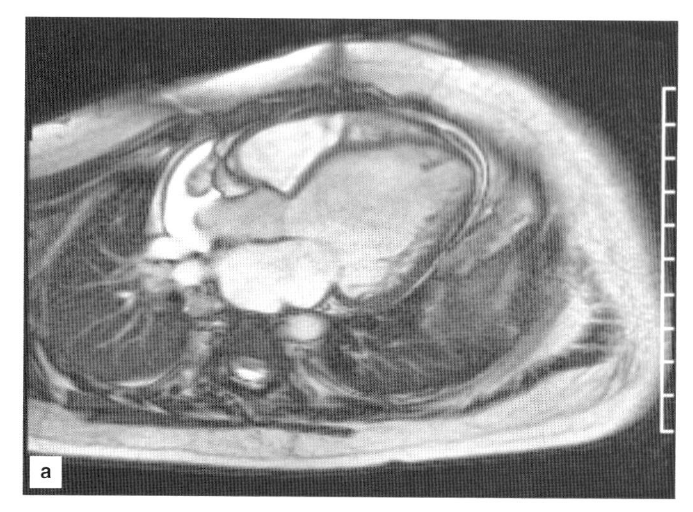

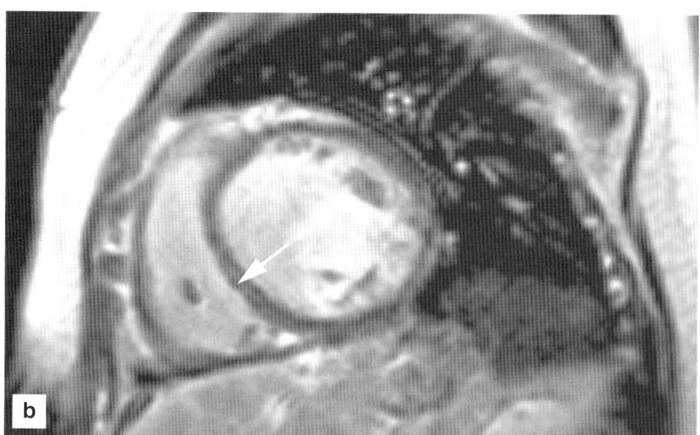

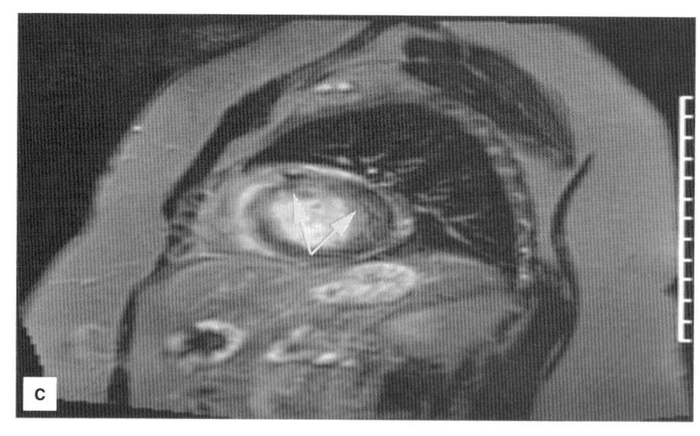

FIGURE 8-1 Cardiac MRI in a woman with end-stage heart failure and severe LV dilation in case presentation (A), who presented with cardiogenic shock requiring multiple inotrope infusions and eventually mechanical circulatory support. Mild mid-wall fibrosis on late post-gadolinium imaging (B, yellow arrow) is consistent with nonischemic etiology of heart failure, which is more common in women with cardiomyopathy. (C) Note the difference when compared to an ischemic etiology of cardiomyopathy with transmural hyperenhancement on late post-gadolinium imaging (green arrows) in a 27-year-old woman with history of 2 left anterior descending artery stents, lupus anticoagulant with hypercoagulable state, and severe LV dysfunction, LVEF of 24%. MRI shows extensive, mostly transmural scar involving the septum and anterior wall consistent with nonviable myocardium in the LAD distribution.
All images from Ohio State University Medical Center noninvasive imaging laboratory.

cardiotoxicity.[30] The pathophysiology resulting in increased cardiomyopathy and heart failure in women is not well elucidated, but a proposed mechanism is related to cardiac damage because of free radicals.[31] Concomitant treatment with dexrazoxane reduces the risk of cardiac toxicity through iron chelation and reduction in free radical production. Current strategies to minimize cardiotoxicity are focused on dose titration and altering treatment regimens to include dexrazoxane and liposomal anthracycline formulations to reduce free radicals.

The toxic effects of heavy alcohol intake on cardiomyocytes stem from esterification of nonesterified fatty acids resulting in fatty acid ethinyl esters that collect in the mitochondria, altering energy utilization.[32] Alcohol ingestion stimulates catecholamine release, which raises blood pressure and heart rate, while also causing a negative inotropic effect. Alcoholic cardiomyopathy accounts for up to one-third of nonischemic cardiomyopathy cases in the Western world and 4-year mortality is nearly 50% if abstinence is not practiced.

Women suffer an increased burden of cardiomyopathy and heart failure from equivalent doses of alcohol compared to men.[33] In contrast to chronic heavy ingestion, light to moderate alcohol consumption has recently been associated with protection from all-cause and vascular mortality, peripheral arterial disease, ischemic stroke, heart failure, and recurrent ischemic events. However, the definition of "light-to-moderate" alcohol consumption is different for men and women. In otherwise healthy individuals, safe alcohol drinking is defined as 2 standard drinks per day for men and 1 standard drink per day for nonpregnant women. In addition, the benefits of safe alcohol consumption on heart disease and heart failure appear to exceed the risk of cancer, and daily light-to-moderate drinking appears to have greater benefit than drinking heavier on 1 to 2 nights per week. The patients with preexisting heart failure and/or cardiomyopathy from other causes, or with other significant comorbid conditions that increase their risk of heart failure, are cautioned to avoid alcohol consumption.

Pregnancy and peripartum cardiomyopathy can cause distinct risks to women's cardiac health. Unique hemodynamic alterations are associated with pregnancy, which begin in the first trimester, peak, and then remain constant during the second trimester until delivery.[34] Cardiovascular changes include up to a 50% increase in cardiac output. Water and sodium are retained, which result in increases in blood volume and decreases in both systemic blood pressure and systemic vascular resistance. The maternal heart rate may increase by up to 15 beats per minute compared to prepregnancy baseline. Certainly, women with a diagnosis of heart failure from any cause carry increased risk during pregnancy, as the hemodynamic changes caused by pregnancy may result in cardiac decompensation.

Although rare, peripartum cardiomyopathy can be deadly. It occurs in approximately 1 in every 4000 live births in the United States.[35] It is defined as clinical heart failure and cardiac decompensation most often occurring in the last month of pregnancy and up to 5 months after birth.[35,36] As previously noted, cardiovascular alterations associated with normal pregnancy may result in symptoms and signs similar to that of heart failure (eg, fatigue, dyspnea, edema), diagnostic acumen is critical with imaging techniques such as echocardiogram or cardiac MRI. Use of computed tomography scans or nuclear medicine-based imaging, with their associated radiation exposure, should in

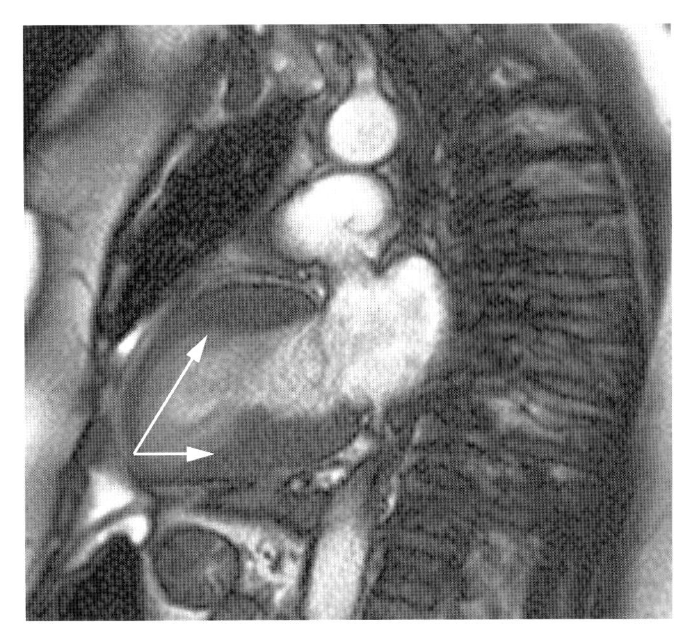

FIGURE 8-2 Cardiac MRI of woman who presented with chest pain, fatigue, and dyspnea with findings of apical ballooning of the left ventricle (arrows); overall LVEF 42%. No myocardial infarct scar or infiltrate and marked edema of mid and apical segments is visible on T2 imaging. This pattern along with apical ballooning and absence of scar is typical for takotsubo cardiomyopathy.

general be avoided in pregnant women. Other causes of cardiomyopathy must be ruled out prior to diagnosis of peripartum cardiomyopathy. Over 70% of cases are diagnosed postpartum, usually in the first month, and about 45% of initial presentations occur within the first week after delivery. Some pregnant patients may initially present with heart failure but also in the setting of other known risk factors (eg, diabetes), which can make differentiating between peripartum cardiomyopathy and cardiomyopathy from other causes difficult. In such a case (first presentation of a pregnant women with known diabetes in acute heart failure) more than one etiology may exist. Risk factors for peripartum cardiomyopathy are numerous: multiparity, multiple gestations, pregnancy-induced hypertension or pre-eclampsia, prolonged tocolytic use, obesity, maternal age >30 years, non-Caucasian ethnicity, and prepregnancy systemic hypertension.[35,37] Predictors of major adverse events are lower ejection fraction (≤25%) and non-Caucasian race along with delay in diagnosis.[38] Similar to other cardiomyopathies, no clear description of the pathophysiology of peripartum cardiomyopathy has yet to be widely accepted; however, several factors have been identified with a possible role including latent viral antigens, immune system–activated cytokine release, increased adrenergic tone, preceding myocarditis, abnormal hormonal balance, high prolactin levels, and genetic inheritance.[37]

Patients with peripartum cardiomyopathy are treated with standard heart failure therapies, including diuresis in the setting of volume overload and β-blockade. Due to the risk of potential fetal birth defects, angiotensin-converting enzyme (ACE) inhibitors and angiotensin receptor blockers (ARBs) are contraindicated during pregnancy and carry a Food and Drug Administration label of Pregnancy Category D due to adverse fetal risk. Overall, peripartum cardiomyopathy carries a better prognosis than other forms of cardiomyopathy, with approximately half of patients recovering left ventricular systolic function within 6 months of initial presentation.[39] Unfortunately, one-fifth of peripartum cardiomyopathy patients will experience progressive heart failure, requiring advanced heart failure therapies such as cardiac transplantation or ventricular assist devices, or need a palliative approach.

For those patients whose ejection fraction recovers, debate exists as to whether to continue evidence-based heart failure therapies (β-blockers, ACE inhibitors, or ARBs) indefinitely or whether it is possible to stop their use safely; this is a particularly relevant question given the young age of most patients diagnosed with this condition. Again, no large, prospective, randomized, controlled trial has been undertaken to address these treatment and prognostic questions. Regardless, most patients who survive peripartum cardiomyopathy are strongly cautioned against future pregnancies, with evidence suggesting a continued decline in cardiac function with future pregnancies even in those with recovered ejection fraction. Ejection fraction is the most important prognostic indicator in these patients.[39] Newer therapies suggesting benefit in ejection fraction and clinical outcome, such as bromocriptine in a pilot study of severe peripartum cardiomyopathy, will warrant further investigation.[40]

TREATMENT

Until recently, in-hospital outcomes and quality of care in women hospitalized for heart failure were understudied. A recent analysis of over 99,000 inpatient admissions for heart failure at over 200 hospitals participating in the American Heart Association's Get With The Guidelines-Heart Failure Registry examined these issues.[41] Compared to men, women accounted for approximately half of all heart failure admissions and were older on presentation (mean age 74±14 vs 69±14 years). They were more likely to have systemic hypertension and less likely to have coronary artery disease or chronic kidney disease. Similar to other registries,[15] women presented with higher blood pressures (by 7 mmHg) and left ventricular ejection fraction (by about 10%) with the rest of admission symptoms similar to men. Quality of care was similar in many aspects, but gender differences in treatment included lower likelihood of measuring left ventricular function, prescribing anticoagulation for atrial fibrillation, and defibrillator implantation for women during the admission.[41] Similar quality measures were appropriate discharge instructions, smoking cessation counseling, and use of evidence-based therapy (ACE inhibitors, ARBs, β-blockers). In terms of outcome measures, no sex difference was found regarding in-hospital survival, but women had a longer length of stay. Further analysis of the Get With the Guidelines-Heart Failure Registry showed higher implantable cardioverter defibrillator (ICD) use for larger hospitals and those equipped for more advanced care (percutaneous intervention, coronary bypass surgery, and transplant); these facilities also had higher compliance with guidelines.[42]

Quality measures in the outpatient setting were followed in the Registry to Improve the Use of Evidence-Based Heart Failure Therapies in the Outpatient Setting (IMPROVE HF).[43] This was a prospective cohort study in chronic heart failure with LVEF ≤35%, N = 15,381 and, consistent with inpatient registries, men were younger than women (age 70 vs 72 years, p <0.001). Seven measures of care were reported (Figure 8-3A) and significant gender-based differences were noted for lower use of anticoagulation for atrial fibrillation, device therapy (ICD and cardiac resynchronization therapy [CRT]), and heart failure education in women. Stratification of the measures of care by age and sex found underutilization in older women with the largest differences documented for aldosterone antagonist, CRT, and ICD/CRT-D (cardiac resynchronization therapy combined with defibrillator) in older females (Figure 8-3B). The study concluded the following: (a) women and the elderly were less likely to receive certain guideline-based therapy, (b) women received less heart failure education and device-based therapy in the outpatient setting, and (c) sex was independently associated with differences in the use of anticoagulation for atrial fibrillation, ICD, CRT-D, and heart failure education. Evidence-based therapy has historically been underutilized in women, with some improvement in the past years, but no gender-specific guidelines exist due to the lack of women's representation in studies related to the efficacy of these guidelines. Therefore, guidelines for management of heart failure in women are similar to men[44,45] (Table 8-3).

Gender may also predict differential responses to therapy. In particular, sex hormones are known to regulate β-receptors, which are a key target of heart failure therapy. Unfortunately, women comprise only one-fifth of enrollment in the major β-blocker trials. Analysis of 3 major studies (Cardiac Insufficiency Bisoprolol Study II [CIBIS II], Carvedilol Prospective Randomized Cumulative Survival Trial [COPERNICUS], and Metoprolol CR/XL Randomized Intervention Trial in Heart Failure [(MERIT-HF]) demonstrated that

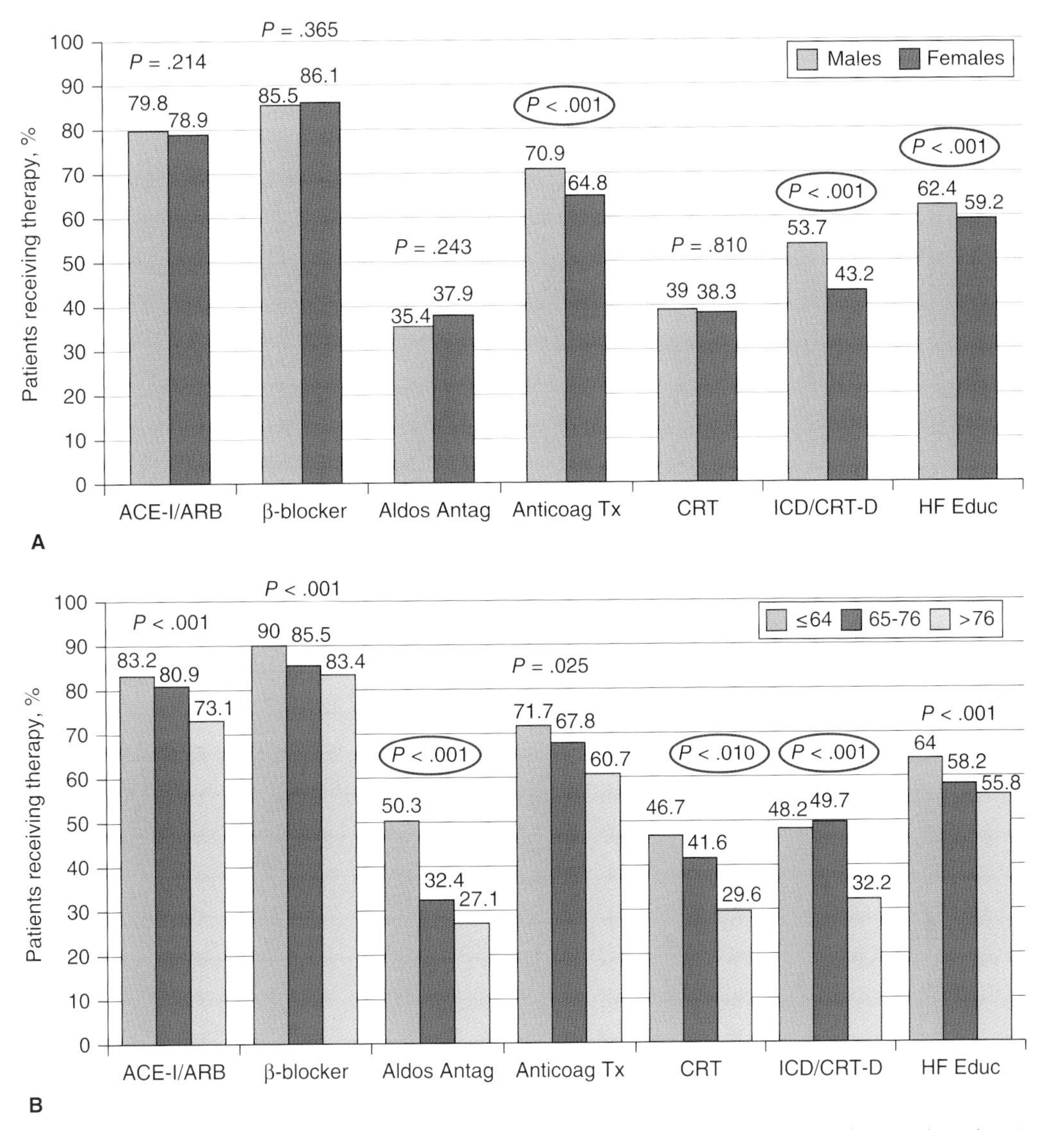

FIGURE 8-3 Heart failure therapies based on gender—results from the IMPROVE HF study, a prospective cohort study in chronic heart failure with LVEF ≤35% in outpatient care.[43] (A) Seven care measures were reported and significant gender-based differences were noted for use of anticoagulation for atrial fibrillation, device therapy, and heart failure education (circled). (B) Heart failure therapies in women based on age. Stratification of the care measures by age and sex found underutilization in older women with the largest differences documented for aldosterone antagonist, CRT, and ICD/CRT-D therapy in older females.
CRT, cardiac resynchronization therapy; ICD: implantable cardioverter defibrillator; LVEF, left ventricular ejection fraction.

β-blocker therapy resulted in similar improvements in mortality for both genders.[10] When these trials were analyzed individually, a similar mortality benefit in women was not found. It is only when these studies were combined that a strong need for greater enrollment of women in trials was felt.

ACE inhibitor therapy is another cornerstone of evidence-based heart failure treatment, and again data are limited in regards to gender differences, particularly benefit-risk analysis in women. In 2003, a meta-analysis of the 12 largest randomized clinical trials of ACE inhibitors and β-blockers showed that women with symptomatic left ventricular dysfunction likely benefit from ACE inhibitor therapy, but asymptomatic women with left ventricular dysfunction may not receive mortality benefit.[46] A proposed mechanism relates to the loss of estrogen after menopause: estrogen provides cardio-protection by inhibiting the renin-angiotensin-aldosterone system.

Aldosterone antagonists are one of the more recent class of medications that provide proven benefit in the overall heart failure patient population; however, the specific benefits in women are not entirely clear. Two major studies examining the benefit of aldosterone antagonism, the Eplerenone Post-myocardial infarction Heart failure Efficacy and Survival Study (EPHESUS) and the Randomized ALdactone Evaluation Study (RALES), enrolled only 25% to 30% women.[47,48] These studies showed equal gender benefit with this therapy.

Prior to current evidence-based therapy, digoxin was the mainstay of heart failure treatment. In 1997, the Digitalis Investigation Group reported that digoxin reduced hospitalizations but did not decrease overall mortality in heart failure patients with reduced left ventricular systolic function.[49] Gender differences were not analyzed in the initial report. In 2002, a post hoc subgroup analysis was performed to examine possible sex-based differences in the 6800 patients that were involved in the initial study.[50] An increased mortality was found in women despite a smaller reduction in rehospitalization rates. This analysis introduced a significant finding, which provided an early indication of basing treatment decisions for heart failure on gender.

Device therapy is another critical component of heart failure treatment for primary prevention in both ischemic and nonischemic cardiomyopathy patients with left ventricular ejection fraction below 30% to 35%.[51] Less than 50% of all eligible patients have an ICD placed and women are even less likely than men to receive such therapy, although there appears to be no gender difference in the survival benefit provided by ICD therapy.[41]

In 2005, the CArdiac REsynchronization-Heart Failure (CARE-HF) demonstrated the benefit of cardiac resynchronization, or biventricular pacing, in New York Heart Association (NYHA) Class III and ambulatory Class IV heart failure patients with left ventricular dysfunction and cardiac dyssynchrony.[52] CRT was shown to improve symptoms and quality of life and also reduce risk of death beyond the benefits of evidence-based medical therapy. Gender utilization of CRT from the Healthcare Cost and Utilization Project database revealed the overall number of CRT device implantations, either with or without an ICD, was significantly lower for women compared to men every year over a 3-year period with significantly larger difference occurring in CRT-D patients (those with combined biventricular pacing and defibrillator therapy who are by definition at a more advanced stage of heart failure).[53]

More recent trial data emphasize the gender difference in response to CRT and the need to improve use of device therapy in qualifying patients. The Multicenter Automatic Defibrillator Implantation Trial with Cardiac Resynchronization Therapy (MADIT-CRT) studied the role of CRT in milder heart failure symptoms or NYHA Class I, II ischemic and NYHA Class II nonischemic patients, who had LVEF $\leq$30%, QRS $\geq$130 ms; patients were randomized to ICD versus CRT-D.[54] The primary endpoint of all-cause mortality or nonfatal heart failure event was significantly reduced in the CRT-D group by 34% (HR 0.66 [0.52-0.84], $p = 0.001$). Gender differences in CRT benefit were suggested in the earlier MIRACLE trials and confirmed with MADIT-CRT (Figure 8-4). Factors associated with reverse remodeling after biventricular pacing in MADIT-CRT that can be used to predict clinical response to the such therapy are: female gender, nonischemic etiology, left bundle branch block (LBBB), QRS

TABLE 8-3 Under-representation of women in heart failure clinical trials

Inadequate participation for women in many landmark trials

- *DIG, Consensus, SAVE, TRACE, US Carvedilol, MERIT-HF, CIBIS II* (18% to 32% women)
- *CARE-HF, MADIT CRT, REVERSE, MADIT II, SCD-HeFT* (≤25% enrollment for women)

ACC/AHA heart failure guidelines: *Class I* recommendation to *all* patients qualifying for a specific heart failure therapy[44]

- Treat specific populations similar to broader population, in absence of evidence directing otherwise
- Including women and elderly, even if underrepresented in clinical trials
- Recognize that older patients may not metabolize or tolerate medications as well

The underrepresentation of women in heart failure clinical trials is possibly due to selection bias, age, or declined participation. Many women have diastolic heart failure and preserved ejection fraction, which would exclude them from studies of systolic dysfunction. These include Class I indications for β-blocker and ACE inhibitor use for women after an MI or LV dysfunction, whether symptomatic or asymptomatic, and ARB in those who are ACE intolerant with these indications. ACE inhibitors are also recommended in women with diabetes mellitus. Aldosterone blockade is recommended in women with symptomatic heart failure, LVEF <40%, and no significant renal dysfunction or hyperkalemia.

Abbreviations: ACC/AHA, American College of Cardiology/American Heart Association; ACE, angiotensin-converting enzyme inhibitor; LV, left ventricular; LVEF, left ventricular ejection fraction; MI, myocardial infarction.

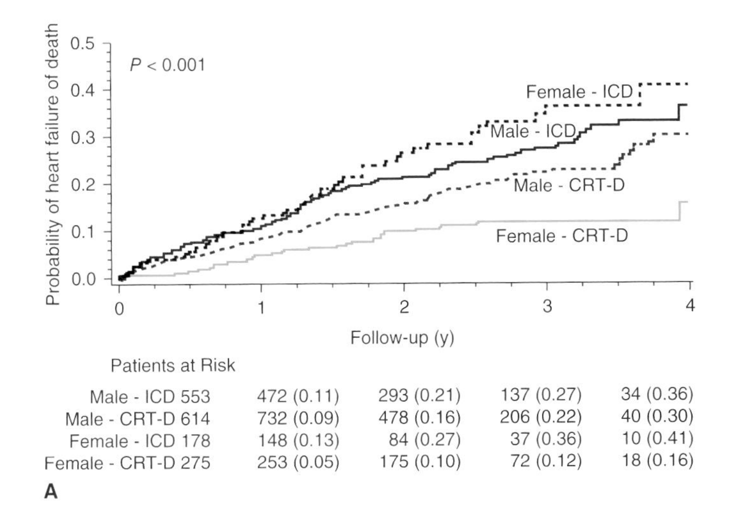

Baseline characteristics by gender in MADIT-CRT

Women
- More likely to have nonischemic etiology
- Greater number of LBBB
- Baseline use of β-blocker

Men
- More likely to have ischemic etiology (history of revascularization)
- Atrial fibrillation present
- Greater number of RBBB
- Chronic kidney disease with creatinine ≥1.4 mg/dL

*All variables with $P < 0.01$ when comparing genders.

B

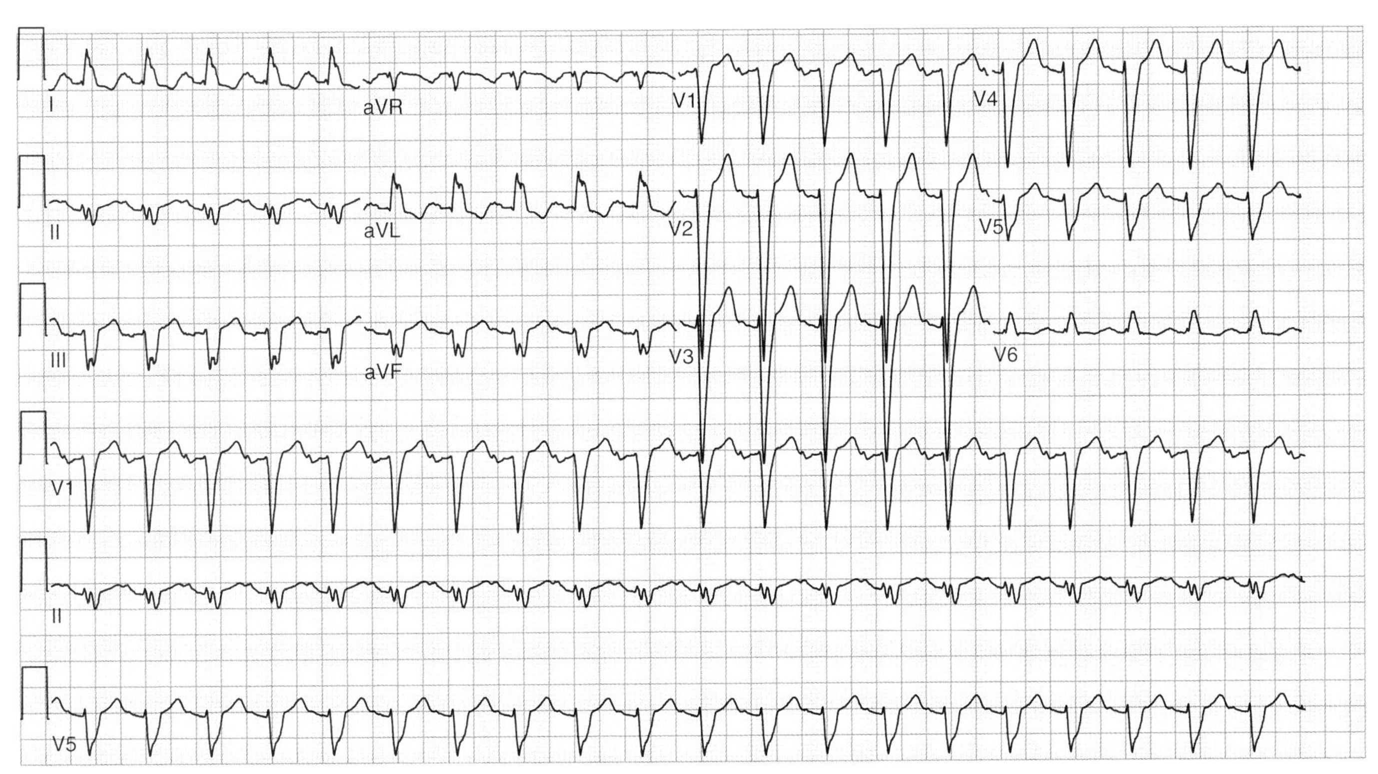

ECG from Ohio State University noninvasive laboratory.

C

FIGURE 8-4 Recent CRT trials have evaluated expanding indications for biventricular pacing to the milder heart failure population. Gender differences in CRT benefit were suggested in the MIRACLE trials and confirmed with MADIT-CRT.[55] A, Women assigned to CRT-D had the lowest risk of death or a heart failure event, whichever came first. A greater reduction in all-cause mortality was noted for women, which was substantially larger if women had LBBB or QRS >150 ms. B, Explanations for the gender differences with CRT benefit are likely related to the baseline differences in etiology and presence of dyssynchrony. Significantly more women had a nonischemic etiology and wider QRS or presence of LBBB, both markers of CRT response. Men were more likely to be ischemic and have RBBB, which are both markers of nonresponse. Atrial fibrillation and chronic kidney disease are also poor prognostic indicators. C, Example of LBBB in a patient with cardiomyopathy.

Abbreviations: CRT, cardiac resynchronization therapy; CRT-D, cardiac resynchronization therapy combined with defibrillator; LBBB, left bundle branch block; RBBB, right bundle branch block.

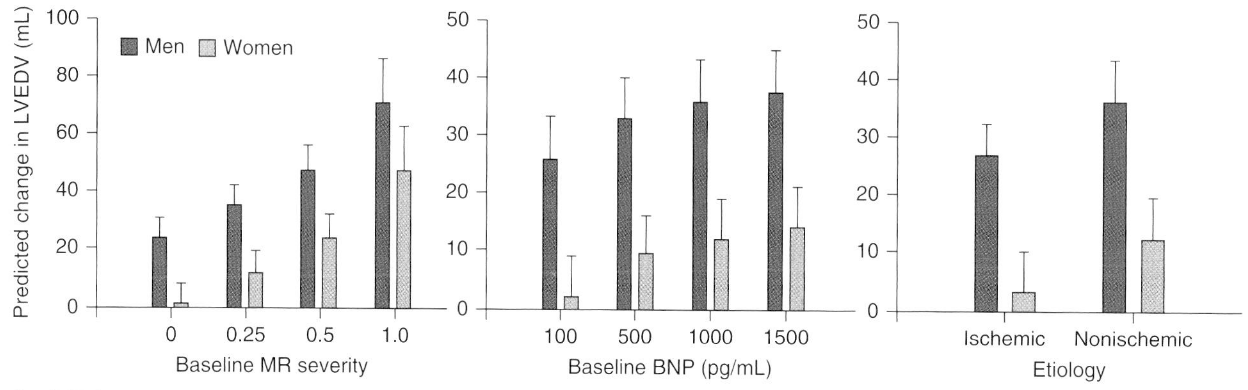

FIGURE 8-5 Gender differences in remodeling from the MIRACLE trials.[56] Men (red) showed more prominent LV remodeling across increasing levels of BNP and mitral regurgitation and regardless of etiology when compared to women (blue).

duration on ECG >150 ms, prior hospitalization for heart failure, left ventricular end-diastolic volume >124 mL/m^2, and left atrial volume <40 mL/m^2. Women had a greater reduction in all-cause mortality, which was substantially larger if women had LBBB or QRS >150 ms.[55] Women are more often diagnosed with nonischemic cardiomyopathy and LBBB compared to men, suggesting CRT-D should be utilized more aggressively in women and, at the very least, should be used at the same rate as in men.

Gender differences in remodeling or worsening of LV function seem to play a role in development of heart failure, as indicated from the MIRACLE trials. Compared to women, men showed more prominent LV remodeling regardless of etiology and across increasing levels of BNP and mitral regurgitation.[56] (Figure 8-5). Possible explanations include the following: (a) gender-specific remodeling response, such as concentric remodeling in women versus dilation in men, (b) protective effect of estrogen and/or an adverse effect of testosterone, (c) smaller body size in women results in higher effective dose of evidence-based therapy, and (d) gender difference in compensatory mechanisms, for example, aldosterone release.

ADVANCED HEART FAILURE THERAPIES

For patients with end-stage heart failure not responding to the aforementioned medical and device therapies, that is, NYHA Class IV or American College of Cardiology/American Heart Association (ACC/AHA) Stage D heart failure, advanced therapies including cardiac transplantation and ventricular assist devices (VADs) provide options for improved mortality, morbidity, quality of life, and functional status.

The 2012 Registry of the International Society for Heart and Lung Transplantation (ISHLT) included data on gender differences for the patients undergoing cardiac transplantation. Between 2006 and 2011, only 23.7%, nearly a quarter, of patients receiving a heart transplant were women, which is trending up in recent years; survival rates were similar between genders[57] (Table 8-4). Multiple explanations

TABLE 8-4 Data published by the international society for heart and lung transplantation (ISHLT) registry[57]

Characteristics and Outcomes of Women After Heart Transplantation
Factors affecting 1-year mortality rate in women vs men
• Parous women are more likely to be allosensitized
• Elevated panel reactive antibodies
• Higher risk of antibody-mediated rejection
Postpartum etiology of heart failure as indication for transplantation
• Worse outcomes
• Younger, higher allosensitization, more rejection within first year, higher pretransplant acuity

for this low rate of transplantation for women have surfaced. One obstacle lies in higher levels of reactive antibodies in women who have given birth, which contributes to a lower likelihood of finding an appropriately matched donor. Smaller body size of women may also lead to more difficulty in matching donors. Additionally, an earlier single-center study concluded that women are less likely to agree to cardiac transplant compared to men (self-refusal by 29% vs 9% patients).[58]

Another limiting factor when listing appropriate patients for cardiac transplant is the use of peak oxygen uptake (VO_2) obtained from cardiopulmonary exercise stress testing. Traditional studies have determined that a peak $VO_2 \leq 14$ mL/kg/min signifies worsening prognosis, and this value is used as a criteria to determine transplant eligibility. Baseline VO_2 values vary between genders with women having lower mean values.[59,60] Women also have improved survival rates at all levels of exercise capacity.[59] Several factors used to calculate VO_2 contribute to this phenomenon, including lower baseline metabolic rate, lower hemoglobin, higher average age at time of transplant evaluation (women present with heart failure in general at an older age), and different levels of muscle mass in women compared to men. Due to these differences, the ISHLT has recommended using a different and more accurate measure in evaluating women for cardiac transplantation: predicted peak VO_2 percentage. A value of 50% or less is now considered a prognostic marker when evaluating for cardiac transplant candidacy. Again, further study is needed to best determine gender differences in prognostic markers and best treatment approaches for women with end-stage heart failure.

For end-stage heart failure patients waiting for cardiac transplant and those who are ineligible for transplant, VAD is a developing therapy providing survival and clinical benefit—benefiting survival by nearly a factor of 4[61] (Figure 8-6). Initially, women were poorly enrolled at a rate of >20% in the first-generation VAD trials due to the large size of these pulsatile-flow devices. Observational data showed that women had poorer survival than men on VAD and a lower rate of successful bridging to transplantation, both at least partly explained by the fact that women were also found to present in a more advanced or critically ill stage of heart failure.[62] VAD technology continues to improve through the years with second-generation devices offering smaller sizes with continuous-flow mechanisms.[63] Survival rates in women increased from the previous generation models to equal those of men (73% survival at 18 months for both genders, $p = 0.855$), but less than one-fourth of end-stage heart failure patients receiving these newer devices were women. Again, fewer women proceeded to transplant compared to men (40% and 55%, respectively), likely due to previously mentioned differences in evaluation and eligibility for cardiac transplant (Figure 8-7). Adverse event rates were similar, except for hemorrhagic stroke, which occurred more frequently in women, an observation that matched the registry data revealing female sex was associated with shorter time to first neurologic event.[64] These 2 studies differ in infection rates, with men more likely to develop device-related infections in one[63] compared to no gender difference in time to first infection in the other.[64] Quality-of-life scores and functional capacity at 6 months post-LVAD implantation were significantly improved in both genders. Table 8-5 lists a few gender differences from the most recent INTERMACS (interagency registry for mechanically assisted circulatory support

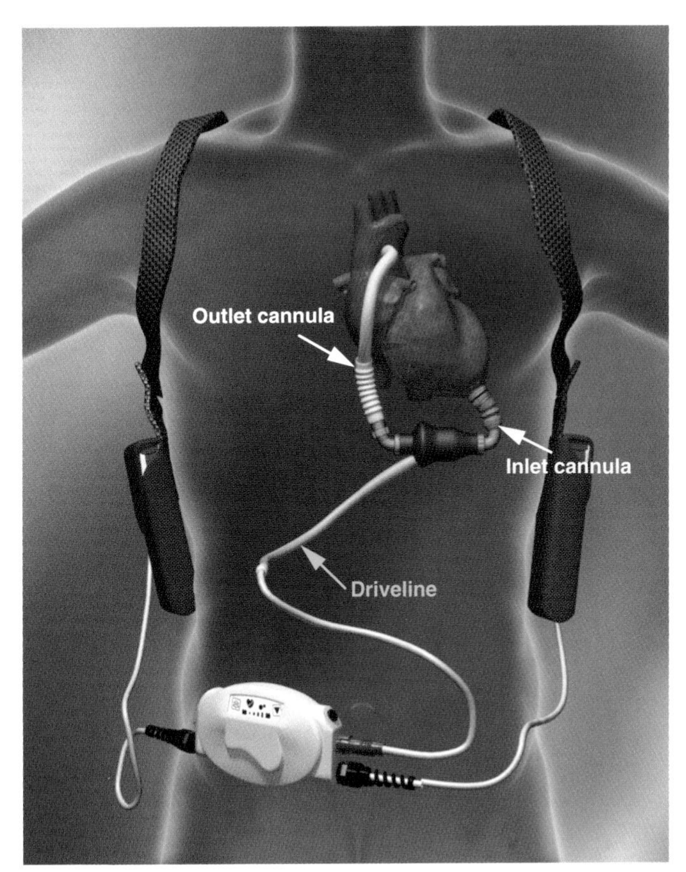

a

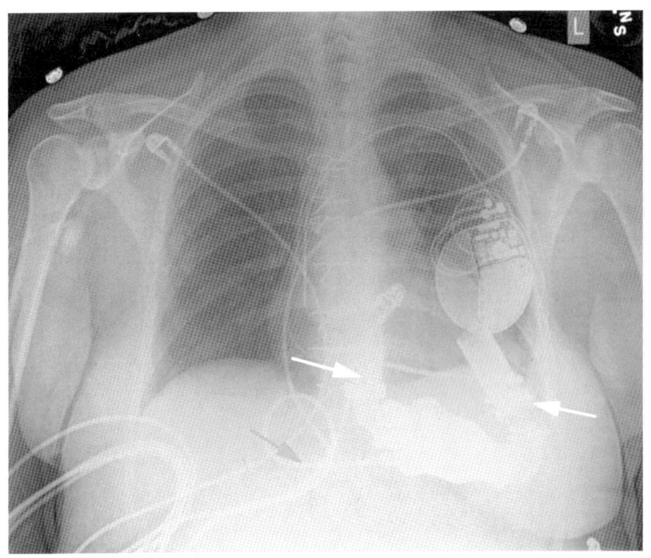

Chest x-ray obtained from Ohio State University Wexner Medical Center.

b

FIGURE 8-6 Example of Heartmate II ventricular assist device components (A) and implanted device in a woman with end-stage heart failure (B). The inlet cannula (yellow arrow) is implanted in the left ventricular apex, connected to the rotary pump. The outlet cannula (white arrow) is placed in the ascending aorta. The controller and batteries provide power to the device through the driveline (green arrow), which exits the skin to connect to the controller.

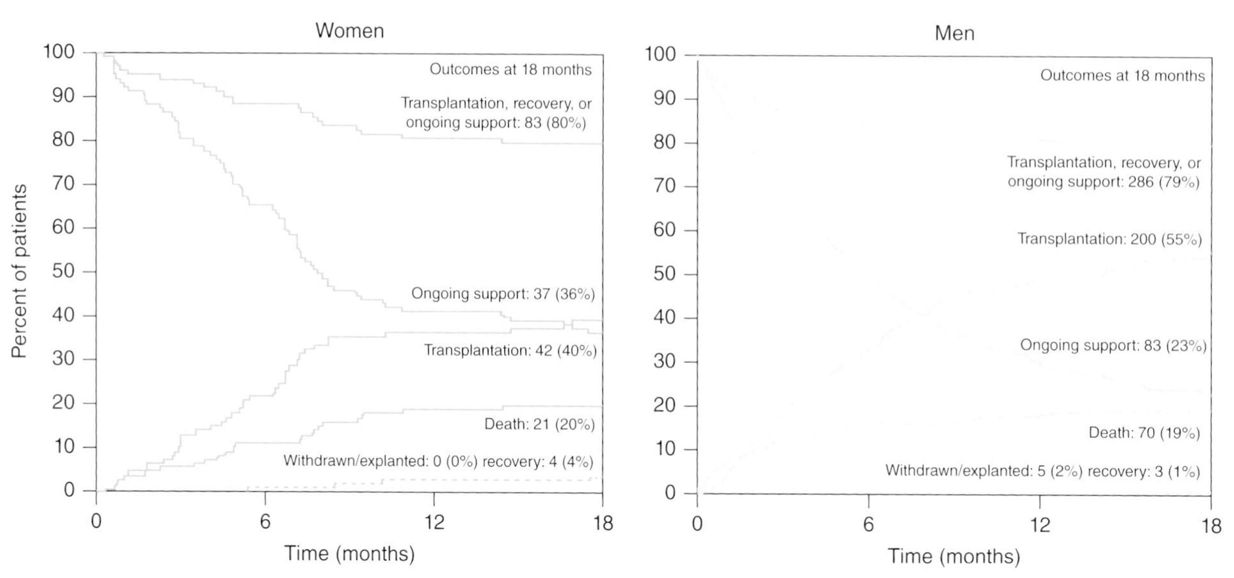

FIGURE 8-7 In the Heartmate II bridge to transplantation trials, more men than women were transplanted, therefore resulting in a larger percentage of women who remained on long-term ventricular assist device support compared to men.[63] These data are consistent with the ISHLT database in which 76% of heart transplant recipients from 2006 to 2011 were men.[57] Lower transplant rates in women may be partly related to higher sensitization or levels of panel-reactive antibodies in parous women, which limits the possibility of suitable donors and leads to higher rates of antibody-mediated rejection. Smaller BSA, a greater number of women than men with BSA <1.5 m^2, and lower referral rates in women also contribute to lower transplantation rates.
Abbreviations: BSA, body surface area; ISHLT, International Society for Heart and Lung Transplantation.

registry) database report.[64] As LVAD technology improves, both genders will receive survival and quality-of-life benefit, yet more women should be evaluated for candidacy and offered LVAD therapy.

CONCLUSION

Heart failure is a complex clinical syndrome and becoming a large burden on our society with increasing prevalence, incidence, expense, and readmission rates—it is now the leading cause of inpatient admissions. Women account for half the heart failure cases but have been underrepresented in clinical trials, with more recent studies indicating gender differences in etiology of heart failure, morbidity, and response to remodeling triggers. Gender differences in response to medical therapy have no strong basis due to limited data on this subject. Utilization of evidence-based medical therapy has improved through more recent years and lessened the gender gap that existed, but we are now dealing with a substantial gender gap in utilization of defibrillator and cardiac resynchronization therapy along with advanced therapies such as cardiac transplantation and ventricular assist devices. Recent data indicate women have a better response rate to biventricular pacing related to a higher likelihood of nonischemic cardiomyopathy and presence of significant dyssynchrony, yet such therapy remains underutilized in them. More men undergo cardiac transplantation and ventricular assist device therapy, which is multifactorial and nonetheless a discrepancy in therapy. Future focus on underlying gender differences in mechanisms of heart failure development, clinical course and response to medical and device therapy, and methods to improve utilization of advanced therapies is a necessity to tailor therapy based on sex-related differences and further impact heart failure outcomes.

TABLE 8-5 Gender differences in utilization of mechanical circulatory support in advanced heart failure patients

Characteristics of Women vs Men Receiving VAD
Younger (50.9 y vs 54.1 y)
Smaller BSA (1.91 vs 2.14 m^2, p <0.0001)
Fewer women are Caucasian (59% vs 71%)
More likely to have urgent implant
INTERMACS level 1, defined as cardiogenic shock (26% vs 19%, p = 0.01)
No difference in use of VAD as bridge to transplant
Similar preimplant hemodynamics, IABP, inotrope use, ventilator
Similar use of ICD

Data was collected from baseline characteristics of patients prospectively enrolled in the INTERMACS registry between June 23, 2006, and March 31, 2010 (N = 1936 implants at 89 sites, including 401 women or 21% of total enrollment).[64] The implanted devices consisted primarily of continuous flow support devices.
Abbreviations: BSA, body surface area; IABP, intra-aortic balloon pump; ICD, implantable cardiac defibrillator; INTERMACS, interagency registry for mechanically assisted circulatory support; VAD, ventricular assist device.

REFERENCES

1. Koelling TM, Chen RS, Lubwama RN, et al. The expanding national burden of heart failure in the United States: the influence of heart failure in women. *Am Heart J.* 2004;147(1):74-78.
2. Roger VL, Go AS, Lloyd-Jones DM, et al. Heart disease and stroke statistics—2012 update: a report from the American Heart Association. *Circulation.* 2012;125:188-197.
3. Rathore SS, Foody JM, Wang Y, et al. Race, quality of care, and outcomes of elderly patients hospitalized with heart failure. *JAMA.* 2003;289(19):2517-2524.
4. Heiat A, Gross CP, Krumholz HM. Representation of the elderly, women, and minorities in heart failure clinical trials. *Arch Intern Med.* 2002;162(15):1682-1688.
5. Schirmer S, Hohl M, Böhm M. Gender differences in heart failure: paving the way towards personalized medicine? *Eur Heart J.* 2010;31:1165-1167.
6. Heidecker B, Lamirault G, Kasper E, et al. The gene expression profile of patients with new-onset heart failure reveals important gender-specific differences. *Eur Heart J.* 2010;31:1188-1196.
7. Ginghina C, Botezatu CD, Serban M, et al. A personalized medicine target: heart failure in women. *J Med Life.* 2011;15;4(3):280-286.
8. Braunstein JB, Anderson GF, Gerstenblith G, et al. Noncardiac comorbidity increases preventable hospitalizations and mortality among Medicare beneficiaries with chronic heart failure. *J Am Coll Cardiol.* 2003;42:1226-1233.
9. Ghali JK, Krause-Steinrauf HJ, Adams KF, et al. Gender differences in advanced heart failure: insights from the BEST study. *J Am Coll Cardiol.* 2003;42(12):2128-2134.
10. Shin JJ, Hamad E, Murthy S, et al. Heart failure in women. *Clin Cardiol.* 2012 March;35(3):172-177.
11. Adams KF, Jr, Fonarow GC, Emerman CL, et al. Characteristics and outcomes of patients hospitalized for heart failure in the United States: rationale, design, and preliminary observations from the first 100,000 cases in the Acute Decompensated Heart Failure National Registry (ADHERE). *Am Heart J.* 2005;149(2):209-216.
12. Zhang P, Engelgau MM,Valdez R, et al. Costs of screening for prediabetes among US adults: a comparison of different screening strategies. *Diabetes Care.* 2003;26(9):2536-2542.
13. Meta-analysis Global Group in Chronic Heart Failure (MAGGIC). The survival of patients with heart failure with preserved or reduced left ventricular ejection fraction: an individual patient data meta-analysis. *Eur Heart J.* 2012;33(14):1750-1757.
14. Deswal A, Bozkurt B. Comparison of morbidity in women versus men with heart failure and preserved ejection fraction. *Am J Cardiol.* 2006;97:1228-1231.
15. Galvao M, Kalman J, DeMarco T, et al. Gender differences in in-hospital management and outcomes in patients with decompensated heart failure: analysis from the Acute Decompensated Heart Failure National Registry (ADHERE). *J Card Fail.* 2006;12:100-107.
16. Gottlieb SS, Khatta M, Friedmann E, et al. The influence of age, gender, and race on the prevalence of depression in heart failure patients. *J Am Coll Cardiol.* 2004;43(9):1542-1549.
17. Nieminen MS, Harjola VP, Hochadel M, et al. Gender related differences in patients presenting with acute heart failure. Results from EuroHeart Failure Survey II. *Eur J Heart Fail.* 2008;10:140-148.
18. Eaton CB, Abdulbaki AM, Margolis KL, et al. Racial and ethnic differences in incident hospitalized heart failure in postmenopausal women: The Women's Health Initiative. *Circulation.* 2012;126(6):688-696.
19. Olivia RV, Bakris GL. Management of hypertension in the elderly population. *J Gerontol A Biol Sci Med Sci.* 2012;67:1343-1351.
20. Iribarren C, Karter AJ, Go AS, et al. Glycemic control and heart failure among adult patients with diabetes. *Circulation.* 2001;103:2668-2673.
21. Kenchaiah S, Evans JC, Levy D, et al. Obesity and the risk of heart failure. *N Engl J Med.* 2002;347(5):305-313.
22. Artham SM, Lavie CJ, Patel HM. Impact of obesity on the risk of heart failure and its prognosis. *J Cardiometab Syndr.* 2008;3(3):155-161.
23. Clark AL, Chyu J, Horwich TB, et al. The obesity paradox in men versus women with systolic heart failure. *Am J Cardiol.* 2012;110(1):77-82.
24. Redberg R, Schiller N. Gender and valvular surgery. *J Thorac Cardiovasc Surg.* 2004;127(1):1-3.
25. Trail TA. Valvular heart disease and pregnancy. *Cardiol Clin.* 2012;30:369-381.
26. Dunlay SM, Roger VL. Gender differences in the pathophysiology, clinical presentation, and outcomes of ischemic heart failure. *Curr Heart Fail Rep.* 2012;9:267-276.
27. Pepine CJ, Anderson RD, Sharaf BL, et al. Coronary microvascular reactivity to adenosine predicts adverse outcome in women evaluated for suspected ischemia results from the National Heart, Lung and Blood Institute WISE (Women's Ischemia Syndrome Evaluation) study. *J Am Coll Cardiol.* 2010;55(25):2825-2832.
28. Neil CJ, Nguyen TH, Sverdlov AL, et al. Can we make sense of takotsubo cardiomyopathy? An update on pathogenesis, diagnosis, and natural history. *Expert Rev Cardivasc Ther.* 2012;10(2):215-221.
29. Zygulska AL, Krzemieniecki K. Cardiological adverse events after oncological treatment in women. *Przegl Lek.* 2012;69(2):87-89.
30. Ng B, Better N, Green MD. Anticancer agents and cardiotoxicity. *Sem in Onc.* 2006;33:2-14.
31. Gennari A, D'Amico M. Anthracyclines in the management of metastatic breast cancer: state of the art. *Eur J Cancer Supplements.* 2011;9:11-15.
32. Skotzko CE, Vrinceanu A, Krueger L, et al. Alcohol use and congestive heart failure: incidence, importance and approaches to history taking. *Heart Fail Rev.* 2009:14:51-55.
33. Di Minno MN, Franchini M, Russolillo A, et al. Alcohol dosing and the heart: updating clinical evidence. *Semin Thromb Hemost.* 2011;37(8):875-884.
34. Ouzounian J, Elkayam U. Physiologic changes during normal pregnancy and delivery. *Cardiol Clin.* 2012;30(3):317-329.
35. Elkayam U, Jalnapurkar S, Barakat M. Peripartum cardiomyopathy. *Cardiol Clin.* 2012;30(3):435-440.

36. Pearson GD, Veille JC, Rahimtoola S, et al. Peripartum cardiomyopathy: National Heart, Lung, and Blood Institute and Office of Rare Diseases (National Institutes of Health) workshop recommendations and review. *JAMA.* 2000;283(9):1183-1188.

37. Ntusi NB, Mayosi BM. Aetiology and risk factors of peripartum cardiomyopathy: a systematic review. *Int J Cardiol.* 2009;131:168-179.

38. Goland S, Modi K, Bitar F, et al. Clinical profile and predictors of complications in peripartum cardiomyopathy. *J Card Fail.* 2009;15(8):645-650.

39. Abboud J, Murad Y, Chen-Scarabelli C, et al. Peripartum cardiomyopathy: a comprehensive review. *Int J Cardiol.* 2007;118:295-303.

40. Sliwa K, Blauwet L, Tibazarwa K, et al. Evaluation of bromocriptine in the treatment of acute severe peripartum cardiomyopathy: a proof-of-concept pilot study. *Circulation.* 2010;121(13): 1465-1473.

41. Klein L, Grau-Sepulveda MV, Bonow RO, et al. Quality of care and outcomes in women hospitalized for heart failure. *Circ Heart Fail.* 2011;4:589-598.

42. Shah B, Hernandez AF, Liang L, et al. Hospital variation and characteristics of implantable cardioverter-defibrillator use in patients with heart failure: data from the GWTG-HF (Get With the Guidelines-Heart Failure) registry. *J Am Coll Cardiol.* 2009;53(5):416-422.

43. Yancy CW, Fonarow GC, Albert NM, et al. Influence of patient age and sex on delivery of guideline-recommended heart failure care in the outpatient cardiology practice setting: findings from IMPROVE HF. *Am Heart J.* 2009:157(4):754-762.

44. Jessup M, Abraham WT, Casey DE, et al. ACCF/AHA guidelines for the diagnosis and management of heart failure in adults. *J Am Coll Cardiol.* 2009;53(15):e1-e90.

45. Mosca L, Banka CL, Benjamin EJ, et al. Evidence-based guidelines for cardiovascular disease prevention in women: 2007 update. *Circulation.* 2007;115(11):1481-1501.

46. Shekelle PG, Rich MW, Morton SC, et al. Efficacy of angiotensin converting enzyme inhibitors and beta-blockers in the management of left ventricular systolic dysfunction according to race, gender, and diabetic status: a meta-analysis of major clinical trials. *J Am Coll Cardiol.* 2003;41(9):1529-1538.

47. Pitt B, Zannad F, Remme WJ, et al. The effect of spironolactone on morbidity and mortality in patients with severe heart failure. Randomized Aldactone Evaluation Study Investigators. *N Engl J Med.* 1999;341(10):709-717.

48. Pitt B, Williams G, Remme W, et al. The EPHESUS trial: eplerenone in patients with heart failure due to systolic dysfunction complicating acute myocardial infarction. Eplerenone Post-AMI Heart Failure Efficacy and Survival Study. *Cardiovasc Drugs Ther.* 2001;15(1):79-87.

49. Garg R, Gorlin R, Smith T, et al. for the Digitalis Investigation Group. The effect of digoxin on mortality and morbidity in patients with heart failure. *N Engl J Med.* 1997;336:525-533.

50. Rathore SS, Wang Y, Krumholz HM. Sex-based differences in the effect of digoxin for the treatment of heart failure. *N Engl J Med.* 2002;347(18):1403-1411.

51. Epstein AE, DiMarco JP, Ellenbogen KA, et al. ACC/AHA/HRS 2008 guidelines for device-based therapy of cardiac rhythm abnormalities: executive summary. *Circulation.* 2008;117(21):2820-2840.

52. Cleland JG, Daubert JC, Erdmann E, et al. The effect of cardiac resynchronization on morbidity and mortality in heart failure. *N Engl J Med.* 2005;352(15):1539-1549.

53. Alaeddini J, Wood MA, Amin MS, et al. Gender disparity in the use of cardiac resynchronization therapy in the United States. *Pacing Clin Electrophysiol.* 2008;31(4):468-472.

54. Goldenberg I, Moss AJ, Hall WJ, et al. Predictors of response to cardiac resynchronization therapy in the Multicenter Automatic Defibrillator Implantation Trial with Cardiac Resynchronization Therapy (MADIT-CRT). *Circulation.* 2011;124(14):1527-1536.

55. Arshad A, Moss AJ, Foster E, et al. Cardiac resynchronization therapy is more effective in women than in men: the MADIT-CRT (Multicenter Automatic Defibrillator Implantation Trial with Cardiac Resynchronization Therapy) Trial. *J Am Coll Cardiol.* 2011;57(7):813-820.

56. Cappola TP, Harsch MR, Jessup M, et al. Predictors of remodeling in the CRT era: influence of mitral regurgitation, BNP, and gender. *J Card Fail.* 2006;12(3):182-188.

57. Stehlik J, Edwards LB, Kucheryavaya AY, et al. The registry of the International Society for Heart and Lung Transplantation: 29th official adult heart transplant report—2012. *J Heart Lung Transplant.* 2012;31(10):1052-1064.

58. Aaronson KD, Schwartz JS, Goin JE. Sex differences in patient acceptance of cardiac transplant candidacy. *Circulation.* 1995;91(11):2753-2761.

59. Elmariah S, Goldberg LR, Allen MT, et al. Effects of gender on peak oxygen consumption and the timing of cardiac transplantation. *J Am Coll Cardiol.* 2006;47(11):2237-2242.

60. Pina IL, Kokkinos P, Kao A, et al. Baseline differences in the HF-ACTION trial by sex. *Am Heart J.* 2009;158(4 suppl):S16-S23.

61. Kilic A, Ailawadi G. Left ventricular assist devices in heart failure. *Expert Rev Cardiovasc Ther.* 2012;10(5):649-656.

62. Morgan JA, Weinberg AD, Hollingsworth KW, et al. Effect of gender on bridging to transplantation and posttransplantation survival in patients with left ventricular assist devices. *J Thorac Cardiovasc Surg.* 2004;127(4):1193-1195.

63. Bogaev RC, Pamboukian SV, Moore SA, et al. Comparison of outcomes in women versus men using a continuous-flow left ventricular assist device as a bridge to transplantation. *J Heart Lung Transplant.* 2011;30(5):515-522.

64. Hsich EM, Naftel DC, Myers SL, et al. Should women receive left ventricular assist device support?: findings from INTERMACS. *Circ Heart Fail.* 2012;5(2):234-240.

9 ARRHYTHMIAS IN WOMEN

Lana Alghothani, MD
Molly Sachdev, MD, MPH

BRADYARRHYTHMIAS

Bradyarrhythmias occur when the heart rate is <60 beats per minute (bpm); can be physiologic, such as in young individuals and in well-trained athletes, or pathologic and symptomatic. Typically, symptoms occur when the heart rate is <40 beats per minute.

DIAGNOSIS

Location of Disease	Name of Disorder	ECG Findings
SA nodal disease	Sinus pause	Transient absence of sinus P wave
AV nodal disease	First-degree AV block	Prolonged PR interval (>200 ms)
	Mobitz Type I second-degree AV block (Wenckebach phenomenon)	PR interval prolongs until a nonconducted P wave is seen; (Figure 9-1)
	Third-degree (complete) block with narrow escape rhythm	P's and QRS's are dissociated; QRS complexes are narrow (Figure 9-2)
Infranodal disease	Mobitz Type II second-degree AV block	PR interval constant and see intermittent nonconducted P waves
	Third-degree (complete) block with wide escape rhythm	P's and QRS's are dissociated; QRS complexes are wide

Abbreviations: AV node, atrioventricular node; SA node, sinoatrial node.

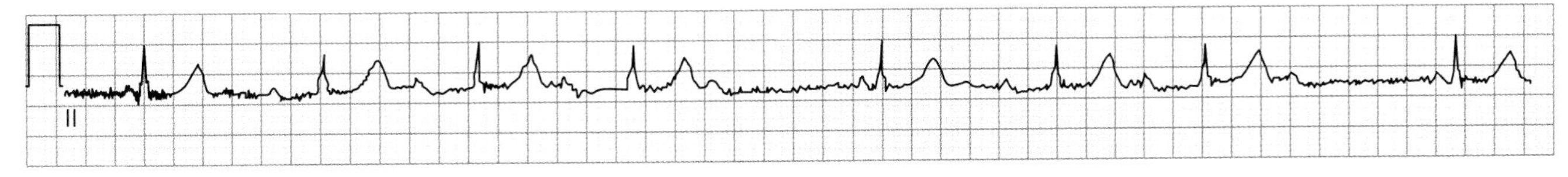

FIGURE 9-1 Mobitz Type I second-degree AV block, also known as Wenckebach phenomenon.

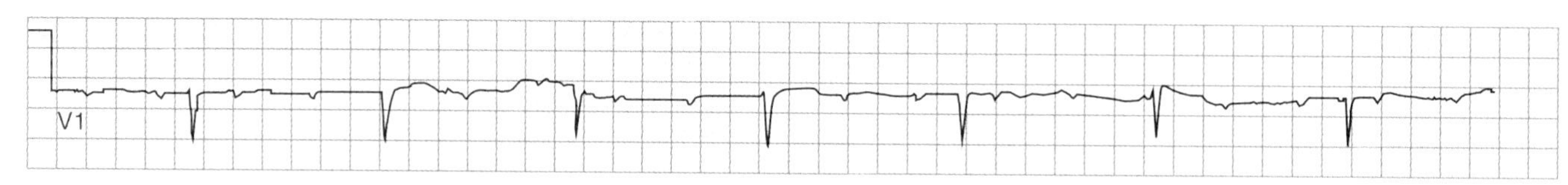

FIGURE 9-2 Complete heart block with a narrow escape.

TREATMENT

- In the setting of a reversible cause, the only treatment indicated is to avoid the inciting cause.
- Indications for permanent pacing include evidence of infranodal disease or symptomatic bradycardia at any level (SA node, AV node, or infranodal) that is spontaneous or secondary to the need for advancement of medical therapy (β-blocker, calcium channel blocker, etc); symptoms include dizziness, fatigue, syncope, poor exercise tolerance, and so on.

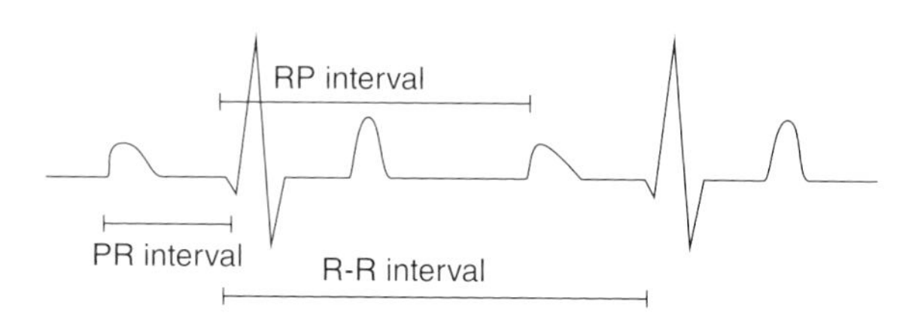

FIGURE 9-3 The figure demonstrates the relationship of the intervals that can be used to distinguish the different SVTs.

TACHYARRHYTHMIAS

Tachyarrhythmias occur when the heart rate is >100 beats per minute and are divided into narrow QRS complex and wide QRS complex tachyarrhythmias.

NARROW QRS COMPLEX

This can be further divided into supraventricular tachyarrhythmias (SVT), atrial fibrillation (AF), and atrial flutter.

Supraventricular Tachyarrhythmias

Diagnosis

Supraventricular Tachycardia	ECG Findings
Sinus tachycardia	Sinus P waves at a rate >100 bpm
AVNRT	Narrow-complex tachycardia with no obvious P waves; short RP interval (Figure 9-3)
ORT	Narrow-complex tachycardia; P waves often not visible, but if visible, then mid-RP interval
Atrial tachycardia	Narrow-complex tachycardia with long RP interval
PJRT	Narrow-complex tachycardia with long RP interval

Abbreviations: AVNRT, AV nodal reentrant tachycardia; ORT, orthodromic reciprocating tachycardia; PJRT, persistent junctional reciprocating tachycardia.

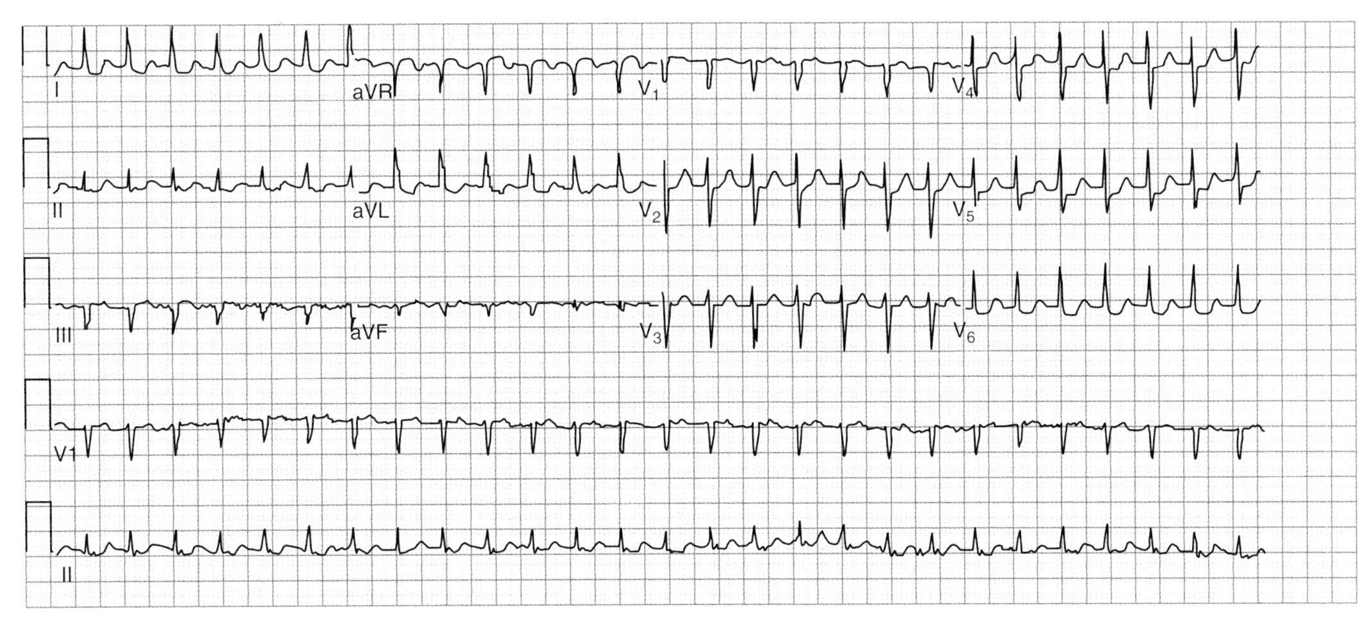

FIGURE 9-4 Supraventricular tachycardia, pseudo R waves are seen in lead V_1 and pseudo S waves in lead II. These likely represent P waves buried in the QRS complex, that is, short RP tachycardia or AVNRT.

- It is often difficult to diagnose the type of SVT based solely on surface ECG findings. Most often, electrophysiology (EP) study is required for definitive diagnosis. However, evaluating the RP interval (Figure 9-4) can be helpful; if the RP interval is short (less than one-half the R-R interval), then the rhythm is usually that of a typical AVNRT or atrioventricular reciprocating tachycardia (AVRT). If the RP interval is long (greater than one-half the R-R interval), then the rhythm is either atrial tachycardia or atypical AVNRT or PJRT.

Treatment

- Acute therapy involves vagal maneuvers and carotid sinus massage; adenosine can be used if vagal maneuvers fail. Cardioversion should also be considered in the setting of hemodynamic instability if the SVT fails to terminate with adenosine.
- Definitive therapy consists of either antiarrhythmic medications or catheter ablation; all patients with SVT should be referred to electrophysiologists for consideration of an EP study and ablation. Catheter ablation is generally associated with a high cure rate and a very low complication rate.

Gender Differences

- Physicians are more likely to attribute symptoms of paroxysmal SVT in women specifically, as compared to men, to panic, anxiety, and stress rather than correctly diagnosing the arrhythmia. This often leads to delay in therapy and a higher likelihood of women not being treated for their arrhythmia.
- Women are not referred for curative ablation as often as men. This is specifically problematic as SVT ablation is associated with a very high cure rate and many of the medications used to suppress SVT are highly toxic.
- A cyclical variation of SVT occurs in women; those with a history of paroxysmal SVT have a higher incidence of episodes during the luteal phase of their menstrual cycle and this is likely secondary to increased progesterone, decreased estrogen, and increased sympathetic activity.[1]

- Women have a 2-fold greater risk of AVNRT as compared to men. AVNRT is one of the most common types of SVT and has a very high cure rate with ablation.

Atrial Flutter and Atrial Fibrillation

Diagnosis

Rhythm	ECG Findings
Atrial flutter	Classic sawtooth pattern on ECG; (Figure 9-5), atrial flutter waves are generally regular and of consistent cycle length
Atrial fibrillation	No clear P waves with irregularly irregular rhythm (Figure 9-6)

Treatment

- Typical atrial flutter (classic sawtooth pattern on ECG) has a very high cure rate with catheter ablation, often >90%, and low rate of complications. Typical flutter is often difficult to treat with antiarrhythmic drugs and has a high rate of recurrence post cardioversion. For these reasons, patients with typical flutter should be referred for catheter ablation as first-line therapy.[2]
- For patients with AF, the physician must decide whether a rate-control versus a rhythm-control strategy should be employed. Rate control implies simply controlling the heart rate when in the arrhythmia. Rhythm control involves attempts at restoring and maintaining sinus rhythm.
- Younger patients who face a lifetime risk of atrial fibrillation or patients with highly symptomatic atrial fibrillation at diagnosis should be referred for a rhythm-control strategy. Rate control should be reserved for asymptomatic, elderly patients for whom rhythm control may be difficult to achieve.
- In patients for whom a rate-control strategy is preferred, nodal blockers such as diltiazem, verapamil, or metoprolol should be prescribed. If these are ineffective, then an AV node ablation can be considered along with implantation of a permanent pacemaker.

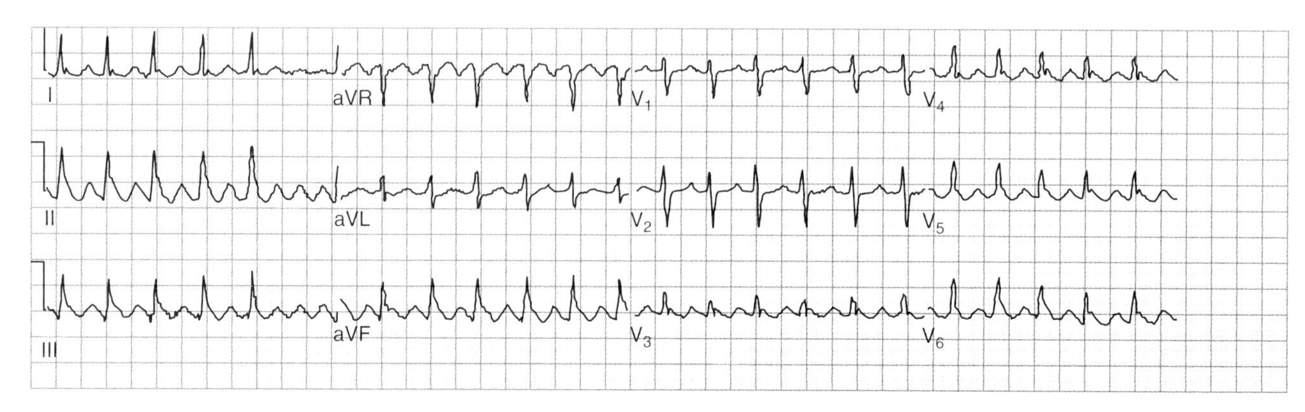

FIGURE 9-5 ECG demonstrating classic sawtooth pattern of atrial flutter.

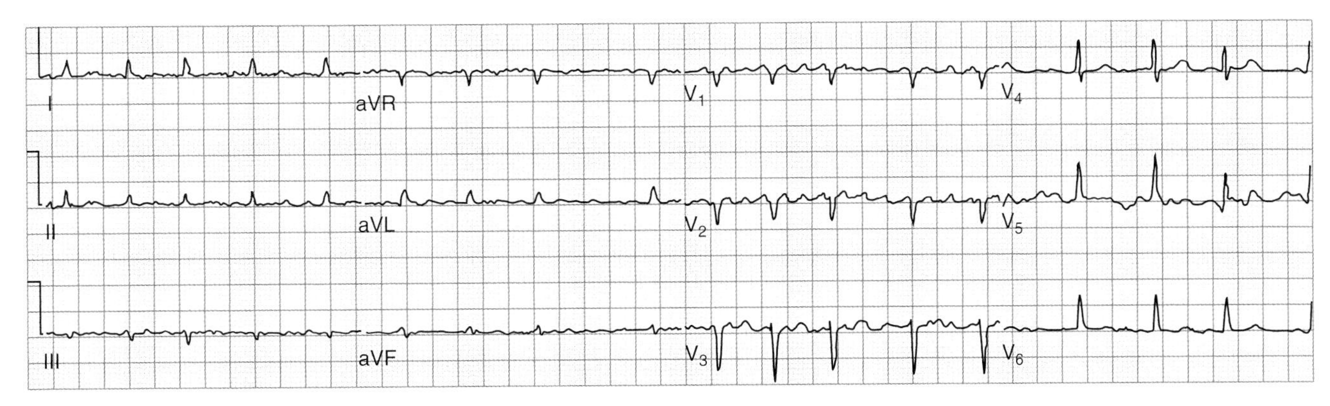

FIGURE 9-6 ECG demonstrating atrial fibrillation with rapid ventricular response.

- In patients for whom a rhythm control strategy is opted, a variety of antiarrhythmic drug options exist. These include the Class IC antiarrhythmics such as propafenone and flecainide and the Class III antiarrhythmics such as sotalol, dofetilide, and amiodarone. The choice of drug depends on the presence of structural heart disease, renal function, hepatic function, and baseline ECG parameters such as the presence of conduction system disease and/or a prolonged QT interval.
- Patients who fail at least one antiarrhythmic drug or in whom antiarrhythmic medications are not an option should be referred for catheter ablation.

Gender Differences

- The incidence of atrial fibrillation increases with age and given the increased longevity of women, the absolute number of women, older than 75, with atrial fibrillation is higher than the number of affected men in this age group.[3]
- Obesity is a known risk factor for development of AF. Recently, obesity has been shown to be a powerful predictor of the development of AF among young women.[4]
- Women with atrial fibrillation have a reduced quality of life as compared to men as they experience longer and more symptomatic episodes. On average, an episode lasted 89.8 minutes in women as compared to 50.5 minutes in men.[5]
- Women experience more frequent recurrences and higher heart rates (120 vs 112 bpm) than men.[5]
- Copenhagen City Heart Study demonstrated a higher cardiovascular mortality rate in women.[6]
- Women are referred for curative ablation less often and on average 28 months later than men, despite suffering worse symptoms. Furthermore, there are no significant differences in success rates, complications, or recurrence rates among men and women that undergo ablation.[7]
- SPAF (Stroke Prevention in Atrial Fibrillation) trials and ATRIA (AnTicoagulation and Risk factors In Atrial fibrillation) study demonstrated an increased risk of stroke in women with atrial fibrillation as compared to men.[8,9] To this end, female sex is included as a risk factor in the $CHADS_2$-Vasc2 score for risk stratification of stroke.

- Yet, the Canadian Registry of Atrial Fibrillation (CARAF) demonstrated that women were 54% less likely than men to receive warfarin, but twice as likely to receive aspirin.[10]
- There have been contradictory studies assessing the risk of hemorrhage in anticoagulated women with atrial fibrillation. The CARAF and SPORTIF (Stroke Prevention Using an Oral Thrombin Inhibitor in Atrial Fibrillation) studies demonstrated that women on warfarin were more likely than men to experience a major bleed;[11,12] however, the ATRIA study and SPAF trials demonstrated a similar bleeding risk among the genders.[9] The sum of the evidence suggests that women likely do not bleed more than men. Therefore, given their definite increase in risk for stroke as compared to men, they should be anticoagulated.

WIDE COMPLEX TACHYARRHYTHMIA

Diagnosis

Wide Complex Tachycardia	ECG Findings
Ventricular tachycardia	Atrioventricular disassociation; lack of fixed relationship between P waves and QRS complexes (Figure 9-7)
SVT with aberrancy	Baseline ECG may have bundle branch block. However, the arrhythmia does not originate in the ventricle; often difficult to distinguish from VT based on ECG criteria alone
Antidromic reciprocating tachycardia	Wide QRS with regular ventricular rhythm
Torsades de pointes	Prolonged QT interval with twisting of the QRS complexes around the isoelectric baseline

Treatment

- Hemodynamically unstable patients should be cardioverted immediately.
- Electrolyte values should be checked.
- Patients with wide-complex tachycardias should not be given nodal blockers or adenosine, with rare exception, as this could potentially exacerbate hypotension and lead to hemodynamic compromise.

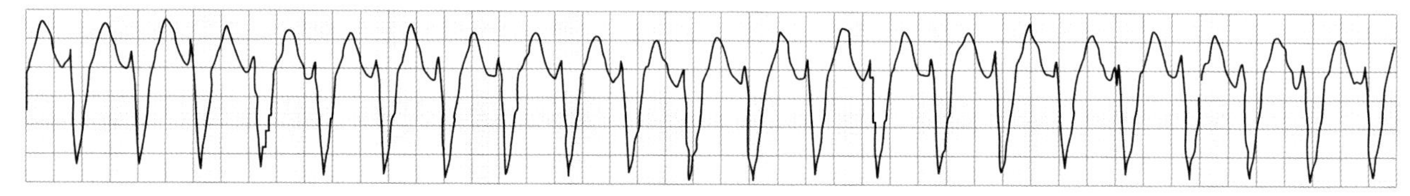

FIGURE 9-7 Wide-complex tachycardia consistent with VT, given the presence of AV dissociation.

- Sustained ventricular tachycardia, lasting for >30 seconds, should be treated with an implantable cardioverter defibrillator (ICD).
- All patients with an ejection fraction of ≤35% should also be considered for an ICD.

LONG QT SYNDROME

Long QT syndrome can either be acquired, from drug therapy or electrolyte imbalances, or congenital; it is associated with an increased risk of developing torsades de pointes as well as an increased risk of sudden cardiac death (SCD).

Diagnosis

- The normal value of QTc is <430 ms in men and <450 ms in women.[13]

Treatment

- Treatment of acquired long QT syndrome involves strict avoidance of the inciting drug as well as optimal electrolyte replacement, with prompt management of hypokalemia and/or hypomagnesemia.
- In patients with long QT syndrome, acquired or congenital, a thorough family history accompanied by ECG screening of the immediate family members is recommended to screen for genetic associations.

GENDER DIFFERENCES

- Men with long QT syndrome are associated with a higher risk of sudden cardiac death before the age of 15 as compared to women; after the age of 15, there is a gender risk reversal.[14]
- The increased risk of QT prolongation and cardiac events after puberty correlate with the effects of sex hormones;[15] for example, the QT interval length decreases in men after puberty secondary to the effect of testosterone.
- Females with long QT syndrome are at a 3-fold higher risk of cardiac events as compared to males.[14]
- Certain medications are known to prolong the QT interval; women have a greater risk of developing torsades de pointes when given drugs that prolong cardiac repolarization.[16]

Gender Differences in Ventricular Arrhythmias and Sudden Cardiac Death

- The incidence of SCD increases with age in both genders, with the incidence in women lagging behind about 20 years.[17]
- Of all out-of-hospital arrests, women more often present with asystole and pulseless electrical activity, whereas men are more likely to present with ventricular tachycardia and ventricular fibrillation.[18]

Gender Differences in the Use and Response to Implantable Cardioverter Defibrillators

- ICDs decrease the mortality when used for both primary and secondary prevention of SCD.
- The AVID (Antiarrhythmics Versus Implantable Defibrillators) trial demonstrated a similar mortality in women (14.4%) and men (15.5%) who received an ICD after a life-threatening ventricular arrhythmia, as compared to 24.4% in control group.[19]
- The SCD-HeFT (Sudden Cardiac Death in Heart Failure Trial) looked at the use of ICDs for primary prevention in patients with heart failure and LVEF<35% as compared to amiodarone or placebo; ICD therapy was associated with significantly reduced mortality. This study also demonstrated a significant decrease in mortality rates in men but not in women, a finding likely related to the small number of women enrolled in these trials.[20]
- Women are less likely to have an ICD placed. Of patients who met Medicare criteria for ICD implantation for primary prevention of SCD, 8.6/1000 women received ICD as compared to 32.3/1000 men within 1 year of diagnosis.[21]

Gender Differences in Cardiac Resynchronization Therapy

- Multiple studies have demonstrated cardiac resynchronization therapy to be as effective in women as compared to men.[22]
- The Multicenter InSync Randomized Clinical Evaluation (MIRACLE) trial demonstrated significant improvement in time to first hospitalization for heart failure and decreased death in women who received CRT as compared to women who were not treated with CRT; furthermore, men who received CRT did not demonstrate benefit to the same degree.[23]

ARRHYTHMIAS IN PREGNANCY

- There is an increase in the resting heart rate by 10 beats per minute in pregnant women.[24]
- There is a leftward shift of axis that is attributed to an enlarged uterus.[25]
- There is an increased incidence of new-onset SVTs and exacerbation of preexisting SVTs during pregnancy, likely related to the change in hormones associated with pregnancy.[26]

REFERENCES

1. Rosano GM, Leonardo F, Sarrel PM, et al. Cyclical variation in paroxysmal supraventricular tachycardia in women. *Lancet*. 1996;347:786-788.
2. Bertaglia E, Zoppo F, Bonso A, et al. Long term follow up of radiofrequency catheter ablation of atrial flutter: clinical course and predictors of atrial fibrillation occurrence. *Heart*. 2004;90(1):59-63.
3. Feinberg WM, Blackshear JL, Laupacis A, et al. Prevalence, age distribution, and gender of patients with atrial fibrillation. *Arch Intern Med*. 1995;155:469-473.
4. Karasoy D, Gislason G, Torp-Pedersen C, et al. Obesity is a powerful predictor of atrial fibrillation in fertile women. *Eur Heart J*. 2012;33(Abstract Supplement):969-970.
5. Hnatkova K, Waktare JE, Murgatroyd FD, et al. Age and gender influences on rate and duration of paroxysmal atrial fibrillation. *Pacing Clin Electrophysiol*. 1998;21(11 pt 2):2455-2458.

6. Friberg J, Scharling H, Gadsboll N, et al. Copenhagen City Heart Study. Comparison of the impact of atrial fibrillation on the risk of stroke and cardiovascular death in women versus men (The Copenhagen City Heart Study). *Am J Cardiol*. 2004;94:889-894.
7. Dagres N, Clague JR, Breithardt G, et al. Significant gender-related differences in radiofrequency catheter ablation therapy. *J Am Coll Cardiol*. 2003;42:1103-1107.
8. Hart RG, Pearce LA, McBride R, et al. Factors associated with ischemic stroke during aspirin therapy in atrial fibrillation: analysis of 2012 participants in the SPAF I-III Clinical Trials. *Stroke*. 1999;30:1223-1229.
9. Fang MC, Singer DE, Chang Y, et al. Gender differences in the risk of ischemic stroke and peripheral embolism in atrial fibrillation: the AnTicoagulation and Risk factors In Atrial fibrillation (ATRIA) study. *Circulation*. 2005;112:1687-1691.
10. Humphries KH, Kerr CR, Connolly SJ, et al. New-onset atrial fibrillation: sex differences in presentation, treatment, and outcome. *Circulation*. 2001;103:2365-2370.
11. Olsson SB. Executive Steering Committee of the SPORTIF III Investigators. Stroke prevention with the oral direct thrombin inhibitor ximelagatran compared with warfarin in patients with non-valvular atrial fibrillation (SPORTIF III): randomized controlled trial. *Lancet*. 2003;362:1691-1698.
12. Rienstra M, Van Veldhuisen DJ, Hagens VE, et al. Gender-related differences in rhythm control treatment in persistent atrial fibrillation: data of the Rate Control Versus Electrical Cardioversion (RACE) study. *J Am Coll Cardiol*. 2005;46(7):1298-1306.
13. Dagres N, Clague JR, Breithardt G, et al. Significant gender-related differences in radiofrequency catheter ablation therapy. *J Am Coll Cardiol*. 2003;42:1103-1107.
14. Moss AJ. Measurement of the QT interval and the risk associated with QTc interval prolongation: a review. *Am J Cardiol*. 1993;72:23B.
15. Locati EH, Zareba W, Moss AJ, et al. Age- and sex-related differences in clinical manifestations in patients with congenital long-QT syndrome: findings from the International LQTS Registry. *Circulation*. 1998;97:2237-2244.
16. Curtis AB, Narasimha D. Arrhythmias in women. *Clin Cardiol*. 2012 March;35(3):166-171.
17. Antzelevitch C, Shimizu W. Cellular mechanisms underlying the long QT syndrome. *Curr Opin Cardiol*. 2002;270:2590-2597.
18. Wolf PA, Abbott RD, Kannel WB. Atrial fibrillation as an independent risk factor for stroke: the Framingham Study. *Stroke*. 1991;22:983-988.
19. Wigginton JG, Pepe PE, Bedolla JP, et al. Sex-related differences in the presentation and outcome of out-of-hospital cardiopulmonary arrest: a multiyear, prospective, population-based study. *Crit Care Med*. 2002;30(4 suppl):S131-S136.
20. The Antiarrhythmics versus Implantable Defibrillators (AVID) Investigators. A comparison of antiarrhythmic-drug therapy with implantable defibrillators in patients resuscitated from near-fatal ventricular arrhythmias. *N Eng J Med*. 1997;337(22):1567-1583.
21. Bardy GH, Lee KL, Mark DB, et al for the Sudden Cardiac Death in Heart Failure Trial (SCD-HeFT) Investigators. Amiodarone or an implantable cardioverter-defibrillator for congestive heart failure. *N Eng J Med*. 2005;352:225-237.
22. Ghanbari H, Dalloul G, Hasan R, et al. Effectiveness of implantable cardioverter-defibrillators for the primary prevention of sudden cardiac death in women with advanced heart failure: a meta-analysis of randomized controlled trials. *Arch Inern Med*. 2009;169:1500-1506.
23. Curtis AB. Are women worldwide under-treated with regard to cardiac resynchronization and sudden death prevention? *J Interv Card Electrophysiol*. 2006;17(3):169-175.
24. Woo GW, Petersen-Stejskal S, Johnson JW, et al. Ventricular reverse remodeling and 6-month outcomes in patients receiving cardiac resynchronization therapy: analysis of the MIRACLE Study. *J Intervent card Electrophysiol*. 2005;12:107-113.
25. Wenger NK, Hurst JW, Strozier VN. Electrocardiographic changes in pregnancy. *Am J Cardiol*. 1964;13:774-778.
26. Tawam M, Levine J. Mendelson M, et al. Effect of pregnancy on paroxysmal supraventricular tachycardia. *Am J Cardiol*. 1993;72:838-840.

10 HEART DISEASE AND PREGNANCY

Grace Ayafor, MD
Sharon L. Roble, MD

INTRODUCTION

Less than 5% (0.2%-4%) of pregnancies in the western world are complicated by cardiovascular diseases;[1] however, the incidence of cardiovascular disease in pregnancy is increasing. This increase is due in part to the increasing prevalence of cardiovascular risk factors such as obesity, hypertension, and diabetes, as well as increasing age at first pregnancy and improved survival of patients with congenital heart disease, with many of these patients now reaching childbearing age. Because of this, cardiovascular disease is now one of the major causes of nonobstetric maternal mortality in the western world.

PHYSIOLOGIC CHANGES IN PREGNANCY

Several physiologic changes occur during a normal pregnancy to accommodate increasing metabolic demands of the mother and fetus. Hemodynamic changes include blood volume expansion, increase in cardiac output, and decrease in systemic vascular resistance. There are also changes in cardiac anatomy and blood vessels. These changes can put additional strain on patients with underlying heart disease or cardiovascular risk factors (Table 10-1).

HEMODYNAMIC CHANGES

Pregnancy

Cardiac output increases by 30% to 50% in normal pregnancy. This increase in cardiac output starts around the 5th gestational week and plateaus around 20 weeks. Early in pregnancy, cardiac output increases primarily due to an increase in stroke volume

TABLE 10-1 Hemodynamic changes of pregnancy

Parameter	First Trimester	Second Trimester	Third Trimester	Labor and Delivery
Blood volume	↑	↑↑	↑↑↑	↑
Stroke volume	↑	↑↑↑	↑	↑
Heart rate	↑	↑↑	↑↑ to ↑↑↑	↑ to ↔
Cardiac output	↑	↑↑ to ↑↑↑	↑↑↑	↑↑↑
Systolic blood pressure	↔	↓	↔	↑ to ↔
Diastolic blood pressure	↓	↓↓	↓	↑ to ↔
Pulse pressure	↑	↑↑	↔	↑ to ↔
Vascular resistance	↓	↓↓↓	↓↓	↔

(Figure 10-1). However, in the third trimester, increases in heart rate contribute more to cardiac output as stroke volume plateaus. Heart rate increases throughout pregnancy by about 15 beats per minute, starting at around 20 weeks' gestation and increasing to up to 32 weeks' gestation. The heart rate stays high until 2 to 5 days postpartum and then gradually decreases. Late in pregnancy, cardiac output can be affected by posture, likely due to mechanical compression of the inferior vena cava by the gravid uterus, resulting in decreased venous return and, in turn, decreased stroke volume. Moving from the left lateral decubitus to supine position can decrease cardiac output by as much as 25% to 30%. This is felt to be the mechanism of supine hypotensive syndrome, a syndrome of hypotension, bradycardia, and occasionally syncope in pregnant women when supine.

Blood pressure and total peripheral resistance decrease during pregnancy. Mean blood pressure starts decreasing early in gestation, with a nadir in the second trimester. However, in the third trimester, blood pressure starts rising and may reach prepregnancy levels. Several mechanisms have been suggested for this fall in vascular resistance including: (1) uteroplacental circulation providing a low resistance circuit, (2) increased nitric oxide production leading to vasodilation, (3) increased endothelial prostaglandin production, and (4) decreased aortic stiffness.

Plasma volume increases by about 45% above nonpregnant values. The exact mechanism is not known but it is thought that it may be in part due to renin-angiotensin-aldosterone system being stimulated by nitric oxide vasodilation. This increase is possibly adaptive in reducing hemodynamic instability after blood loss. Red cell mass also increases during pregnancy. However, plasma volume increases more than red cell mass, leading to the physiologic anemia of pregnancy. This physiologic anemia is likely adaptive as it causes a decrease in blood viscosity, which may counteract the increased thrombotic risk in pregnancy and may also improve intervillous perfusion.

There are also structural cardiac changes that occur during pregnancy. Echocardiographic studies have shown a mild increase in the dimensions of all cardiac chambers. End diastolic volume of the left ventricle increases, but the end systolic volume remains stable, which results in an increase in stroke volume. With dilatation of ventricular cavities comes dilation of valve annuli, and there may be some amount of mitral, tricuspid, and pulmonic regurgitation. There also appears to be an increase in left ventricular mass and wall thickness in normal pregnancy, primarily during the first trimester.

Labor and Delivery

Several factors of labor and delivery have significant effects on the cardiovascular system including pain, anxiety, bleeding, physical exertion, uterine contraction, and anesthesia. Cardiac output increases during labor due to increases in both stroke volume as well as heart rate. Stroke volume increases during labor because blood from uterine sinusoids is pushed into the systemic circulation with each contraction. During active labor, cardiac output further increases due to the physical exertion of delivery. Immediately after delivery, autotransfusion from uterine involution can result in an increase in cardiac output by up to 80%. Increases in heart rate due to pain, anxiety, and blood loss can further increase cardiac output during labor (Figure 10-2).

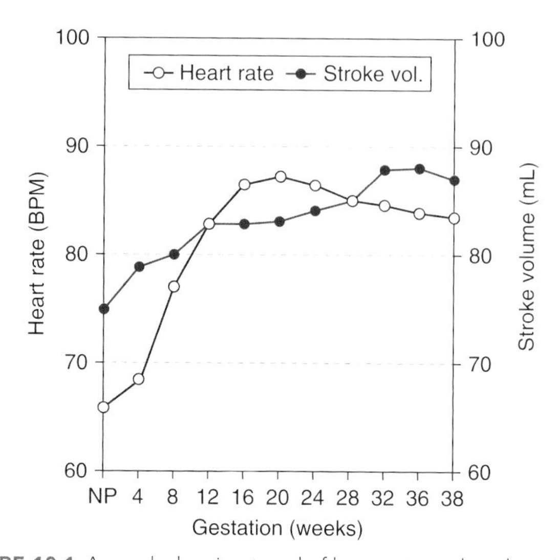

FIGURE 10-1 A graph showing trend of heart rate and stroke volume throughout pregnancy. Note that up to 26 to 28 weeks' gestation, the increase in cardiac output is primarily due to stroke volume.

From Creasy and Resnik's *Maternal–Fetal Medicine*. Figure 7-1.

Adapted from Robson SC, Hunter S, Boys RJ, et al. Serial study of factors influencing changes in cardiac output during human pregnancy. *Am J Physiol*. 1989;256:H1060.

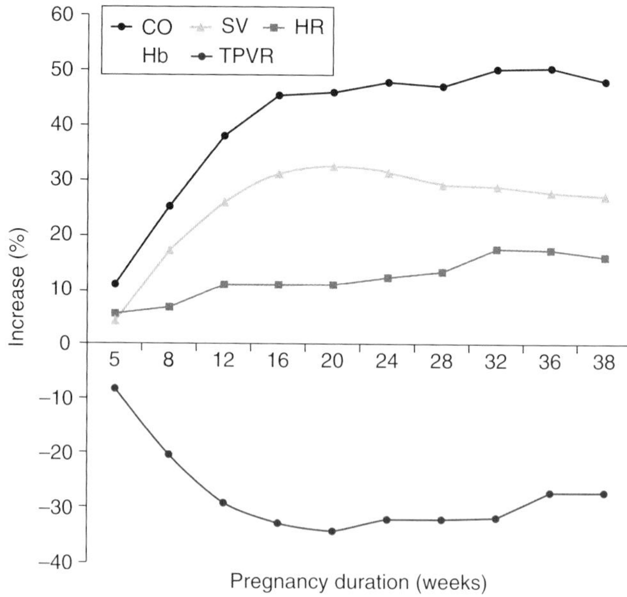

FIGURE 10-2 A graph showing percent changes in cardiac output, stroke volume, hemoglobin, and peripheral vascular resistance (TPVR) throughout pregnancy.

Abbreviations: CO, cardiac output; Hb, hemoglobin; HR, heart rate; SV, stroke volume; TPVR, total peripheral vascular resistance.

Reproduced with permission from Roos-Hesselink JW. et al. *Heart*. 2009;95:680-686.

Both systolic and diastolic blood pressure also increase during labor and delivery and are related to the magnitude of contractions, position of the patient, amount of pain, and anxiety. Analgesia, specifically spinal epidural anesthesia, may cause a marked decrease in systemic vascular resistance with a compensatory increase in stroke volume and heart rate.

Postpartum

The early postpartum period is associated with a high risk of cardiac decompensation because of further intravascular volume loading in a relatively short period of time. There is a significant increase in preload within 10 minutes after delivery, which can result in significant volume overload. As mentioned earlier, there is autotransfusion of blood from the involuting uterus back into the systemic circulation. Additionally, the gravid uterus is no longer compressing the inferior vena cava allowing for a rapid increase in venous return. In the absence of cardiovascular disease, this increase in preloads results in an increase in stroke volume and cardiac output. In the presence of cardiomyopathy and/or fixed heart obstruction, this increase in preload can lead to volume overload or pulmonary edema and decreased cardiac output. Within a week of delivery, postpartum autodiuresis of 2 to 5 L occurs. During the next several weeks, hemoglobin begins to increase, heart rate and stroke volume gradually decrease resulting in a decrease in cardiac output, and vascular resistance increases. These changes result in hemodynamics gradually returning to a prepregnancy state by 8 to 12 weeks postpartum, although some studies suggest this may take up to 6 months postpartum.

VASCULAR CHANGES

Hormone-induced changes occur in the vascular system as early as the fifth gestational week. Histologic changes in the aortic media that have been reported include smooth muscle hypertrophy and hyperplasia, loss of normal corrugation of elastic fibers, and fragmentation of reticular fibers. These changes lead to increased compliance of the vascular system, which is further accentuated by the vasodilatory effects of endogenous progesterone and prostaglandins produced during pregnancy. This is of particular importance in patients with aortopathies as they are at higher risk of aneurysm formation and dissection during pregnancy as well as labor and delivery. These changes may also contribute to the increased risk of spontaneous coronary artery dissection in pregnancy and the immediate postpartum period.

CHANGES IN COAGULATION FACTORS

Pregnancy is a hypercoagulable state due to changes in the concentration and effects of particular coagulation factors. Protein S decreases and resistance to protein C develops in the second and third trimesters. Other coagulation factors including factors I, II, V, VII, VIII, X, and XII increase in concentration. These changes lead to an approximately 20% reduction in prothrombin and partial thromboplastin times. The hypercoagulable state of pregnancy is adaptive in that it leads to less bleeding during delivery and in the immediate postpartum period. However, this also puts patients at risk for serious thromboembolic events.

ASSESSMENT OF RISK IN PATIENTS WITH PREEXISTING HEART DISEASE

The physiologic changes previously discussed are usually well tolerated in healthy women. However, these changes may be less well tolerated in patients with preexisting heart disease and may lead to adverse maternal and fetal outcomes. As such, assessment of cardiovascular risk in women with preexisting heart disease is paramount. Risk stratification should ideally occur prior to conception, although many women present for evaluation when they are already pregnant. It is important to note that a woman's risk may change over time during pregnancy, labor, delivery, and the postpartum period depending on her underlying heart condition.

There are no standardized, evidence-based guidelines to aid in maternal risk stratification. However, several factors have been shown to increase maternal risk in women with preexisting heart disease. These factors have been evaluated in a few studies and have been used to come up with various risk-scoring models in an attempt to accurately predict the risk of maternal adverse cardiovascular events. The 2 largest studies include CARPREG and ZAHARA.

The CARPREG study was a prospective multicenter study of 562 women with congenital and acquired heart disease in Canada who underwent 599 term pregnancies between 1994 and 1999. There was a 98% live birth rate. Only 27% of patients underwent a cesarean section with the vast majority of C-sections (96%) being for obstetric reasons. Primary cardiac events, defined as cardiac death, cardiac arrest, stroke, symptomatic arrhythmia requiring treatment, or pulmonary edema, occurred in 13% of the study population. Only 55% of primary cardiac events occurred prior to delivery, confirming that labor, delivery, and the postpartum periods are also associated with significant cardiovascular risk. Three deaths occurred in this study.[1]

In this study, there were 4 main predictors of maternal cardiovascular risk. These were prior cardiac event (arrhythmia, cerebrovascular event, heart failure), cyanosis or functional status (NYHA class > II), left heart obstruction, and myocardial dysfunction (ejection fraction <40%, hypertrophic or restrictive cardiomyopathy). One point was assigned to each of these predictors, and a risk index was developed to predict the level of risk. A score of 0 correlated with an estimated risk of a maternal cardiovascular event of <5%, a score of 1 with 27%, and a score of >1 with an approximately 75% risk of a maternal cardiac event.[1]

The CARPREG study also suggested predictors of adverse neonatal events, including NYHA class > II or cyanosis, maternal left heart obstruction, smoking, multiple pregnancies, and use of anticoagulants during pregnancy.[1]

More recently, the ZAHARA study retrospectively looked at pregnancy outcomes in women with congenital heart disease. The study population included 1802 women with congenital heart disease who had completed pregnancies between 1980 and 2007. In this population, the incidence of maternal cardiovascular and neonatal events was 7.6% and 25%, respectively. Several predictors of adverse outcomes in this study were noted to be similar to the findings of CARPREG. New associations included the presence of moderate to severe AV valve regurgitation, the presence of a mechanical valve prosthesis, and cyanotic heart disease. Based on ZAHARA data, a more complex scoring system was developed to predict maternal and neonatal risk, which included 13 variables (Table 10-2).[2]

While the above scoring systems help categorize patients into low-, intermediate, or high-risk groups, it is still very important to consider the risk associated with specific cardiac conditions as well as functional status and make management recommendations on a case-by-case basis.

TABLE 10-2 ZAHARA I scoring system

Risk Factor	Points
History of arrhythmias	1.5
Cardiac medications prior to pregnancy	1.5
NYHA > II prior to pregnancy	0.75
Left-sided obstructive lesions (mitral, aortic, LVOT) with peak gradient >50 mm Hg or valve area <1 cm^2	2.5
Moderate or severe systemic AV valve regurgitation	0.75
Moderate or severe pulmonic AV valve regurgitation	0.75
Mechanical valve prosthesis	4.25
Cyanotic heart disease (corrected or uncorrected)	1
Total	13

MANAGEMENT OF PREGNANT PATIENTS WITH UNDERLYING HEART DISEASE

PREGNANCY

Management of pregnant patients with underlying cardiovascular disease depends on their underlying condition. It is imperative that these patients be managed collaboratively, involving high-risk obstetricians, cardiologists specializing in pregnancy or adult congenital heart disease, and anesthesiologists in order to coordinate patient care and improve outcomes. Depending on the underlying disease process, patients may require medical therapy not traditionally required during pregnancy. They may also require more invasive procedures such as cardiac catheterizations, cardioversions, or, rarely, surgical intervention.

Patients with congenital heart disease should be offered genetic counseling as well as a fetal echocardiogram between 24 and 28 weeks' gestation to evaluate for any significant structural abnormalities prenatally. Fetal echocardiograms should be performed by pediatric cardiologists with expertise in fetal imaging. This affords a consultation with the pediatric cardiologist if an anomaly is identified and allows for coordination of care in the postpartum period.

LABOR AND DELIVERY

As outlined earlier, significant hemodynamic changes occur during labor and delivery that can have a significant impact on the cardiovascular system. These cardiovascular changes occur frequently and more rapidly as labor progresses. As with pregnancy, management of the cardiovascular system during labor is dependent on the underlying cardiac issues.

One of the most important questions often asked of cardiologists is regarding the safest mode of delivery from a cardiovascular standpoint. While a C-section may reduce the large hemodynamic changes associated with a vaginal delivery as well as the anxiety and pain associated with a prolonged labor, there are significant cardiovascular risks as well. The amount of anesthesia required for a C-section is much higher than that given during a vaginal delivery. This can result in significant changes in systemic and pulmonary vascular resistance and affect cardiac output. Blood loss is typically higher with a C-section as compared to a vaginal delivery (1000 mL with C-section versus 500 mL with vaginal delivery), which may affect stroke volume and, in turn, cardiac output. In addition, acute blood loss can lead to tachycardia that can further impact cardiac output. Certain cardiac lesions such as right ventricular myocardial dysfunction, hypertrophic cardiomyopathy, and left ventricular outflow tract (LVOT) obstruction are dependent on preload to maintain cardiac output, and significant blood loss will result in a decrease in preload, in turn decreasing cardiac output. Compensatory tachycardia due to blood loss further decreases ventricular-filling time in certain lesions, which can further decrease cardiac output.

POSTPARTUM

Significant hemodynamic changes begin to occur immediately after delivery. There is autotransfusion of uterine blood, which occurs with involution of the uterus. This can result in significant volume overload in patients with ventricular dysfunction or fixed obstructive lesions that are unable to tolerate large fluid shifts. Large fluid shifts can also result in electrolyte disturbances that may lead to arrhythmias in patients with underlying heart disease. In addition, there is a relatively rapid increase in both the pulmonary and systemic vascular resistance within the first 72 hours postpartum. This can lead to life-threatening pulmonary hypertension in patients with underlying pulmonary vascular disease or worsening ventricular function in patients with underlying ventricular dysfunction or significant structural heart disease. Depending on the underlying heart disease, patients may require invasive cardiac monitoring and or telemetry monitoring for a period of time postpartum until hemodynamics stabilize.

HYPERTENSION AND PREGNANCY

Hypertension is the most common medical problem in pregnancy. It occurs in up to 15% of pregnancies and accounts for significant morbidity and mortality, increasing the risk of CVA, abruptio placentae, and DIC in the mother. In the fetus, it increases the risk of prematurity, IUGR, and intrauterine death. Hypertension in pregnancy is defined as SBP ≥140 mm Hg or DBP ≥90 mm Hg. It is classified as mild (140-159/90-109) or severe (≥160/110). Elevated blood pressure in pregnancy may be due to several different etiologies, including:

- Preexisting Hypertension: Blood pressure ≥140/90 mm Hg that presents prior to pregnancy or prior to 20 weeks of gestation. It may be masked in early pregnancy due to the physiologic drop in blood pressure that occurs in the first trimester.
- Gestational Hypertension: Pregnancy-induced hypertension (blood pressure ≥140/90) that develops after the 20th gestational week and usually resolves within 42 days postpartum.
- Preeclampsia/eclampsia: Elevated blood pressure ≥140/90 mm Hg associated with proteinuria (>0.3 g/24 h). Risk factors for preeclampsia include nulliparity, multiple fetuses, diabetes, or hydatidiform mole. Signs and symptoms of eclampsia include right upper quadrant (RUQ) and epigastric pain due to hepatic congestion, headache and visual changes due to cerebral edema, occipital lobe blindness, hyperreflexia, and clonus. Preeclampsia may also present as the HELLP syndrome consisting of hemolysis, elevated liver enzymes, and low platelet count in addition to hypertension and proteinuria. Eclampsia is defined as seizures occurring in the presence of preeclampsia when the seizures cannot be explained by any other condition.

MANAGEMENT

Most women with hypertension in pregnancy have mild hypertension. Nonpharmacologic therapy should be considered in these patients, including limitation of activities and bed rest in the left lateral decubitus position. Salt restriction is not recommended as it may lead to intravascular volume depletion. Also, weight loss during pregnancy is not recommended as it may lead to reduced neonatal weight and slower growth in infants of these patients. However, there are established guidelines for healthy weight gain during pregnancy and these should be emphasized.

Pharmacologic treatment of mild or moderate hypertension in pregnancy is controversial as too aggressive of treatment may result in uteroplacental insufficiency and affect fetal growth and development. However, untreated hypertension may lead to stroke and placental abruption as well as coronary ischemia, heart failure, and volume overload. So need for treatment should be determined based on the risk-benefit ratio of pharmacologic therapy and may require discussion between both high-risk obstetrics and cardiology.

CORONARY ARTERY DISEASE AND PREGNANCY

CASE 1

A 31-year-old G7P4 woman with insulin-dependent (Type I) diabetes mellitus, 3-vessel coronary artery disease, ischemic cardiomyopathy with LVEF 35%, hypertension, and hyperlipidemia presents with non-ST elevation myocardial infarction. Precatheterization pregnancy test was positive and patient was found to be 7 weeks pregnant. Catheterization was postponed and patient was treated medically with heparin, aspirin, β-blockers, hydralazine, and nitrates. Patient was reportedly on an angiotensin-converting enzyme (ACE)-inhibitor, which was discontinued upon results of pregnancy test. Her echocardiogram on admission showed a left ventricular ejection fraction of 30%. Her previous cardiac catheterization images are shown in Figures 10-3 and 10-4.

Patient was counseled on the risks of continuing pregnancy and her medical therapy was optimized for coronary artery disease and ventricular dysfunction in the setting of pregnancy. She suffered a spontaneous abortion at 13 weeks' gestation.

Coronary artery disease remains a rare condition in women of childbearing age; however, given the growing epidemic of obesity, glucose intolerance/diabetes, hypertension, and hyperlipidemia in addition to more women postponing pregnancy until older ages, there are patients of childbearing age with significant underlying coronary atherosclerosis that can contribute to both maternal and fetal morbidity and mortality. Because of the increase in cardiac output and heart rate associated with pregnancy, these patients are at risk for myocardial ischemia due to myocardial oxygen supply-demand mismatch. This is especially concerning during labor and delivery, when cardiac output can increase by 80% in a relatively short period of time. In addition, several of the medications used for treatment of coronary artery disease and plaque stabilization are teratogenic and must be discontinued prior to conception. Ideally, patients with coronary artery disease or significant coronary artery risk factors should have prepregnancy evaluation, including a thorough history, physical, and a stress test to assess for any significant ischemia. Based on the patient's functional status and symptoms, assessment of ventricular function may also be warranted. Optimization of medical therapy with discontinuation of teratogenic drugs is also important as a majority of the teratogenic effects occur in the first trimester during organogenesis. For patients with coronary disease who present after conception, a thorough evaluation of symptoms and optimization of medical therapy would be an appropriate starting point. Based on symptomatology, further functional evaluation with submaximal stress testing may be indicated. Cardiac catheterization can be performed safely during pregnancy with appropriate fetal shielding and should be considered in patients presenting with an acute coronary syndrome or in patients with large areas of ischemia on functional testing.

Coronary artery dissection is a rare event; however, there is a relatively high incidence of spontaneous dissection associated with pregnancy, especially in the postpartum state. The etiology of this is unknown, although suggested hypotheses include alterations in the arterial walls related to endogenous hormonal changes of pregnancy, inflammation, or underlying connective tissue disorders.[3] These patients will present with an acute coronary syndrome and should be treated as such, although thrombolytics should be avoided due to risk of life-threatening hemorrhage.

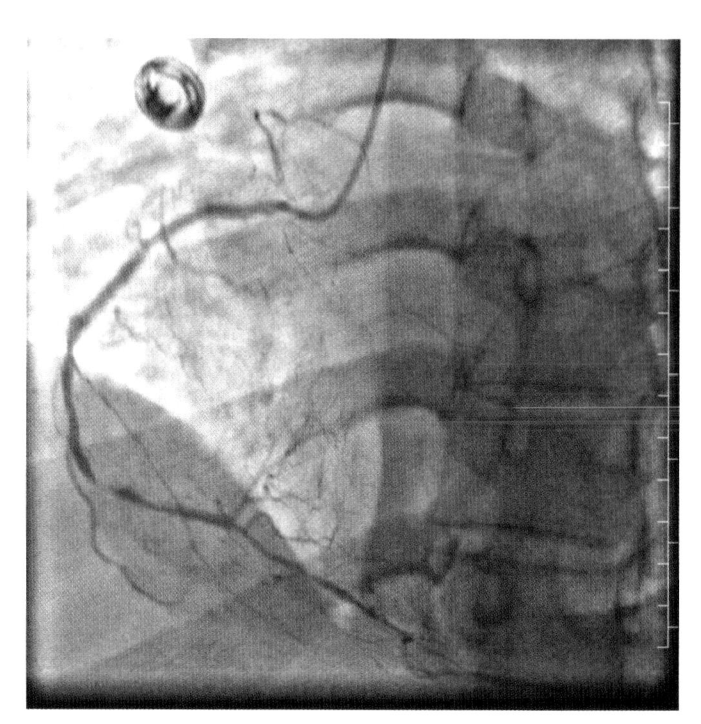

FIGURE 10-3 A selective right coronary artery angiogram showing dominant right coronary artery with severe diffuse disease with collateralization.

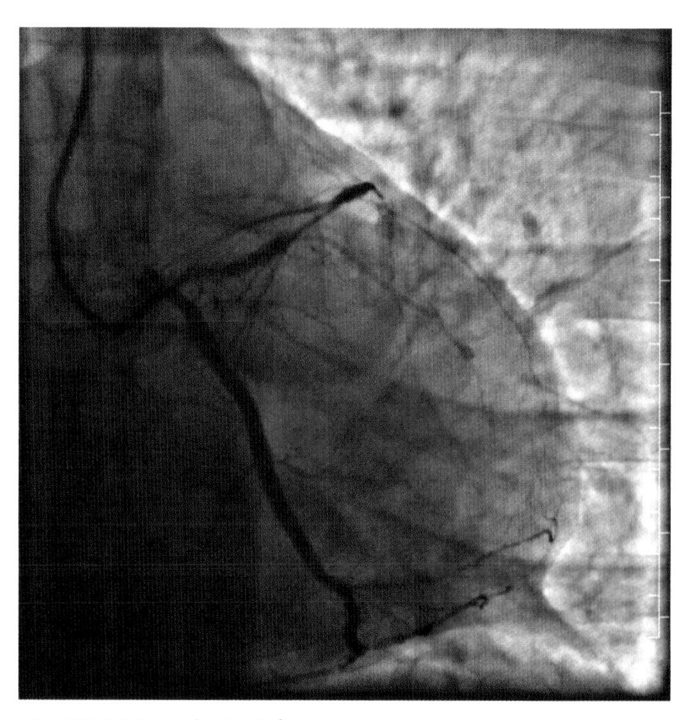

FIGURE 10-4 A selective left coronary artery angiogram showing severe proximal left anterior descending artery (LAD) stenosis and totally occluded mid-LAD stenosis with collateralization. The left circumflex artery is a large-caliber vessel with mild luminal irregularities noted.

CARDIOMYOPATHIES AND PREGNANCY

Cardiomyopathy occurring in pregnancy is rare and of diverse etiology. Careful history taking and physical examination together with echocardiographic evaluation can help distinguish normal physiologic changes of pregnancy from pathologic ventricular dysfunction. Biomarkers may be helpful in making a diagnosis, but do not confirm it. *N*-terminal prohormone of brain natriuretic peptide (NT-proBNP) is reportedly higher in pregnant patients versus nonpregnant controls, but should still fall within the normal range. Levels may be elevated with CHF and preeclampsia. Initial management of ventricular dysfunction during pregnancy is similar to management in nonpregnant patients, starting with medications including β-blockers, nitrates, diuretics, and digoxin. Of note, ACE inhibitors and angiotensin receptor blockers (ARBs) are teratogenic and should not be used during pregnancy. In patients who are on ACE inhibitors or ARBs prior to becoming pregnant, these medications should be stopped immediately upon even the possibility of pregnancy. In severe cases of ventricular dysfunction, advanced heart failure therapies including mechanical assist devices and heart transplant may be necessary.

CASE 2

A 44-year-old G2P1 woman with a past medical history of peripartum cardiomyopathy presents at 8 weeks' gestation for further cardiac evaluation. During her first pregnancy, she presented 1 week postpartum with dyspnea and lower extremity edema. An echocardiogram at that time showed a left ventricular ejection fraction of 25%. She was treated with diuretics, ACE-inhibitors, and β-blockers with improvement in her ventricular function upto 50%. She was counseled on the risk of recurrence and avoidance of future pregnancies. However, she presents 6 years later with an unexpected pregnancy and NYHA class II heart failure symptoms. A baseline echo showed a left ventricular ejection fraction of 55%. During second trimester, she developed orthopnea and lower-extremity edema and an echo showed a decrease in ventricular function to 45%. She was treated with β-blockers and diuretics which improved her symptoms and stabilized her ventricular function.

She was admitted to the hospital 48 hours prior to elective C-section at 38 weeks' gestation for optimization of her volume status prior to delivery. Postoperatively, she was monitored for 72 hours with a central venous catheter to guide optimization of her fluid status.

PERIPARTUM CARDIOMYOPATHY

Peripartum cardiomyopathy (PPCM) refers to idiopathic heart failure in the last month of pregnancy or during the first 5 months postpartum that occurs in the absence of any determinable heart disease. The incidence in the United States is about 1:3000 to 4000, but higher in developing countries.[4,5]

Risk factors for developing PPCM include African American race, maternal age >30, multiparity, twin pregnancy, history of hypertension, preeclampsia and eclampsia.[4] The etiology of peripartum cardiomyopathy is unclear but several mechanisms have been proposed, including inflammatory, autoimmune, and genetic mechanisms. There have been reports of high levels of inflammatory markers, specifically tumor necrosis factor-α (TNFα), interferon-g, interleukin-6, and C-reactive protein (CRP). There is also evidence of increased oxidative stress in these patients.[5] Other studies have reported a high prevalence of active myocarditis in these patients, some with evidence of viral involvement. Another proposed mechanism is that of fetal chimerism, in which some fetal cells settle into the maternal heart, and in the postpartum period when the maternal immune system has improved, an antibody response is triggered. Finally, mutations associated with dilated cardiomyopathy have been identified in patients with PPCM, suggesting a genetic component.[5]

Peripartum cardiomyopathy presents with typical signs and symptoms of heart failure, such as exertional dyspnea, fatigue, orthopnea, peripheral edema, and paroxysmal nocturnal dyspnea. These symptoms may be present in a normal pregnancy, particularly in the third trimester. However, a delay in returning to the prepregnancy state should prompt evaluation for PPCM. Diagnosis is based on clinical and echocardiographic criteria (Table 10-3).

If PPCM occurs during pregnancy, urgent delivery should be considered followed by standard treatment for heart failure. Benazepril, captopril, and enalapril may be used while breastfeeding, with monitoring of the child's weight for at least the first month as an indicator of renal dysfunction. ACE inhibitors, ARBs, and renin inhibitors are contraindicated during pregnancy because of fetotoxicity. Hydralazine and nitrates can be safely used during pregnancy for afterload

TABLE 10-3 Diagnostic criteria for peripartum cardiomyopathy

- Development of heart failure in the last month of pregnancy or within 5 months postpartum
- Absence of any other identifiable cause of heart failure
- Absence of preexisting heart disease
- Echocardiographic criteria
    - Left ventricular ejection fraction <45%
    - Fractional shortening <30%
    - Left ventricle end-diastolic dimension >2.7 cm/m^2

reduction in place of ACE inhibitors/ARBs. Pregnancy and cardiomyopathy both increase the risk of thromboembolism; hence anticoagulation should be considered to prevent systemic embolization. When low molecular weight heparins are used, factor Xa levels should be monitored to ensure adequate anticoagulation.

Advanced heart failure therapies may be necessary in patients with severe symptoms. Because up to 50% of patients may recover LV function, ventricular assist devices may be preferable to emergent heart transplant patients when available. Patients who do not recover ventricular function within 6 months of appropriate medical therapy should be considered for implantable cardioverter-defibrillator (ICD) or resynchronization therapy per guidelines for nonischemic cardiomyopathies. Several small trials have looked at targeted therapies that may be added to standard heart failure therapy to improve outcomes in PPCM. These include intravenous immunoglobulin, pentoxifylline, and bromocriptine. Larger, randomized multicenter trails are needed to further evaluate the efficacy and safety of these therapies.

Recovery from PPCM, defined by an increase in LVEF by >20% or to >50%, usually occurs in about 50% of patients within 3 to 6 months. Negative prognostic factors include baseline LVEF <30%, LV end-diastolic diameter >5.6 cm, and high troponin at baseline. Reported maternal mortality rate in the United States is 6% to 10%. Risk of recurrence in subsequent pregnancies is up to 80% even with previously recovered LV function. As such, current guidelines recommend against subsequent pregnancies, although small studies have suggested that the risk of recurrence may be lower in patients who recover ventricular function within 6 months postpartum.

DILATED CARDIOMYOPATHY

Women with preexisting dilated cardiomyopathy are at a high risk of cardiac complications during pregnancy, with some studies reporting a complication rate of up to 39%. These usually happen around the third trimester or in the postpartum period when the hemodynamic burden of pregnancy is highest. Women with dilated cardiomyopathy are at increased risk for heart failure, arrhythmias, and cerebrovascular events during pregnancy. Risk factors for developing cardiac adverse events include LVEF <40%, NYHA functional class > II, prior history of heart failure, or other cardiovascular event (arrhythmias, cerebrovascular events). Associated adverse fetal events include preterm delivery and low birth weight. Women of childbearing age with dilated cardiomyopathy should be extensively counseled about the risks associated with pregnancy at every visit regardless of their immediate plans for pregnancy.[6] In addition, patients with DCM should undergo an extensive cardiac evaluation prior to pregnancy. Echocardiogram and exercise testing may be useful prior to pregnancy to help in risk stratification. Medications should be evaluated, and teratogenic medications such as ACE inhibitors/ARBs should be discontinued in patients trying to get pregnant. These patients should be followed throughout their pregnancy by a maternal-fetal medicine specialist as well as a cardiologist with expertise in pregnancy or heart failure.

Regular follow up with serial echocardiograms may be necessary during pregnancy, with the frequency of these based on their risk for cardiovascular events and clinical symptoms. β-Blockers may be continued throughout pregnancy with close fetal monitoring to ensure adequate growth on β-blockers. Other potential fetal effects of β-blockers include fetal bradycardia, apnea, and hypoglycemia. Vasodilators like hydralazine and nitrates may be used in place of ACE inhibitors during pregnancy. Loop diuretics may be needed when there are concerns for pulmonary edema, although their use should be minimized due to the risk for uteroplacental insufficiency and fetal electrolyte abnormalities including elevated uric acid.

During labor and delivery, patients with dilated cardiomyopathy require close cardiovascular monitoring dependent upon the severity of their symptoms during the pregnancy. For patients who were asymptomatic during pregnancy with no significant decompensation, monitoring may consist of continuous telemetry monitoring and noninvasive assessment of volume status and cardiac output. More invasive monitoring with pulmonary artery catheterization may be necessary for patients with evidence of decompensated heart failure during pregnancy, severe ventricular function, or those at high risk for decompensation in the immediate postpartum period. Most patients may undergo vaginal delivery, although mode of delivery should be an individualized decision made in conjunction with high-risk obstetrics, anesthesia, and cardiology. Anesthesia with an epidural is recommended as it blunts the increased hemodynamic changes of labor and delivery and may result in a more comfortable and successful delivery. The preload and afterload changes frequently caused by epidural anesthesia may be advantageous in patients with dilated cardiomyopathy. Need for C-section should be individualized to the patient based on the risks and benefits of the procedure and the patient's cardiac status.

CASE 3

A 25-year-old G1P0 with no significant past medical history presents at 7 weeks' gestation with complaints of shortness of breath and chest pain. On physical examination, she is noted to have a hyperdynamic precordium, normal carotid upstrokes and jugular venous pulsation, a grade II/VI harsh systolic ejection murmur at the upper left sternal border which radiates to the apex, a grade III/VI holosystolic murmur at the apex, which radiates to the axilla, and normal peripheral pulses with no brachiofemoral delay. An electrocardiogram (Figure 10-5) and echocardiogram (Figures 10-6 and 10-7) are performed.

She was admitted to the hospital 72 hours prior to delivery and had a pulmonary artery catheter and arterial line placed to monitor her volume status. Her fluid status was optimized and she underwent a forceps-assisted second-stage delivery in the surgical intensive care unit at 38 weeks' gestation. Invasive hemodynamic monitoring was continued for 72 hours postpartum to maintain euvolemia.

HYPERTROPHIC CARDIOMYOPATHY

Hypertrophic cardiomyopathy (HCM) is one of the most common genetic heart diseases, transmitted in an autosomal dominant fashion, and diagnosed in about 1:500 adults. Although it has a variable phenotype, common features include asymmetric left ventricular hypertrophy with wall thickness >15 mm, preserved systolic function, diastolic dysfunction due to impaired relaxation, and a nondilated left ventricular cavity. Nearly 20% of patients have left ventricular outflow obstruction associated with systolic anterior motion of the mitral valve and mitral regurgitation. Pregnant patients with HCM are at

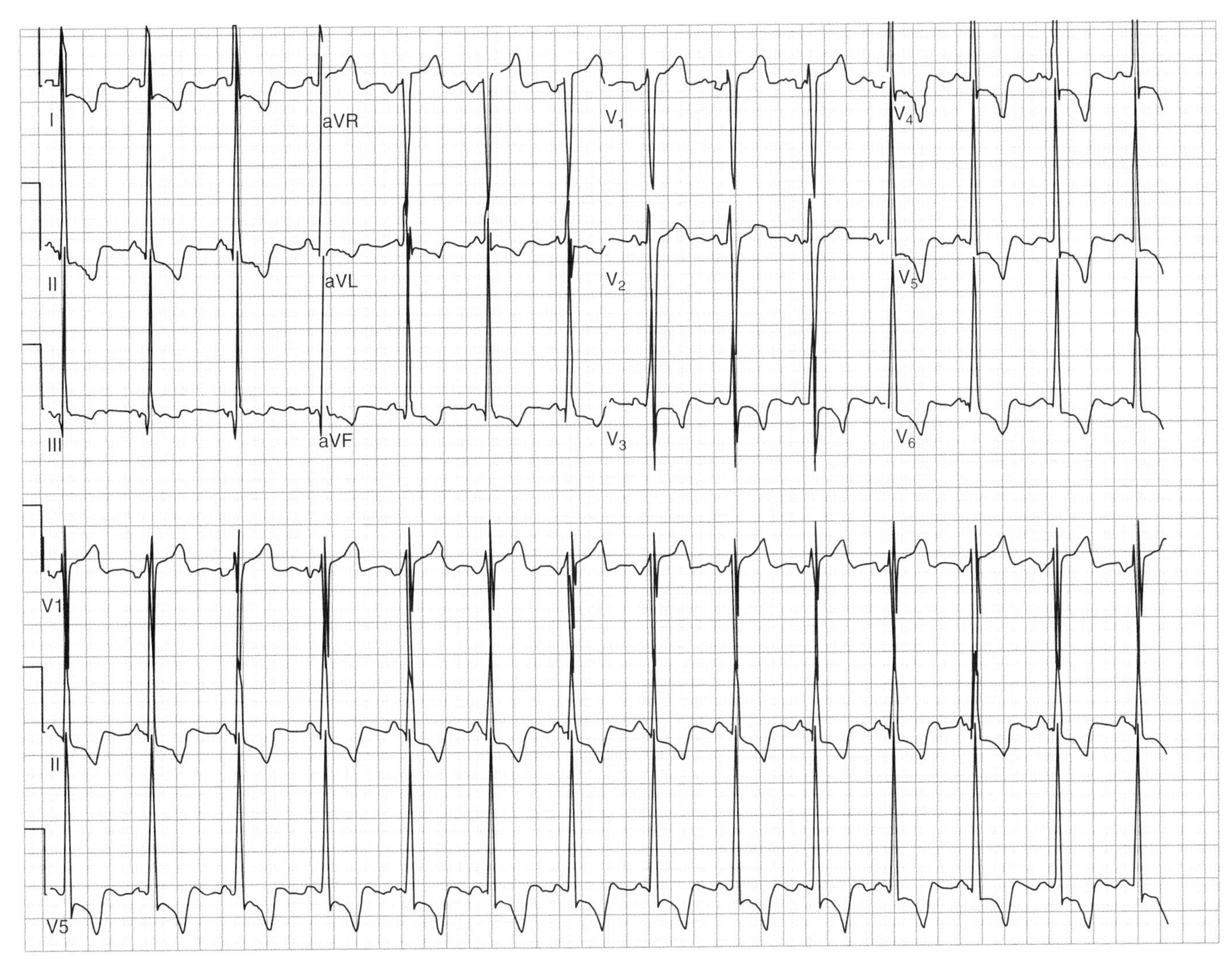

FIGURE 10-5 A 12-lead electrocardiogram showing sinus rhythm with left ventricular hypertrophy and diffuse ST depression and T-wave inversions consistent with hypertrophic cardiomyopathy.

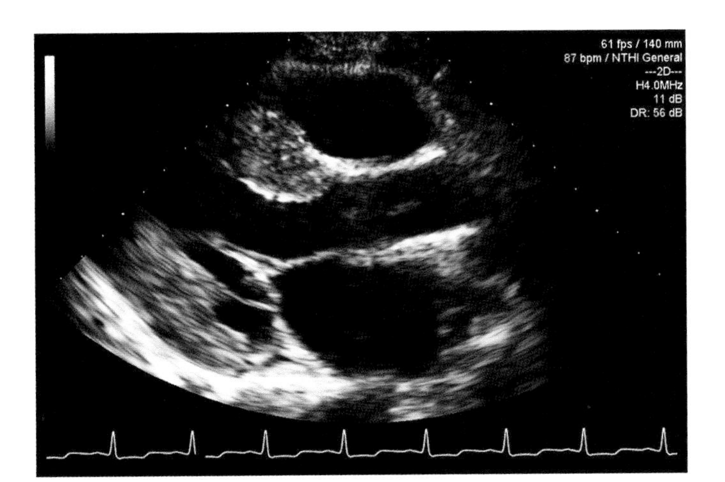

FIGURE 10-6 A two-dimensional echocardiogram in parasternal long-axis view showing severe left ventricular hypertrophy that is most prominent in the basal septum.

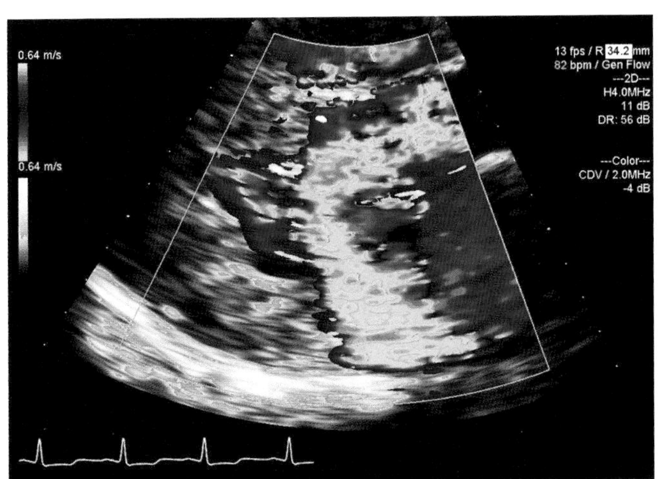

FIGURE 10-7 A color flow Doppler echocardiogram in parasternal long view showing severe, posteriorly directed mitral regurgitation and aliasing of flow across the left ventricular outflow tract consistent with hypertrophic obstructive cardiomyopathy with systolic anterior motion of the mitral valve (SAM).

risk for heart failure, arrhythmias, and sudden cardiac death. Because of the genetics of HCM, all patients with the disease should undergo genetic counseling either prior to or during pregnancy and their offspring will require cardiology evaluation by a pediatric cardiologist during childhood and adolescence.

Clinical presentation is related to the degree of LVH and the gradient across the LVOT. Symptoms that occur during pregnancy are similar to prepregnancy symptoms and include exertional chest pain, dyspnea, fatigue, palpitations, and syncope. Pregnancy is a volume overload state, which may be beneficial as the increased volume that occurs during pregnancy may lead to increased left ventricular end-diastolic diameter, in turn increasing the LVOT diameter and decreasing the LVOT gradient. This decrease in LVOT gradient may actually improve symptoms and likely explain why patients with hypertrophic obstructive cardiomyopathy tend to tolerate pregnancy well.

Management during pregnancy should include the use of β-blockers, particularly in patients with more than mild LVOT obstruction and wall thickness >15 mm. β-blockers are indicated to lower the heart rate and prolong ventricular filling time. Verapamil may be used as a second-line agent. Because atrial arrhythmias are usually not well tolerated in HCM, cardioversion should be considered in any patients with symptomatic recurrent atrial arrhythmias that are not well controlled with medical therapy. Anticoagulation should also be considered in the presence of atrial arrhythmias due to the increased risk of thromboembolism during pregnancy.

The hemodynamic changes during labor and delivery may be detrimental to these patients. Increased circulating catecholamines lead to increased heart rate, which decrease the LV filling time, resulting in decreased preload and hence, increased LVOT gradient. Valsalva maneuver and blood loss both decrease preload as well. Epidural anesthesia may cause vasodilation and hypotension, which can also increase the LVOT gradient. The vasodilatory effects of epidural anesthesia can be counteracted by phenylephrine, which is a pure α-agonist and will not affect ventricular contractility. These patients require close hemodynamic monitoring during labor and delivery, frequently requiring invasive cardiac monitoring to maintain preload and, in turn, cardiac output. Coordination of labor and delivery with high-risk obstetrics, cardiology, and anesthesia is imperative in this patient population.

VALVULAR HEART DISEASE

Valvular heart disease in pregnancy is commonly due to rheumatic disease or corrected congenital heart disease. Asymptomatic and mildly symptomatic (NYHA class I and II) lesions pose lower cardiovascular risk than lesions which are more symptomatic (NYHA III/IV). Symptomatic valvular heart disease prior to pregnancy has a high risk of adverse maternal cardiovascular outcomes. As such, evaluation and management of valvular heart disease should ideally occur prior to conception, with particular attention paid to the severity of the valvular lesion and functional class of the patient. Exercise testing may be necessary in patients with unclear functional capacity. Symptomatic valvular disease diagnosed prior to pregnancy should be treated and/or repaired prior to conception to improve both maternal and fetal outcomes.

CASE 4

A 29-year-old G5P4 woman with rheumatic mitral stenosis requiring valvuloplasty presents during her second trimester with exertional dyspnea. On physical examination, there is a quiet precordium, single S_1, split S_2 with prominent pulmonary component, opening snap, grade II/VI diastolic rumble, grade II/VI holosystolic murmur at the apex, no gallops, normal carotid upstrokes, and jugular venous pulsation. An echocardiogram is shown in Figures 10-8 through 10-10.

She was started on β-blockers with improvement in her symptoms and underwent a forceps-assisted second-stage delivery at 37 weeks' gestation. A pulmonary artery catheter was placed 24 hours prior to delivery to monitor her volume status during delivery and for 48 hours postpartum.

MITRAL STENOSIS

Mitral stenosis is one of the more common valvular lesions in pregnancy, with a majority of cases due to rheumatic heart disease. Mitral stenosis restricts flow from the left atrium to the left ventricle. Because of the fixed stenosis, left ventricular filling is dependent on heart rate. The physiologic increase in heart rate during pregnancy decreases the time it takes for the ventricle to fill in diastole. In addition, the increased volume load of pregnancy leads to an increase in the gradient across the stenotic valve, resulting in elevated left atrial pressure and left atrial dilatation. The pressure is transmitted backward to the pulmonary vasculature and can cause pulmonary edema. Left atrial dilatation can result in disruption of the conduction system causing atrial arrhythmias, particularly atrial fibrillation. As such, many patients with mitral stenosis, including those who were previously asymptomatic, may have some clinical deterioration with pregnancy.

Women with moderate and severe mitral stenosis (mitral valve area <1.5 cm^2) and NYHA class III or IV heart failure have a higher incidence of adverse cardiovascular events including heart failure, arrhythmias (atrial fibrillation and supraventricular tachycardia), or embolic events, although maternal mortality from mitral stenosis is rare (0%-3%).[7]

Patients with severe mitral stenosis who desire pregnancy should undergo balloon valvuloplasty prior to pregnancy, as this may decrease the risk of developing heart failure, as well as the need for medications or diagnostic and therapeutic procedures that may be detrimental to the fetus. Patients with moderate mitral stenosis prior to pregnancy should be considered for valvuloplasty prior to conception based on their symptoms and exercise tolerance.

Initial management of mitral stenosis during pregnancy should be aimed at reducing heart rate and left atrial pressure. Heart rate may be decreased with β-blockers or calcium channel blockers. β-1 selective blockers are preferred as they are theoretically less likely to interfere with uterine relaxation. Atenolol should be avoided as it has been associated with intrauterine growth retardation. Patients may need to be on bed rest. Left atrial pressure may be decreased with diuretics, but close attention should be paid to avoid uterine hypoperfusion from volume depletion.

Optimal medical therapy may not suffice in all patients, and some remain with significant symptoms and elevated pulmonary pressures despite adequate heart rate control. Percutaneous commissurotomy is preferred over open heart surgery during pregnancy, and ideally should be performed after 20 weeks of gestation. Abdominal lead shielding should be used to decrease the radiation dose to the fetus.

Most patients may safely undergo vaginal delivery with assisted second stage of labor. Epidural anesthesia is recommended to decrease the hemodynamic fluctuations that occur with pain during labor and delivery, keeping in mind the risk of hypotension. Invasive hemodynamic monitoring may be necessary depending on severity of stenosis and symptomatology. Cesarean section should be done as needed for obstetric reasons.

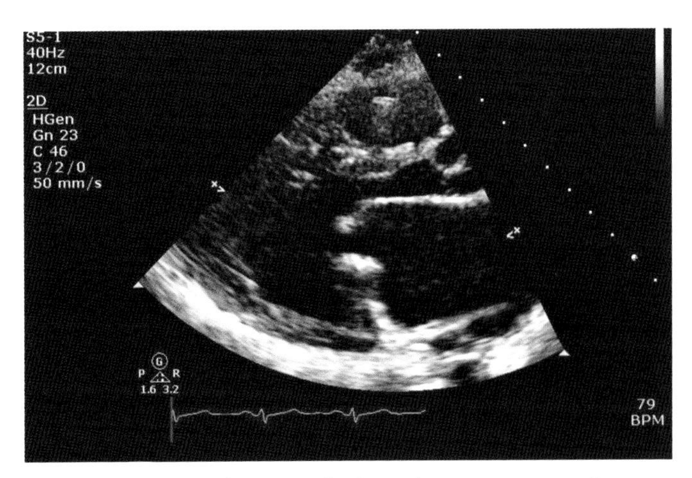

FIGURE 10-8 A two-dimensional echocardiogram, parasternal long-axis view, showing thickened mitral valve with "hockey stick" appearance to anterior mitral valve leaflet consistent with rheumatic mitral valve disease.

CASE 5

A 36-year-old G2P1 woman with a bicuspid aortic valve and mild aortic stenosis presents at 22 weeks' gestation with complaints of exertional dyspnea. On physical examination, she is in no acute distress with normal carotid upstrokes and jugular venous pulsation. There is a quiet precordium, normal first and second heart sounds, systolic ejection click, grade III/IV harsh systolic ejection murmur at the upper left sternal border that radiates to the carotids bilaterally, and no diastolic murmurs or gallops noted. There are 2+ femoral pulses with no brachiofemoral delay noted. An echocardiogram is performed (Figures 10-11 through 10-13).

Because of her echocardiogram findings, a noncontrast MRI was performed (Figure 10-14). The patient underwent a forceps-assisted second-stage vaginal delivery with epidural anesthesia at 37 weeks' gestation, which was uncomplicated. She did not require invasive cardiac monitoring prior to delivery or in the immediate postoperative period.

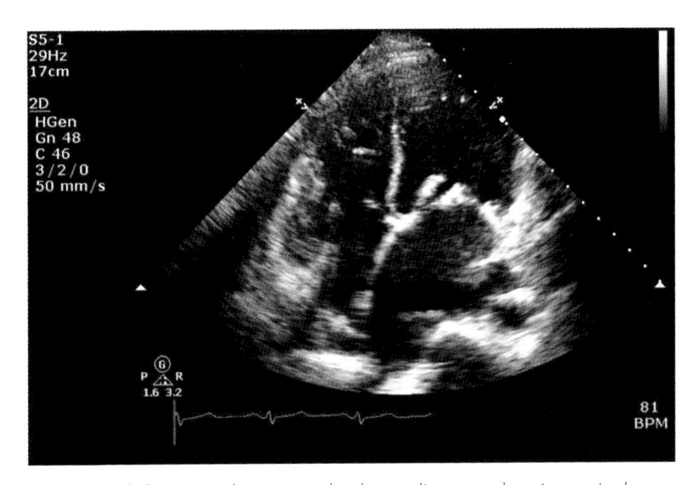

FIGURE 10-9 A two-dimensional echocardiogram showing apical 4-chamber view. Note severe biatrial enlargement and thickened mitral valve leaflets and annulus.

AORTIC STENOSIS

Congenital aortic stenosis occurs in 8 per 1000 live births accounting for 3% to 5% of congenital heart disease. Calcific or degenerative aortic stenosis occurs later in life and is not typically seen in women of childbearing age. Mild or moderate aortic stenosis is typically well tolerated during pregnancy, although left-sided obstructive lesions do confer some risk to both the mother and fetus irrespective of symptoms based on retrospective studies. Because of the increase in blood volume and cardiac output during pregnancy, aortic valve gradients will increase although this does not necessarily correlate to clinical symptoms. Distinguishing symptomatic aortic stenosis from symptoms related to the normal physiologic changes of pregnancy can be challenging. Symptoms include exertional dyspnea, orthopnea, PND, and chest pain. Patients with symptomatic aortic stenosis during pregnancy pose a significant management problem as medical therapy is typically not effective. Treatment options during pregnancy include judicious use of diuretic therapy for volume issues, although care must be given not to cause a significant reduction in afterload as it can worsen symptoms. There is little role for vasodilators in patients with aortic stenosis unless there is hypertension that remains uncontrolled by more conservative measures. While surgical intervention would be a definitive therapy, there continues to be a significant fetal morbidity and mortality associated with cardiopulmonary bypass.

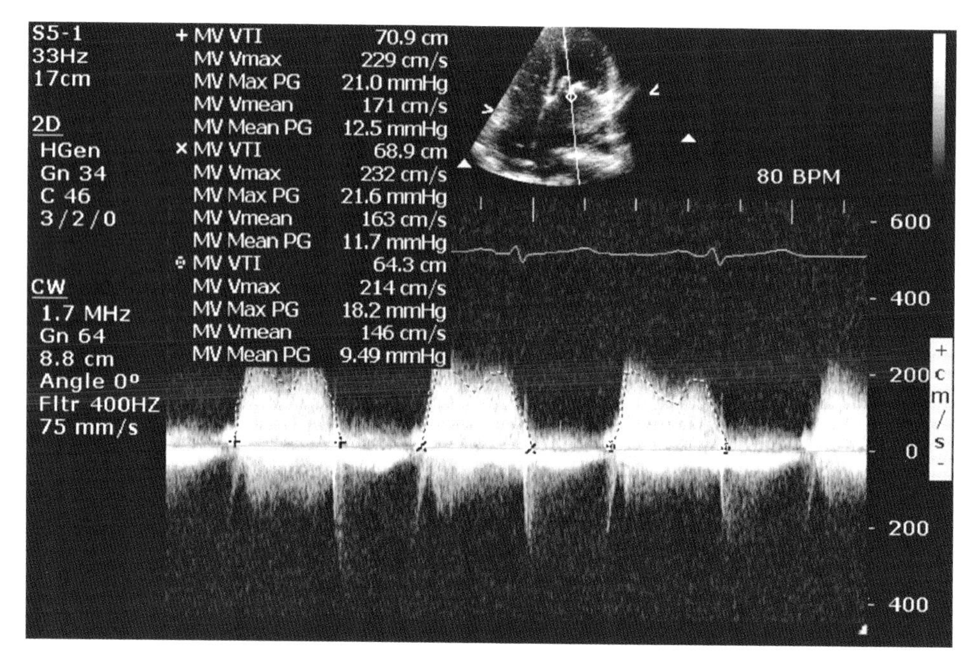

FIGURE 10-10 A continuous-wave Doppler echocardiogram through the mitral valve, showing mean gradient of 10 to 11 mm Hg consistent with moderate-to-severe mitral stenosis.

Balloon valvuloplasty has been performed safely during pregnancy for symptomatic relief and has allowed continuation of the pregnancy with good neonatal and maternal outcomes in several small series. However, the long-term efficacy of balloon valvuloplasty is low and in several case reports, valve replacement was eventually necessary in the midterm. Aortic regurgitation is a contraindication for balloon valvuloplasty and the decision regarding balloon valvuloplasty during pregnancy should be made in conjunction with a pediatric interventional cardiologist, who has extensive experience performing aortic valvuloplasties. Severe aortic stenosis is typically not well tolerated during pregnancy due to the increase in blood volume across the fixed obstruction. Patients with severe aortic stenosis, regardless of symptoms, should be counseled against pregnancy until their underlying valvular disease is addressed.

Patients with congenital aortic valve abnormalities frequently have an aortopathy associated with their valvular disease, which is unrelated to the severity of stenosis. Therefore, all patients with aortic valve disease contemplating pregnancy should have their aorta imaged prior to pregnancy with either an MRI or CT scan. A noncontrast MRI can be safely performed during pregnancy and provides useful information regarding aortic size. Patients with connective tissue disorders, such as Marfan syndrome are at high risk for aortic dissection during pregnancy likely related to vascular changes that occur during pregnancy. This risk is further increased with a vaginal delivery due to increased aortic wall stress with pushing. In these patients, an ascending aortic dimension of more than 4 cm is an indication for elective C-section. In addition, any patient who has a rapid change in their aortic size by more than 1 cm during pregnancy are at risk for dissection due to aortic instability and should undergo a C-section.

Patients with congenital aortic stenosis and/or connective tissue disorders should undergo genetic counseling as part of their routine prenatal care as well as a fetal echocardiogram around 24 to 28 weeks' gestation to assess for any structural abnormalities.

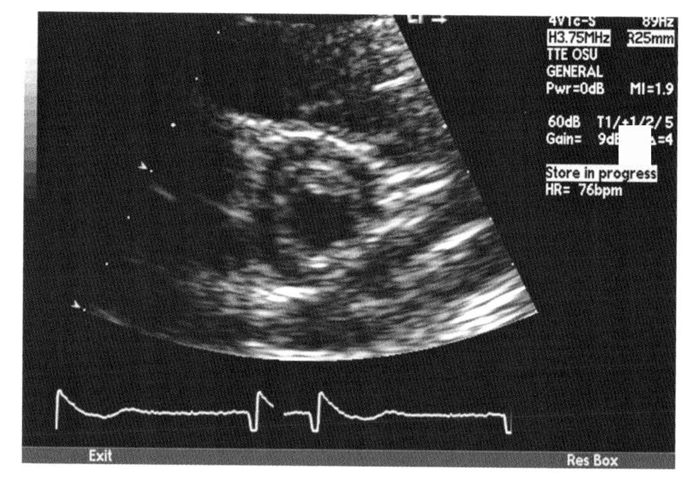

FIGURE 10-11 A two-dimensional echocardiogram, parasternal short-axis view through aortic valve showing classic "fish mouth" opening of a bicuspid aortic valve.

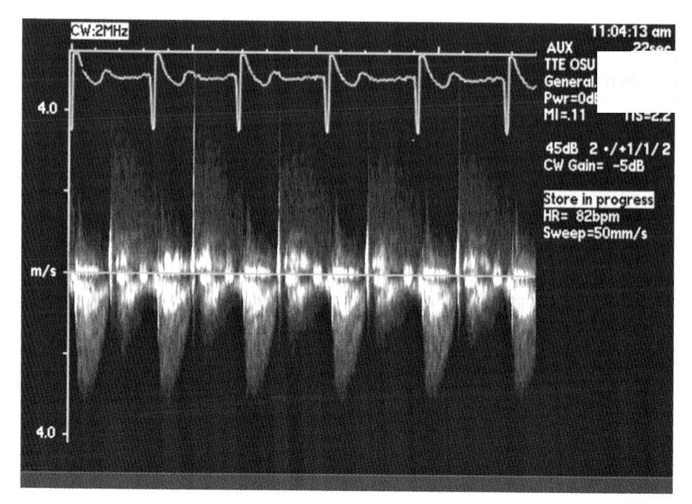

FIGURE 10-12 A continuous-wave Doppler echocardiogram through aortic valve showing both moderate aortic stenosis and regurgitation.

PULMONIC STENOSIS

Pulmonic stenosis is typically well tolerated during pregnancy as the increased blood volume of pregnancy helps maintain forward flow through the pulmonic valve. Right ventricular function does play a role in both maternal and fetal outcomes as patients with right ventricular dysfunction are at risk for volume overload potential requiring medial therapy. In patients who have undergone intervention on the pulmonary valve, there is a risk for arrhythmias that warrants periodic Holter monitoring to evaluate any significant arrhythmias that may impact pregnancy or delivery. If patients are symptomatic during pregnancy, balloon valvuloplasty may be indicated.

Patients with pulmonic stenosis that are minimally symptomatic may undergo either a vaginal delivery or C-section as indicated from an obstetrical standpoint. They do not typically require invasive hemodynamic monitoring during labor and delivery, although if there are concerns about volume issues, then more invasive monitoring may be necessary.

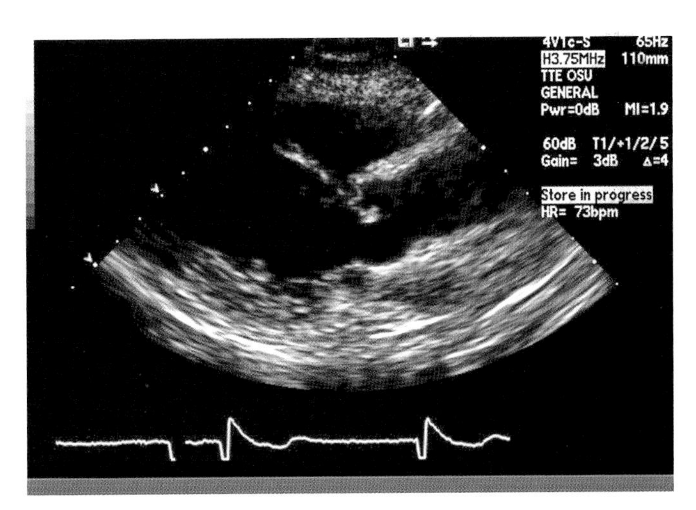

FIGURE 10-13 A two-dimensional echocardiogram, parasternal long-axis view, showing dilatation of the proximal ascending aorta.

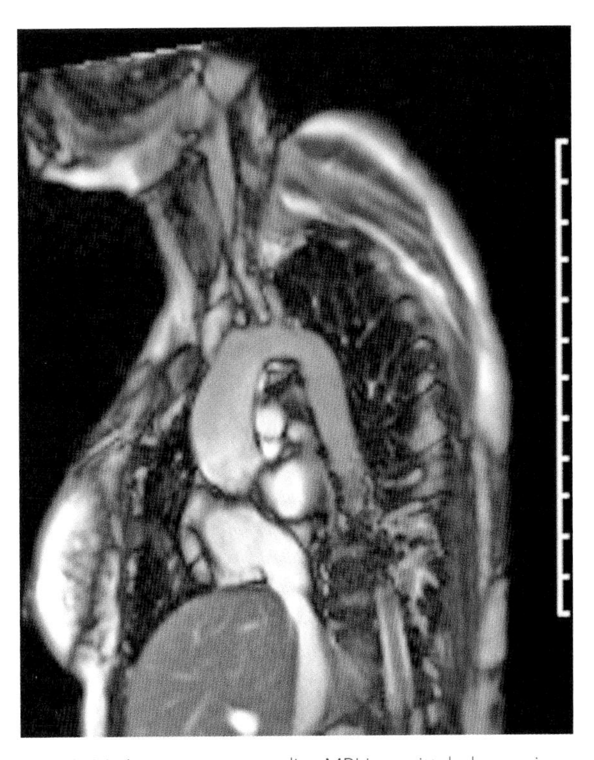

FIGURE 10-14 A noncontrast cardiac MRI in sagittal plane using real-time imaging showing ascending aortic dilatation, no evidence of dissection, and normal-caliber descending aorta.

REGURGITANT LESIONS

In general, regurgitant lesions are better tolerated than stenotic lesions during pregnancy. However, because of the increased blood and plasma volume associated with pregnancy, a majority of these patients will have worsening of the regurgitation noted by echocardiogram. This may not necessarily manifest clinically and, if patients remain symptomatic, then no further treatment or intervention is indicated. Reassessment of the valvular disease in a nonpregnant state 3 to 6 months postpartum can be useful to determine if further cardiovascular monitoring is necessary in the long term. If patients do become symptomatic, treatment with gentle diuresis can provide symptomatic relief, although these should be used judiciously due to potential fetal effects. Patients with regurgitant valvular disease can typically undergo a vaginal delivery without invasive hemodynamic monitoring unless there is coexisting ventricular dysfunction or other associated congenital lesions.

"SIMPLE" CONGENITAL LESIONS

CASE 6

A 40-year-old G5P4 woman presents at 28 weeks of gestation, complaining of palpitations and shortness of breath. Her previous 4 pregnancies were uncomplicated and resulted in normal vaginal delivery of healthy babies. On physical examination, she is in no acute distress. There are normal carotid upstrokes and jugular venous pulsations, quiet precordium, normal first heart sound, fixed split second heart sound, grade II/VI short, systolic ejection murmur along mid-right sternal border, and no gallops or rubs noted. Electrocardiogram shows sinus rhythm with an incomplete right bundle branch block and rightward axis (Figure 10-15). Because of her symptoms and an abnormal RCG, an echocardiogram was done (Figures 10-16 through 10-19). An event monitor was placed showing isolated premature atrial and ventricular complexes and no significant atrial arrhythmias.

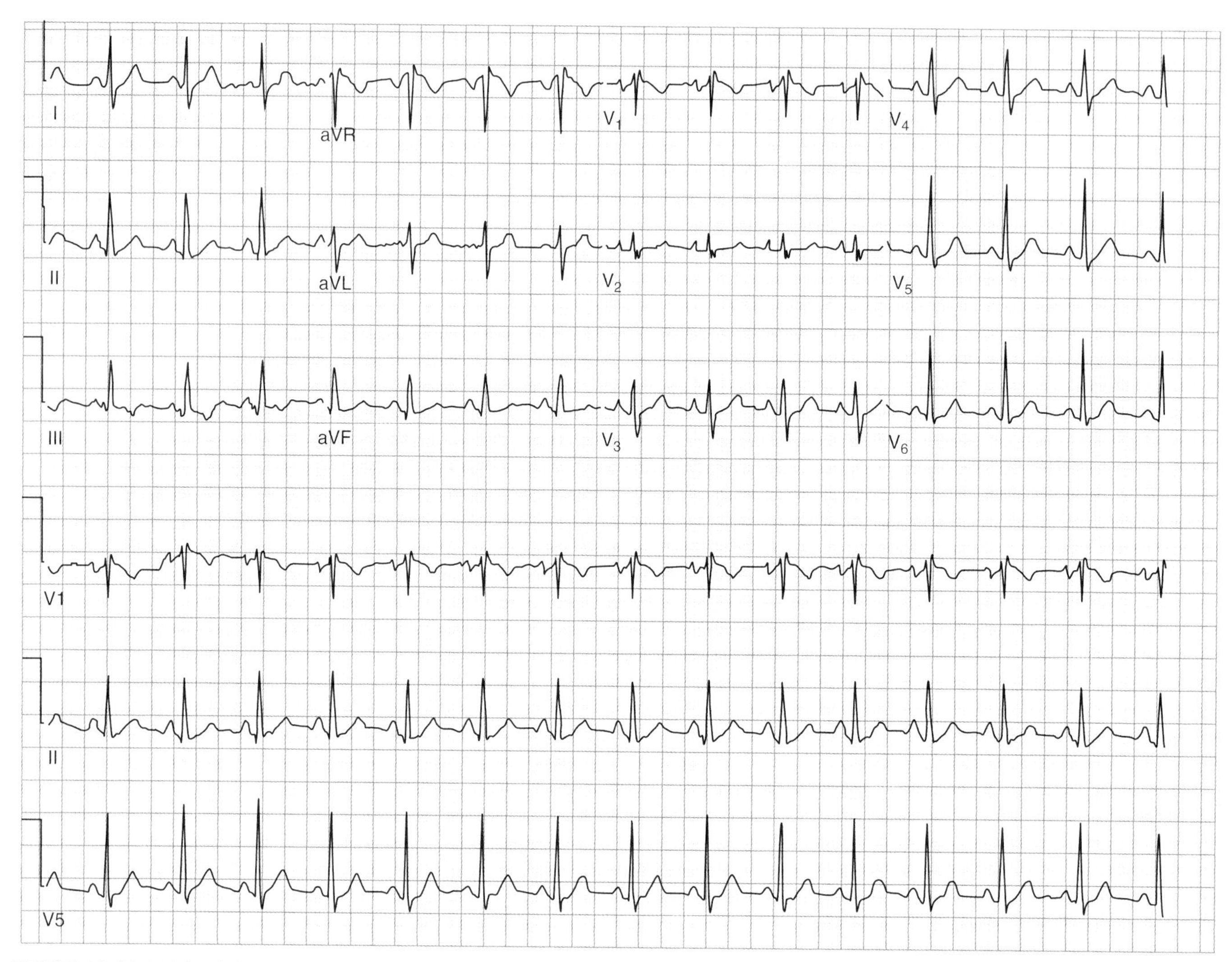

FIGURE 10-15 A 12-lead electrocardiogram showing sinus rhythm, RSR′ in V_1.

The patient was started on aspirin 81 mg daily based on her echocardiogram findings and underwent an elective repeat C-section at 39 weeks' gestation. Six months postpartum, she underwent elective percutaneous ASD device closure.

ATRIAL SEPTAL DEFECTS

Atrial septal defects (ASDs) are the most common congenital heart lesion diagnosed in adults. An ASD occurs when there is a communication between the left and right atria along the interatrial septum. There are 5 types of ASDs depending on where in the septum the defect is located. The types of ASDs are: secundum ASD, primum ASD, sinus venosus ASD, coronary sinus ASD, and a patent foramen ovale. Although the physiology of the ASD is similar regardless of the location of the defect, the long-term effects and outcomes of the various defects are different. Normally, left atrial pressure is higher than right atrial pressure, and as such, oxygenated blood flows from the left atrium to the right atrium. Isolated ASDs are usually asymptomatic. However, if pulmonary blood flow is significantly greater than systemic blood flow (ratio ≥2:1), most patients eventually become symptomatic. Manifestations of ASDs in adulthood include atrial arrhythmias, embolic events such as TIA/CVA or embolic coronary

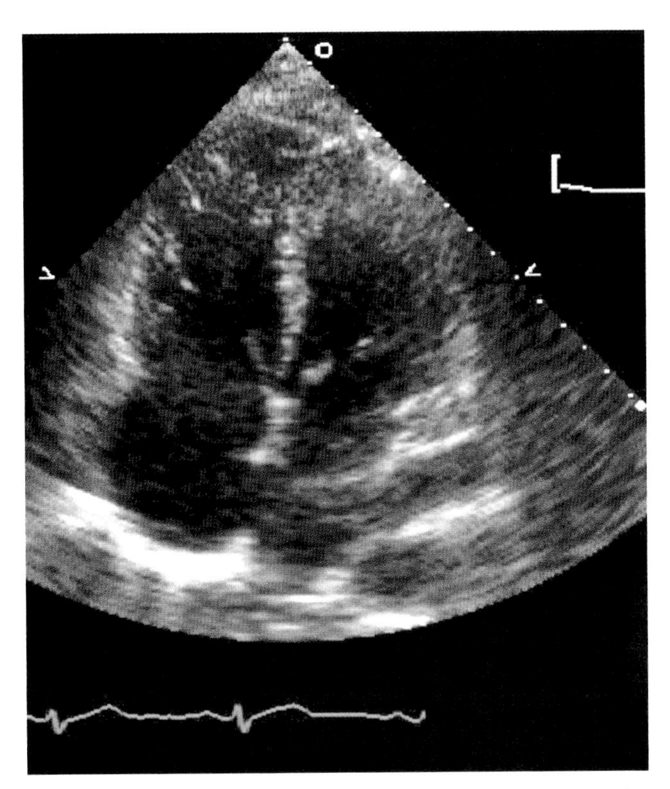

FIGURE 10-16 A two-dimensional echocardiogram showing apical 4-chamber view. Note right ventricular and right atrial enlargement as well as moderate-sized defect within the midportion of the atrial septum.

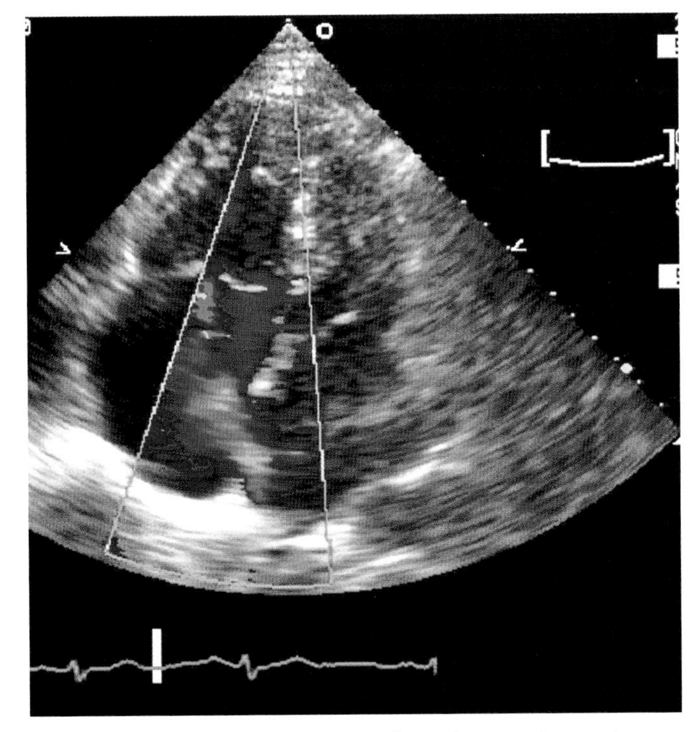

FIGURE 10-17 A color flow Doppler echocardiogram showing large color jet consistent with left-to-right shunting across the atrial septum.

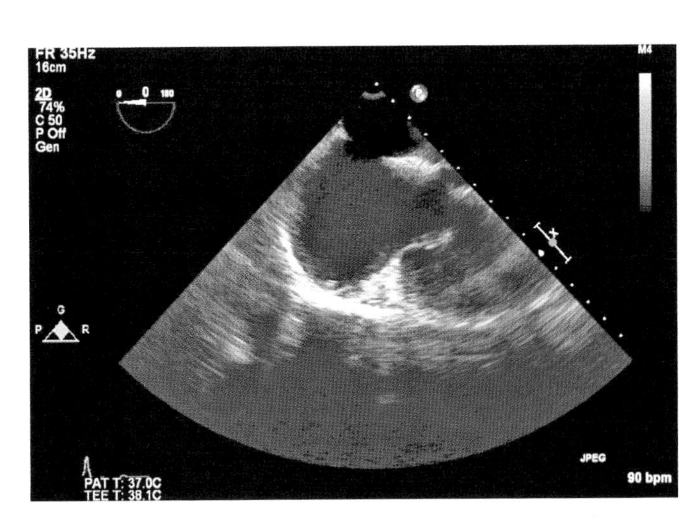

FIGURE 10-18 A two-dimensional transesophageal echocardiogram confirming presence of moderate-to-large-sized secundum atrial septal defect. Note the presence of both inferior and superior "rims" of defect that is important in planning for percutaneous versus surgical closure.

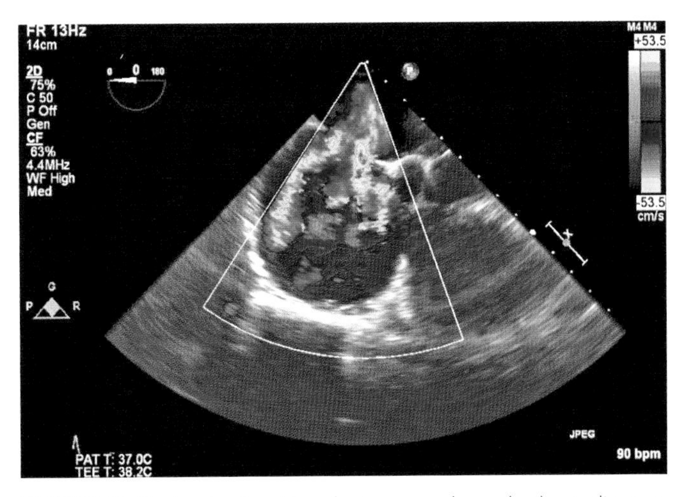

FIGURE 10-19 A color flow Doppler transesophageal echocardiogram showing broad jet of color flow across defect consistent with left-to-right shunting.

events due to paradoxical embolization, and signs of right-sided heart failure such as dyspnea, peripheral edema, and/or decreased exercise tolerance due to right ventricular enlargement and dysfunction. Severe manifestations include pulmonary hypertension and Eisenmenger syndrome, although this is rare in patients with isolated secundum ASDs.

In spite of the increased blood volume, pregnancy is usually well tolerated by most women with ASDs. Hemodynamically significant shunts should ideally be repaired before pregnancy. In pregnant women with an unrepaired ASD who develop refractory symptoms uncontrolled by medications, catheter-based closure may be considered, preferably under echocardiographic guidance to minimize radiation exposure. Although pregnancy is a prothrombotic state, ASD repair to prevent paradoxical embolization is not recommended. However, measures to prevent venous stasis, such as the use of compression stockings, should be implemented. All pregnant patients with intracardiac shunting should, at a minimum, be started on aspirin 81 mg daily to decrease the risk of embolic events. In cases of prolonged immobilization, heparin may be used for prophylaxis. Intravenous (IV) filters are also recommended to decrease the risk of systemic air embolization.

Pregnancy is contraindicated in patients with atrial septal defects who have developed severe pulmonary hypertension or Eisenmenger syndrome which is considered a contraindication to pregnancy with a maternal mortality rate of approximately 50%. Most patients with atrial septal defects, repaired on unrepaired, may undergo a vaginal delivery. A majority of these patients will not require any monitoring at the time of delivery, although need for monitoring may be individualized to the patient based on clinical symptoms.

VENTRICULAR SEPTAL DEFECTS

Ventricular septal defects (VSDs) are the most common congenital heart defects at birth, but as many as 75% will close spontaneously in childhood. Most VSDs that do not close spontaneously are detected in childhood and repaired. As such, unrepaired VSDs are relatively rare in pregnancy.

Repaired VSDs without residual intracardiac shunting or very small, unrepaired VSDs that are hemodynamically insignificant generally do not carry any increased maternal risk. Unrepaired moderate and large-sized VSDs may lead to atrial enlargement and ventricular volume overload. A majority of these patients will develop pulmonary arterial hypertension (PAH) by the time they reach adulthood. Progressive PAH may lead to right ventricular pressures that reach systemic pressures and lead to reversal of the direction of shunt flow, called Eisenmenger syndrome. Eisenmenger syndrome results in chronic cyanosis and is considered a contraindication to pregnancy with mortality rates reaching 50% during pregnancy.

As with ASDs, hemodynamically significant VSDs should ideally be repaired before pregnancy. If not diagnosed before pregnancy, repair should be delayed until after delivery, unless the patient is clinically deteriorating and developing complications such as heart failure or pulmonary hypertension. Spontaneous vaginal delivery without cardiac monitoring is usually appropriate for uncomplicated or repaired VSDs.

CASE 7

A 32-year-old G1P1 woman, who had undergone a patch repair for coarctation of the aorta in childhood, presents for prepregnancy cardiovascular evaluation. She is currently asymptomatic from a cardiovascular standpoint. On physical examination, she has normal carotid upstrokes and jugular venous pulsations. She has a quiet precordium with a well-healed left lateral thoracotomy scar. There are normal first and second heart sounds and grade II/VI harsh systolic murmur noted in posterior lung fields. No diastolic murmurs, gallops, or rubs are noted. 2+ femoral pulses with minimal brachiofemoral delay were found. An echocardiogram and cardiac MRI/MRA were performed (Figures 10-20 through 10-23).

COARCTATION OF THE AORTA

Coarctation of the aorta refers to a narrowing of the aorta that most often occurs distal to the left subclavian artery in the thoracic aorta, but may also occur proximal to the left subclavian artery, or in the abdominal aorta. It may occur in isolation, or in association with other congenital abnormalities. The most common coexisting lesion is a bicuspid aortic valve. The classic presenting sign in adults is hypertension. Other physical examination findings include differential blood pressure in the upper and lower extremities, and a pulse delay in the lower extremities. Long-term complications of coarctation, regardless of repair, include early atherosclerosis and systemic hypertension compared to control subjects.

Pregnancy is typically well tolerated in women with repaired coarctation, but these women are still at increased risk of hypertensive disorders and miscarriages. Blood pressure should be monitored closely and hypertension should be treated appropriately. Care should also be taken to prevent hypotension and placental hypoperfusion. Because the aorta of patients with coarctation is abnormal, these patients are at risk for aortic dilatation due to the physiologic effects of pregnancy on systemic vascular resistance and should have periodic imaging of the aorta during pregnancy, typically with either echo or noncontrast MRI. If a pregnant patient with coarcation of the aorta presents with symptoms concerning aortic dissection, more definitive imaging with contrast CT scan would be indicated.

Pregnant women with unrepaired coarctation or re-coarctation may undergo percutaneous treatment during pregnancy if their hypertension cannot be controlled with medical therapy, keeping in mind that the risk of dissection is higher during pregnancy.

Vaginal delivery with epidural anesthesia is preferred; however, if there is any concern for aortic instability, C-section should be considered.

"COMPLEX" CONGENTIAL LESIONS

CASE 8

A 28-year-old G1P0 woman with tetralogy of Fallot, who had undergone a complete repair at age 2 consisting of VSD closure and right ventricular outflow tract (RVOT) patch presents at 10 weeks' gestation for cardiac evaluation. She is currently asymptomatic from a cardiovascular standpoint with good functional capacity, NYHA class I. On physical examination, there are normal carotid upstrokes and jugular venous pulsation, mild right ventricular lift, single first and second heart sounds, grade II/VI harsh, short, systolic ejection murmur along upper right sternal border and grade III/VI early diastolic murmur in same area. No gallops were noted and an echocardiogram is performed (Figures 10-24 through 10-26).

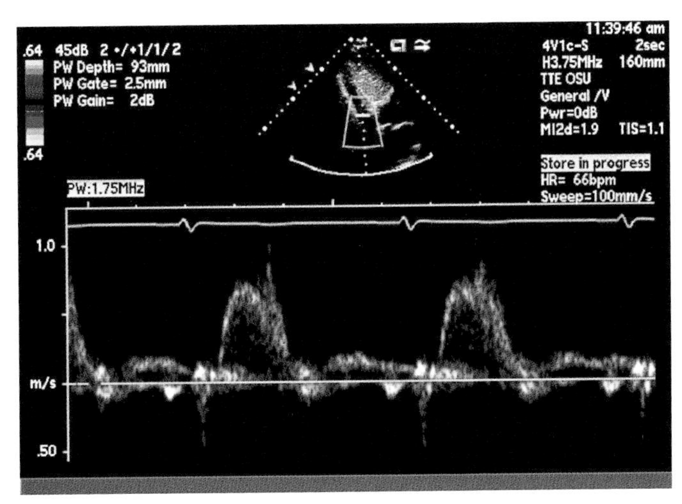

FIGURE 10-20 A pulse-wave Doppler echocardiogram through the descending aorta showing normal aortic pulsatility, which suggests that coarctation site is patent without severe restenosis.

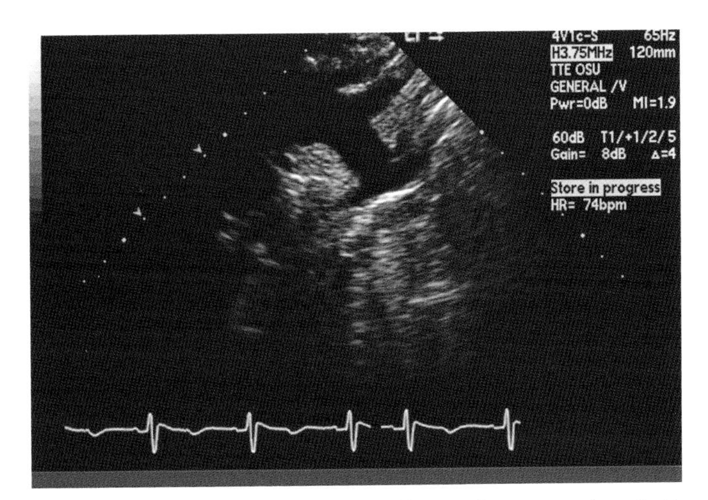

FIGURE 10-21 A two-dimensional echocardiogram showing suprasternal notch view of patent aortic arch. Note narrowing in proximal descending aorta just beyond subclavian artery, which is likely the site of previous coarctation repair.

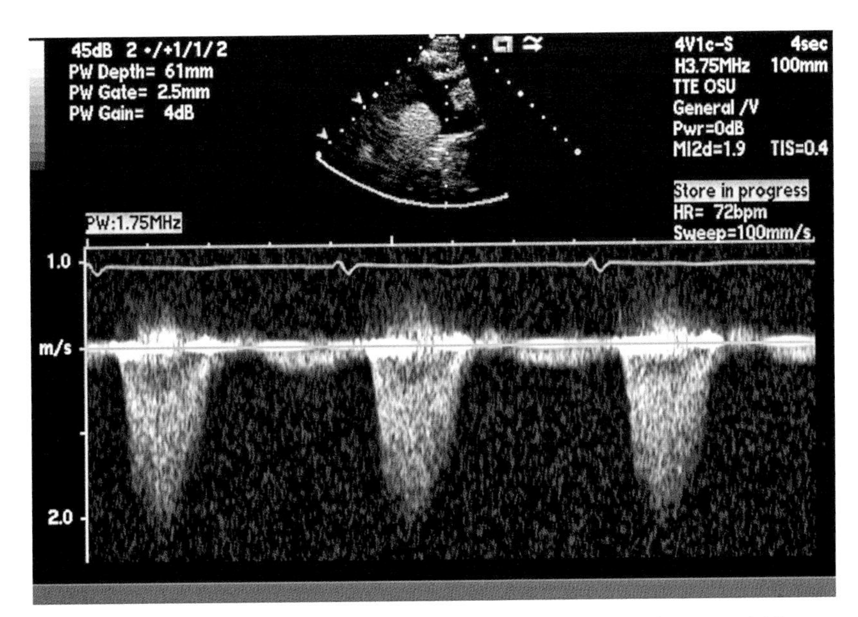

FIGURE 10-22 A continuous-wave Doppler echocardiogram through proximal descending aorta showing mild-flow acceleration across coarctation site with a velocity of just over 2 m/s.

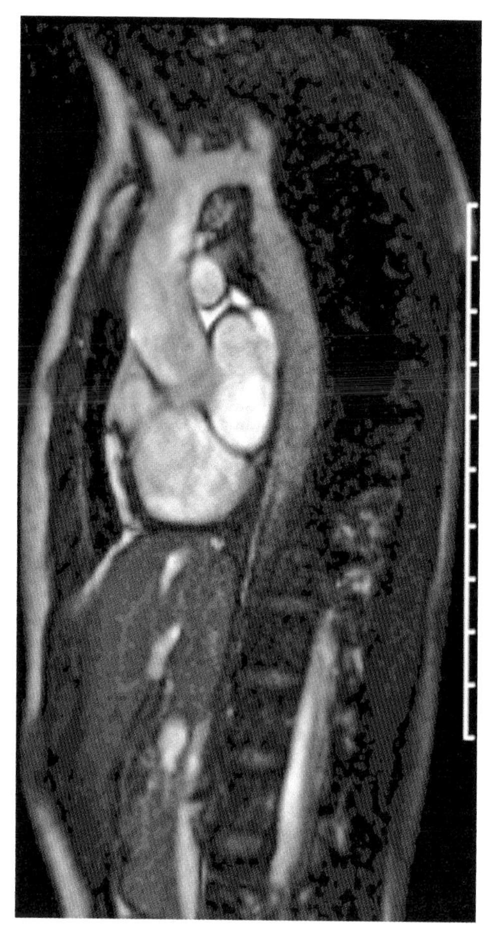

FIGURE 10-23 A noncontrast MRI showing mild narrowing just distal to left subclavian artery at site of previous repair.

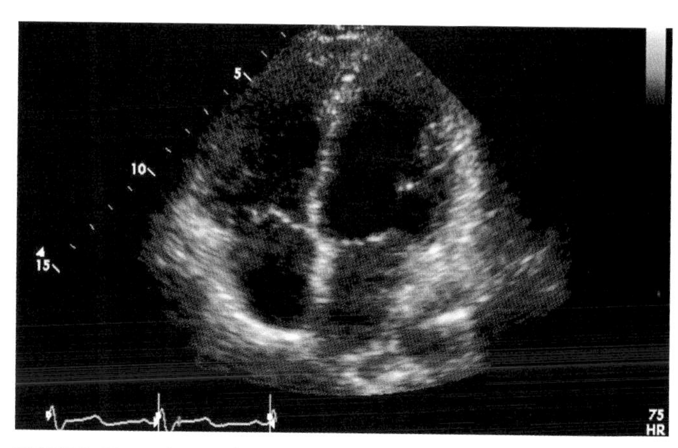

FIGURE 10-24 A two-dimensional echocardiogram, apical view. Note right ventricular enlargement and hypertrophy, intact ventricular septum.

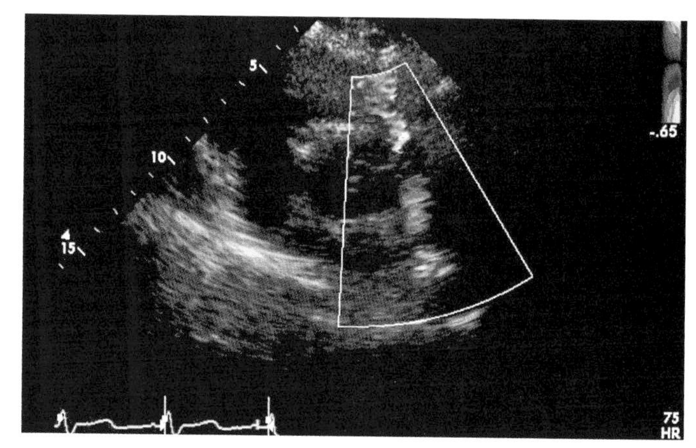

FIGURE 10-25 A color Doppler echocardiogram, parasternal short-axis view of pulmonary artery shows severe (free) pulmonic regurgitation.

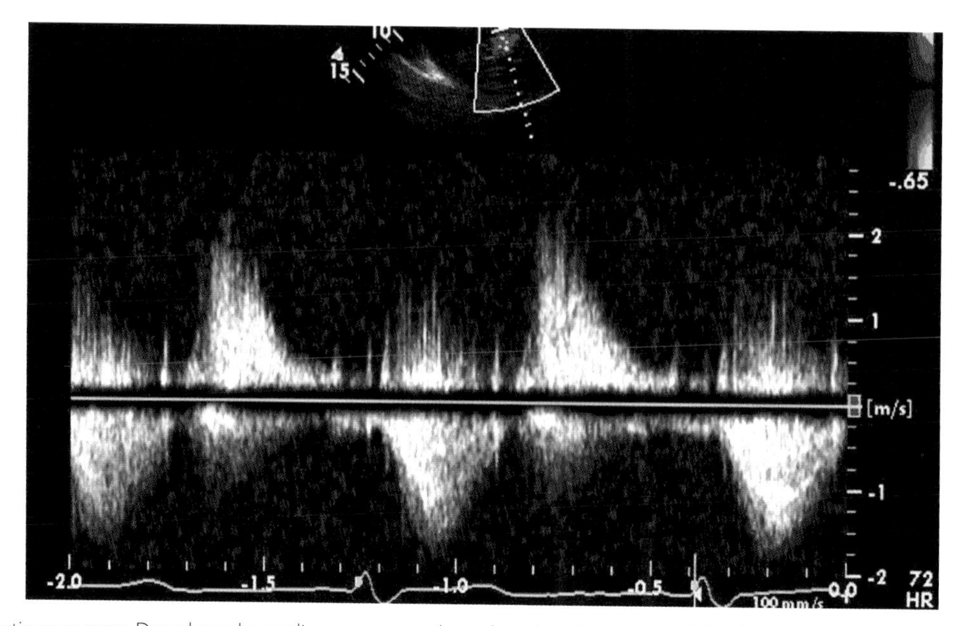

FIGURE 10-26 A continuous-wave Doppler echocardiogram across the pulmonic valve shows mild-pulmonic stenosis with severe regurgitation.

The patient remained asymptomatic throughout her pregnancy and underwent a vaginal delivery at 39 weeks gestation, which was uncomplicated. She was monitored on telemetry during labor and delivery, but did not require invasive cardiac monitoring.

TETRALOGY OF FALLOT

Tetralogy of Fallot is the most common cyanotic congenital heart lesion occurring in 2 to 5 per 10,000 live births. Tetralogy of Fallot consists of a perimembranous ventricular septal defect, pulmonic stenosis, overriding aorta, and right ventricular hypertrophy. Timing of surgical intervention is dependent on the amount of pulmonary blood flow. In patients with severe pulmonic stenosis, initial surgical palliation will occur within the first few weeks of life and typically consists of some type of pulmonary-to-systemic shunt, such as a Blalock-Taussig shunt. Definitive repair most commonly occurs between 18 months and 3 years of age and consists of VSD closure and relief of RVOT obstruction. Relief of RVOT obstruction may be performed via right ventricular patch arterioplasty, which results in severe pulmonic regurgitation or with placement of a right ventricular-to-pulmonary artery conduit. Current 20-year survival rates for tetralogy of Fallot exceed 90%.

Long-term complications of tetralogy of Fallot repair include right ventricular dilatation and/or dysfunction due to long-standing pulmonic regurgitation, residual pulmonary stenosis or regurgitation depending on type of repair, and arrhythmias. Pregnancy outcomes are dependent on the severity of the residual valvular disease, right ventricular dysfunction, history of previous cardiac events, and functional status. In patients with good functional status, preserved right ventricular function and no previous history of adverse cardiovascular events, pregnancy is typically well tolerated. Recommendations regarding pregnancy, labor, and delivery need to be individualized based on the patient's underlying residual defects.

Transposition of the Great Arteries and Single Ventricle Physiology (Fontan)

Patients with more complex congenital heart disease such as transposition of the great arteries, lesions which result in single ventricular physiology, or Eisenmenger syndrome are at significant risk for cardiovascular complications which may affect both maternal and fetal outcomes. These patients should be cared for by a multidisciplinary team consisting of cardiologists with expertise in adult congenital heart disease, high-risk obstetricians, and both obstetric and cardiac anesthesiology.[8] Delivery should occur in a tertiary care center with active involvement by all the necessary subspecialists.[6]

CARDIOVASCULAR DRUGS AND PREGNANCY

Many drugs used for cardiovascular disease have not been extensively studied in pregnant women. Certain medications which are the mainstays of treatment for coronary artery disease, cardiomyopathies, hyperlipidemia, and arrhythmias are contraindicated in pregnancy. It is important to address this issue with all women of childbearing age even if they are not pregnant or planning to become pregnant. Table 10-4 lists common classes of cardiovascular medications and their fetal effects.

Special consideration needs to be given to warfarin (Coumadin), especially for patients with mechanical valves. In the past, warfarin (Coumadin) was absolutely contraindicated for pregnancy and patients who conceived while on this drug were given the option of elective termination. Warfarin crosses the placenta and results in "warfarin embryopathy". The fetal effects of warfarin (Coumadin) include cartilage abnormalities, bone stippling, small, hypoplastic nose, optic atrophy, seizures, and mental retardation. The effects of warfarin (Coumadin) primarily occur between 8 and 11 weeks' gestation. No fetal effects have been reported if the drug is stopped prior to 8 weeks' gestation. The fetal effects appear to be dose dependent and some studies have suggested that these effects are substantially less on doses <5 mg daily.

Warfarin (Coumadin) is accepted to be safe during the second trimester. There is some concern about its use in the third trimester related to immature fetal liver function. Current ACC/AHA guidelines with regards to warfarin (Coumadin) therapy for mechanical valves recommend that the drug be used after 12 weeks' gestation and discontinued at 36 weeks' gestation at which time the patient should be transitioned to intravenous heparin in anticipation of delivery. Should a patient go into labor while on warfarin (Coumadin), a C-section is recommended due to the risk of fetal intracranial bleeding. Postpartum, if there are no significant bleeding issues, heparin should be restarted 4 to 6 hours after delivery in addition to warfarin. The guidelines are less clear as to recommendations during the first trimester when the risk for embryopathy is the highest. It is recommended that patients be given the option of continuing warfarin (Coumadin) versus transitioning to heparin, realizing that there is increased risk of valve thrombosis and bleeding with heparin. In patients who elect to transition to heparin, they should be started on unfractionated heparin IV until they are reinitiated on warfarin (Coumadin). If low-molecular weight heparin is used, Factor Xa levels should be followed; however, there is little data to support the use of low-molecular weight heparin for mechanical valves and patients should be extensively counseled on the potential risk of valve thrombosis.

SUMMARY

Due to advancements in the care of patients with congenital heart disease and women postponing pregnancy until older ages, cardiovascular disease has become one of the major causes of nonobstetric maternal mortality in the western world. Because of this, it has become imperative that cardiologists have an adequate understanding of the normal physiologic changes of pregnancy and their effects on the cardiovascular system in both healthy and diseased states. Management of these patients require a multidisciplinary approach involving high-risk obstetricians, cardiologists with expertise in both pregnancy and adult congenital heart disease, and anesthesiologists in order to optimize both maternal and fetal outcomes.

TABLE 10-4 Cardiovascular drugs and pregnancy

Drug Class	Indications	Fetal Effects	Drug Name and Safety Class
β-blockers	Supraventricular or ventricular arrhythmias, hypertension, cardiomyopathies	Intrauterine growth restriction (IUGR), bradycardia, apnea, hypoglycemia	Sotalol B (reserved for treatment of arrhythmias) Metoprolol C Labetalol C Propranolol C Atenolol D (has been associated with fetal demise)
Calcium channel blockers	Supraventricular arrhythmias, hypertension	Generally safe although tocolytic effects require discontinuation in third trimester	C
Diuretics	Congestive heart failure, pulmonary edema, hypertension	Uteroplacental insufficiency, hypoglycemia, hypokalemia, hyperuricemia, hyponatremia, thrombocytopenia	C
ACE-inhibitors/ARB	Cardiomyopathies, hypertension	Renal anomalies, oligohydramnios, IUGR, hypotension, anemia, limb and skull abnormalities, fetal demise	D
Warfarin (Coumadin)	Anticoagulation	Embryopathy, CNS effects, seizures, fetal hemorrhage	X in first trimester, may be safely used in second and third trimester
Aspirin	Antiplatelet agent	Generally safe at low doses, higher doses have been associated with IUGR, CNS anomalies	No formal class assigned
Clopidogrel (Plavix)	Antiplatelet agent	Generally safe	B
Statins	Hyperlipidemia	Paucity of data, effects are at cellular level in the first trimester. Placental abnormalities, CNS and limb abnormalities have been reported	X
Amiodarone	Supraventricular and ventricular arrhythmias	Thyroid disorders (hypo- or hyperthyroid), IUGR, transient bradycardia, prolonged QT	D
Adenosine	Supraventricular arrhythmias	Generally safe	C
Digoxin	Supraventricular arrhythmias, symptomatic heart failure	Generally safe, used to treat fetal arrhythmias	C
Nitrates	Coronary artery disease, cardiomyopathies in conjunction with hydralazine	Generally safe	C
Hydralazine	Hypertension, cardiomyopathies	Generally safe	C

REFERENCES

1. Siu S, et al. Prospective multicenter study of pregnancy outcomes in women with heart disease. *Circulation.* 2001;104:515-521.
2. Drenthen W, et al. Predictors of pregnancy complications in women with congenital heart disease. *Eur Heart J.* 2010;31:2124-2132.
3. Koul AK, et al. Coronary artery dissection during pregnancy and the postpartum period. *Cathet Cardiovasc Intervent.* 2001;52:88-94.
4. Siu SC, Coleman JM. Heart disease and pregnancy. *Heart.* 2001;85:710-715.
5. Oakley C, Warnes CA, eds. *Heart Disease in Pregnancy.* 2nd ed. Malden, MA: Blackwell Publishing; 2007.
6. Roos-Hesselin JW, et al. Outcome of pregnancy in patients with structural or ischaemic heart disease: results of a registry of the european sociate of cardiology. Eur Heart J. 2013;34:657-665.
7. Opotowsky AR, et al. Maternal cardiovascular events during childbirth among women with congenital heart disease. *Heart.* 2012;98:145-151.
8. Khairy P, et al. Pregnancy outcomes in women with congenital heart disease. *Circulation.* 2006;113:517-524.

11 ARTERIAL VASCULAR DISEASE IN WOMEN

Jean Starr, MD, FACS, RPVI

Peripheral arterial disease (PAD) in women is an under-recognized, understudied, and undertreated disorder. The magnitude of this problem can be realized from the fact that 21% to 67% of documented symptoms or diagnoses upon admission in nursing home residents are consistent with PAD.[1] Nearly 75% to 90% of nursing home residents are women, aged 65 years or older. PAD may therefore be a large contributor to disability in this population. Adding to the problem is the fact that 48% of women aged 65 to 75 years live alone, without readily available, adequate support at home, potentially resulting in the need for an extended care facility. Therefore, it seems it would be in society's best interest, in terms of costs and disability, to prevent, identify, treat, and better study PAD in women.

Women are obviously different from men in terms of anatomy and physiology, but may also differ in terms of clinical presentation of disease states and response to treatment. In general, women tend to have smaller, less-compliant arteries, which may translate into the need for different devices and techniques to treat PAD. Even though less is known about the natural history of PAD in women, none can argue about the disability that it can cause across the genders. Cardiovascular disease is the number 1 cause of death in women and a recent survey showed only 50% of respondents understood this to be true.[2]

Women tend to be underrepresented in clinical studies, but it is unclear if lower prevalence of some subtypes of PAD contributes to this or if there is a true bias against including women. There are few studies aimed at PAD in women alone and fewer that perform significant subgroup analyses of PAD in women. We have yet to elicit whether there is a difference in vascular biology between the genders and whether women react differently to various treatments for vascular disease than men. There may be questions raised if physicians treat women with vascular disease differently than men. Herein, we will review the 3 major subtypes of PAD: carotid atherosclerotic disease (Figure 11-1), lower extremity arterial disease, and aneurysmal disease, specifically in women, with respect to biology, treatment, and outcome.

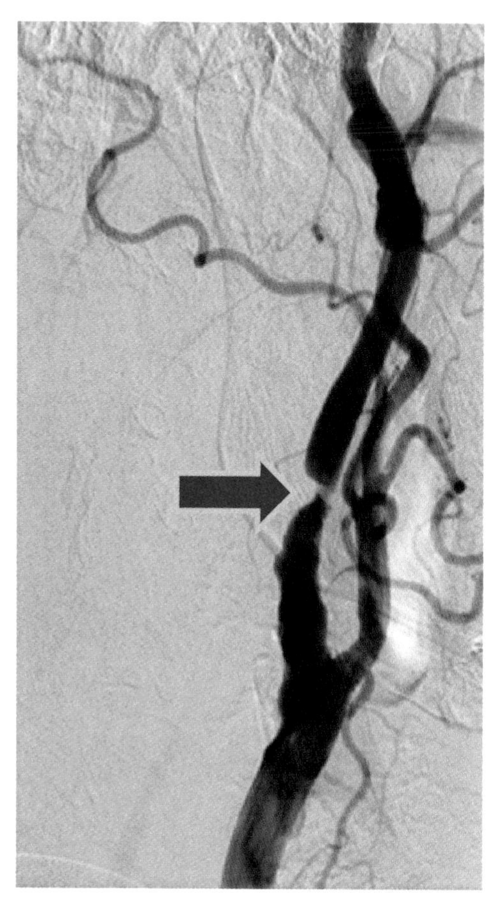

FIGURE 11-1 Carotid angiogram demonstrating severe, focal stenosis (arrow).

CAROTID ARTERY DISEASE

It may prove important to determine the difference between the genders in regards to carotid artery anatomy and physiology. In general, there are differences in carotid artery diameter between women and men from the age 25 years and onward.[3] Both genders, however, experience an increase in diameter as well as a decrease in compliance with age, which most likely contributes to the increased formation of atherosclerotic lesions later in life. In fact, a reduced compliance in women aged 45 to 60 years has been found when compared with men aged 60 to 70 years. Likewise, enlargement of carotid artery diameter with advancing age is less marked in women than in men.

These underlying anatomic differences may make women more vulnerable to increased arterial injury and hence, they may respond differently to traditional treatment therapies. It is unclear if there also exists a hemodynamic difference in women's arterial flow, which may also contribute to gender differences.

Different plaque composition may contribute to the tendency of a lesion to become symptomatic. Histological examinations of surgical specimen of women have suggested that women may possess more fibrous plaque, making it more stable than the more lipid-laden plaque of men[4] (Figure 11-2). MRI examination of plaque also demonstrated that men may possess a thinner or ruptured fibrous cap, have a higher degree of lipid in the core, and experience more subplaque hemorrhage than women[5] (Figure 11-3). In addition to these findings, women may have a lower concentration of inflammatory cells.[6] This may help explain the higher incidence of stroke in men <75 years, as these characteristics may be associated with symptomatic lesions.

In addition to vascular biology, differences may exist between the genders in terms of treatment outcome of carotid artery disease. Several large randomized, controlled trials have suggested this to be the case for both symptomatic and asymptomatic patients.[7-10] Women, in general, were found to have a higher operative risk for carotid endarterectomy (CEA) (Figure 11-4), but a lower risk from medical treatment, making some question the benefit of CEA in women. However, women tended to be underrepresented in these studies.

Data is conflicting as to whether women actually undergo CEA at a lower rate than men with similar degree of stenosis and symptomotology.[11-14] Since the randomized controlled studies cited previously in which women were not specifically studied, several large population studies, retrospective reviews, and database analyses have examined the role of gender in the outcomes after CEA in women versus men. These have shown that CEA can be safely performed in women without significant differences in perioperative stroke and mortality rates.[15-18] Long-term outcomes, including recurrence rates, were also found to be similar; therefore, the net benefit after CEA in women was found to be equivalent to men, whether symptomatic or asymptomatic. In fact, the typical longer life expectancy of women was maintained after CEA, supporting surgical management of carotid artery disease as an established treatment modality for women.[19] Truly, it is difficult to say if women are actually treated differently than men in clinical practice.

With the advent of carotid artery stenting (CAS) (Figure 11-5), there may be questions raised regarding the utility of this procedure in women who naturally have smaller, less-compliant arteries. In general, women as a subgroup were underrepresented in most of the large CAS trials.[20-22] In general, similar perioperative stroke rates after CAS were found in women and men, suggesting stenting to be a viable alternative to CEA in women. Other single-center series suggest the short-term complication rate, as well as long-term outcome after CAS, including restenosis, to be similar between men and women.[23,24] One might question whether stenting might turn out to be better suited for women, in order to avoid manipulating a small vessel and suturing it directly, with the concomitant trauma. Certainly, appropriately sized and designed stents for women may eventually yield better outcomes as well.

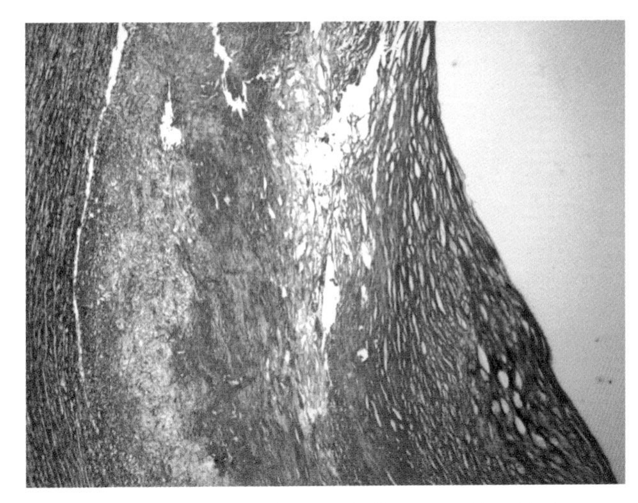

FIGURE 11-2 Combination plaque with fibrous and lipid-laden components.

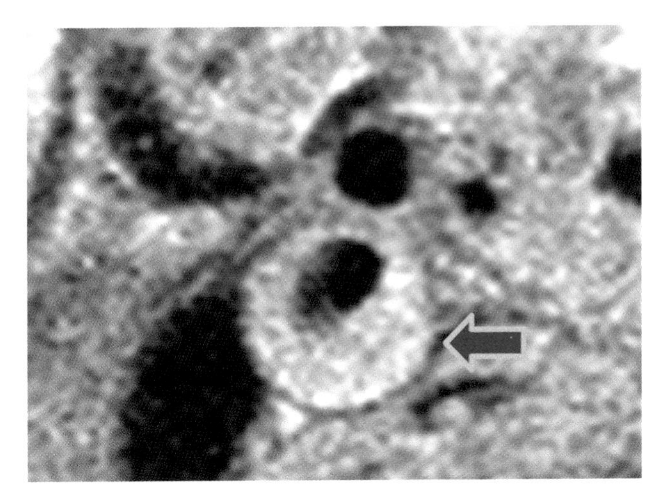

FIGURE 11-3 MRI cross-section of carotid artery with plaque (arrow).

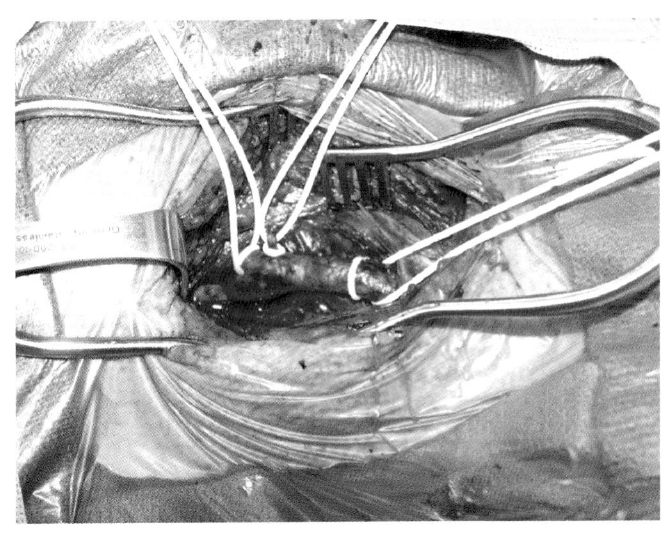

FIGURE 11-4 Surgical exposure of carotid artery in preparation for endarterectomy.

ABDOMINAL AORTIC ANEURYSM

In 2005, the US Preventative Task Force recommended that men aged 65 to 75, who have ever smoked, undergo a screening aortic duplex for abdominal aortic aneurysm (AAA) (Figure 11-6) upon entry into the Medicare program.[25] The Task Force recommended against primary aortic aneurysm screening for women. This recommendation was based on the decreased prevalence of AAA in women versus men and the theoretical increased risk to women undergoing such screening, who might sustain psychological injury or undergo increased number of surgeries with concomitant risks. These recommendations were based on only 4 studies outside of the United States and women were underrepresented in all of them. Any psychological side effects were found to be short lived.[26] Certainly, the prevalence of AAA in women is less than men, but the associations with smoking, age, and family history are similar.[27] Women also tended to have higher associated cerebrovascular disease prevalence. When screening women with multiple other atherosclerotic risk factors, the prevalence of AAA increased significantly, implying that routine AAA screening in women at risk seems justifiable, based on prevalence in this group.[28]

A higher percentage of women compared to men present with ruptured AAA,[29] and these aneurysms tend to rupture aortas in these women tend to rupture at a smaller size than men. In many studies, the 30-day and in-hospital mortality for women is significantly higher than men.[30,31] This may also be related to women being older at the time of presentation than men, with the concomitant increased comorbidities that often come with age.[32] These differences would also support the routine screening for AAA in women at risk; despite the lower prevalence, the increased morbidity and mortality for women specifically justifies identifying the problem in order to decrease the complications and other implications for society.

Modern AAA management involves offering patients open and/or endovascular repair (EVAR) (Figures 11-7 and 11-8). It has been found that endovascular AAA (Figure 11-9) repair lowers the complication rate and 30-day mortality for all-comers over open AAA repair. It is typically preferred by the patients because it results in a shortened hospital stay and recuperation period. Unfortunately, a lower proportion of women than men undergo endovascular repair.[33,34] Many factors may contribute to this discrepancy, including shorter, more angled aneurysm necks just below the renal arteries, where proximal fixation of an endograft is based (Figure 11-10). Women also tend to have smaller diameter iliac arteries with more calcification (Figure 11-11), which may prevent the introduction of a large bore endograft through a smaller access site and into the aorta without trauma to the vessels traversed (Figure 11-12). More EVARs are aborted in women than in men[35] and there is a higher intraoperative complication rate, often related to the need for iliac reconstruction after injury.[36] Despite potential intraoperative challenges, women and men have been found to have similar perioperative morbidity and mortality rates, supporting EVAR as a viable therapy for AAA in women.

With respect to open AAA repair, women with intact AAA tend to undergo repair less frequently than men and present at a more advanced age, in a condition that may be similar to those who have sustained rupture.[37] There may also be a higher inpatient mortality after open AAA in women.[30] While some have suggested women may exhibit a higher 5-year mortality (thought to be related to increased

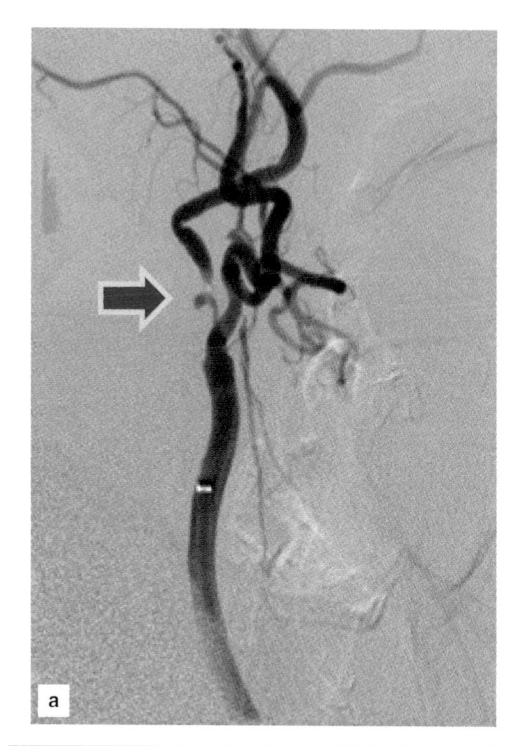

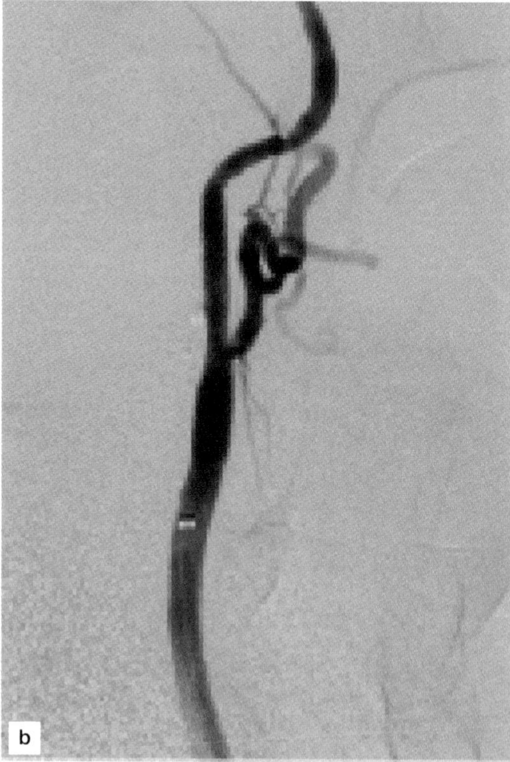

FIGURE 11-5 Carotid stent procedure. (A) Severe carotid stenosis (arrow). (B) After carotid stent placement.

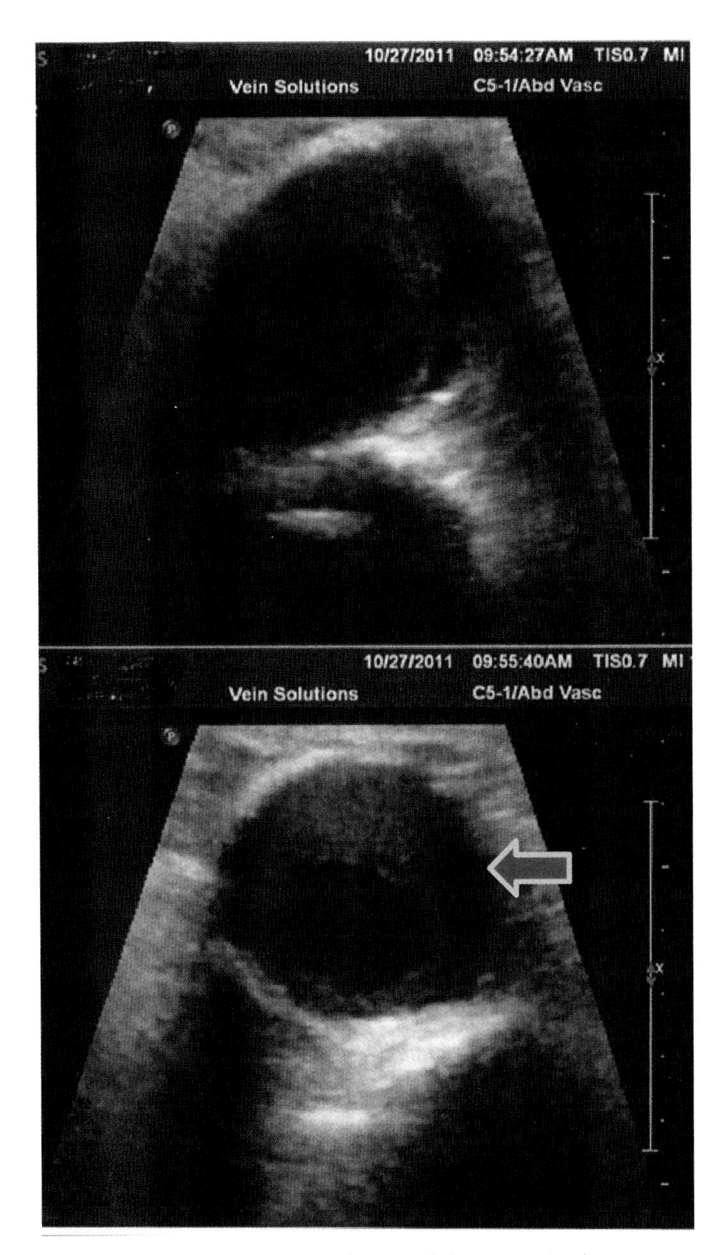

FIGURE 11-6 Transverse aortic ultrasound demonstrating large abdominal aortic aneurysm with thrombus (arrow).

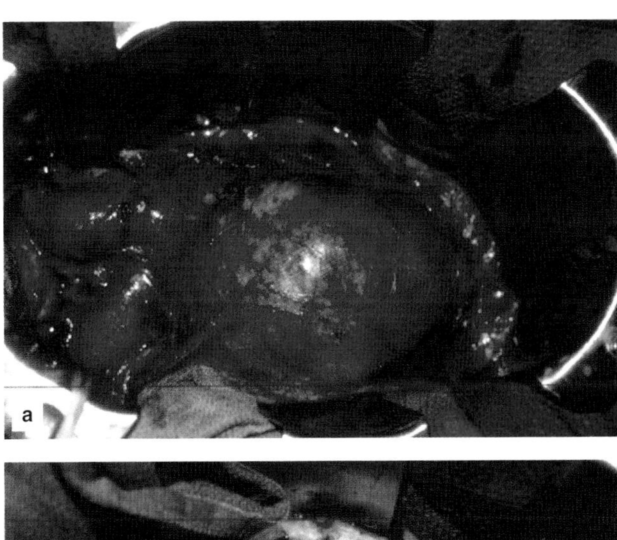

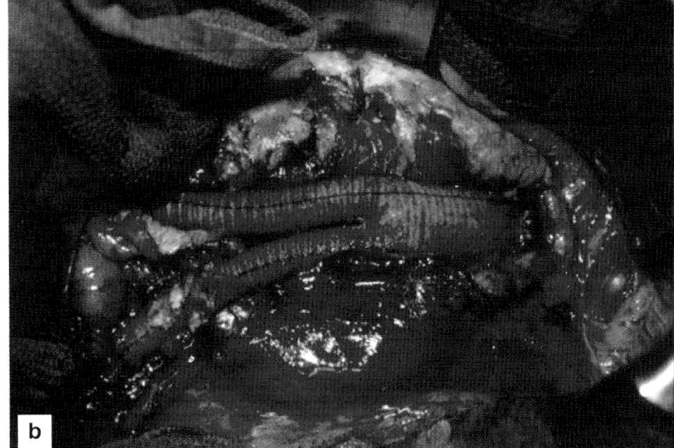

FIGURE 11-7 Open AAA repair. (A) AAA before repair. (B) Graft in place after repair.

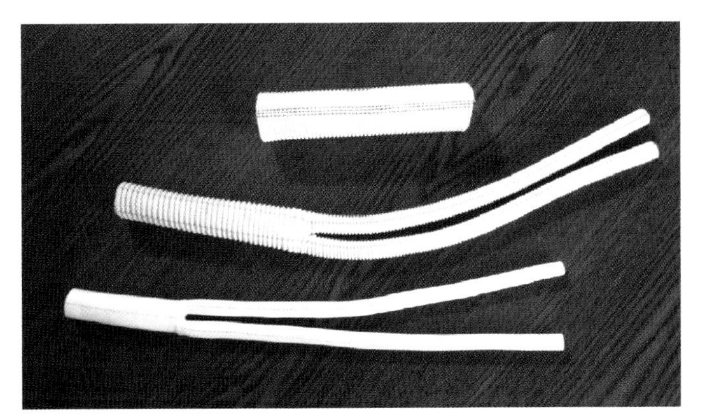

FIGURE 11-8 Polyester and PTFE aortic grafts used in aneurysm repair.

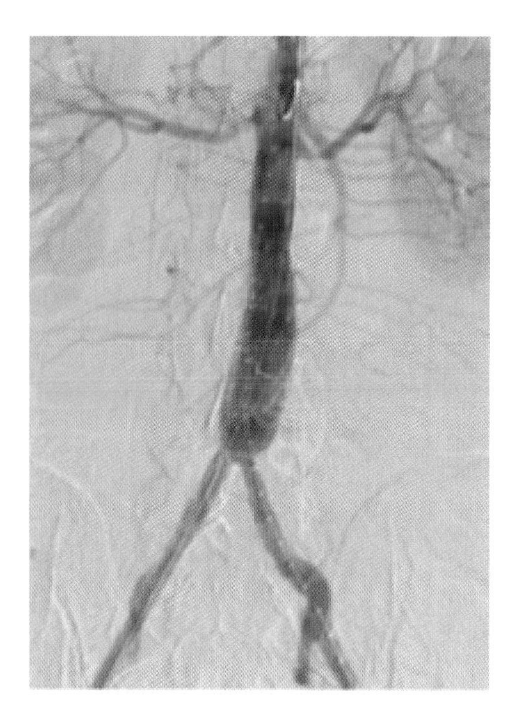

FIGURE 11-9 Angiogram after endovascular abdominal aortic aneurysm repair.

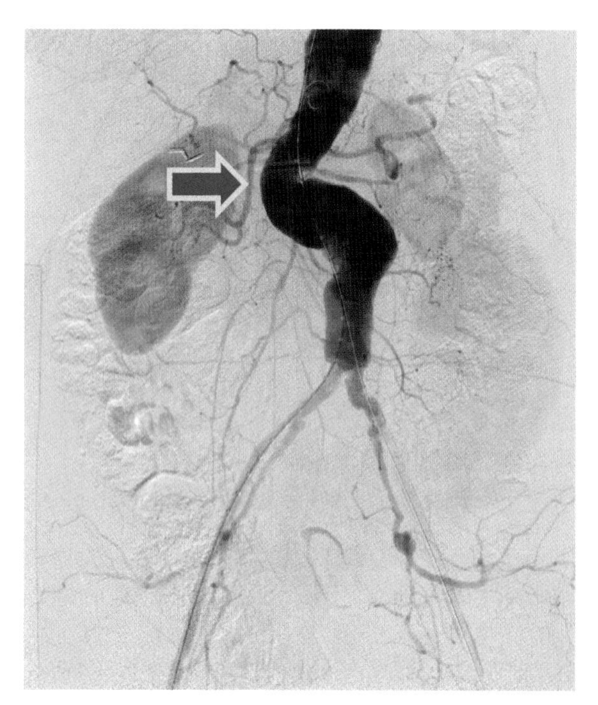

FIGURE 11-10 Angiogram demonstrating extreme proximal aortic neck angulation (arrow).

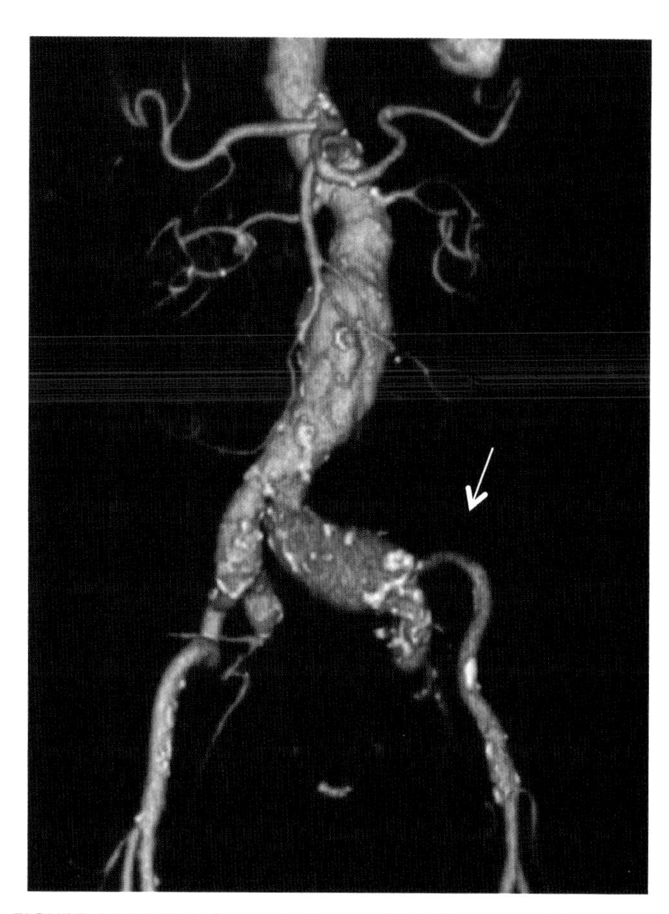

FIGURE 11-11 CTA demonstrating small left iliac artery with calcifications (arrow).

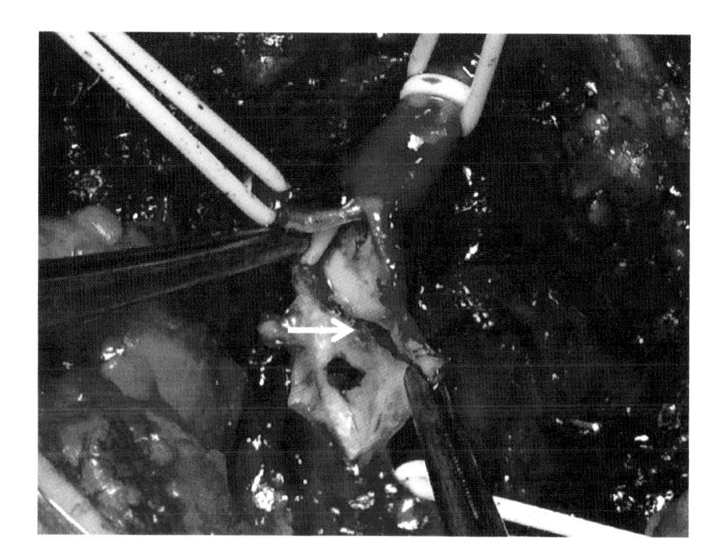

FIGURE 11-12 Intimal damage to femoral artery (arrow), requiring repair.

cardiovascular morbidities),[38] others have suggested the long-term outcome to be similar.[39] It is important to keep in mind that women tend to be underrepresented in many studies. Awareness of potential gender biases may help the medical community better in referring and choosing patients who should undergo either type of AAA repair. Intervening earlier in women may impart survival benefits in the long run.

PERIPHERAL ARTERIAL DISEASE

Peripheral arterial disease can occur in any noncardiac arterial bed, but most frequently affects the lower extremity vasculature. PAD can be manifested by claudication, pain at rest, nonhealing wounds, and gangrenous changes. Nearly 8.5 million Americans are thought to be affected with PAD, including 12% to 20% of those over 60 years, and an additional 1.7 million may have undiagnosed PAD.[40] The higher prevalence in African Americans may also be under-recognized. Only 20% to 30% of all those with known PAD take the recommended antiplatelet or lipid-lowering medications.[41] The risks from PAD extend past the manifestations listed earlier and include coronary and cerebrovascular complications, yet the public is woefully unaware of these associated risks and the economic implications.[42] An ankle–brachial index (ABI) <0.9 is positively associated with an increased cardiovascular and cerebrovascular mortality rate[43] (Figure 11-13).

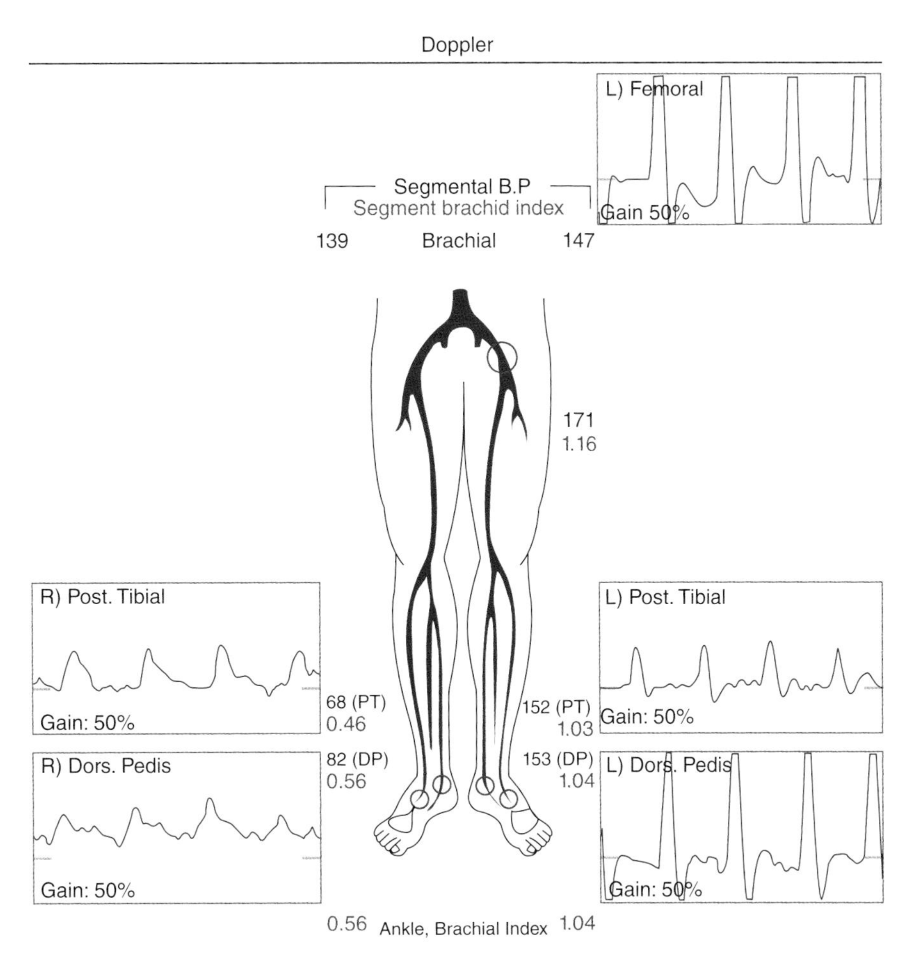

FIGURE 11-13 Diminished ankle–brachial index on the right.

Unlike other vascular diseases, PAD exhibits equal prevalence in men and women,[44] but the disease prevalence greatly increases in postmenopausal women for unknown reasons. More women may not exhibit the earlier, classic symptoms of claudication, including exertional leg pain. Patients with PAD, even though they may not have exertional leg pain, show a decline in lower extremity functioning over time.[45] This may contribute to elderly women needing more assistance to remain at home or require more skilled inpatient care. Indeed, women tend to present later in the course of the disease and are more likely to be admitted on an emergent basis and be discharged to an extended care facility.[46] They have a higher periprocedural mortality rate and tend to be hospitalized at a more advanced stage of their disease, similar to the condition in AAA. Fortunately, the advent of endovascular procedures has reduced the mortality rate due to PAD in women.

PAD sometimes follows a clinical course from claudication to irreversible ischemic changes (Figures 11-14 and 11-15). The management depends on the symptoms at presentation and presence of limb-threatening ischemia. All patients should be managed with best-possible methods (with control of lipids, blood glucose, hypertension, and antiplatelet administration) as well as lifestyle modifications, including smoking cessation, weight loss, diet modifications, and increase in physical activity. Treatment of the underlying vascular lesion depends on the location and extent of the disease; there is much variability among clinicians as to how a specific lesion may be managed. Balloon angioplasty is the oldest form of modern treatment and can include "plain old balloon angioplasty," (Figure 11-16), cutting/molding balloon angioplasty, cryoplasty (Figure 11-17), and drug-coated balloons. Peripheral stenting improved the results in some arterial beds and with certain lesions (Figure 11-18). Stent design has now evolved to include balloon-expandable stents, self-expanding stents, covered stents, and drug-eluting stents (Figure 11-19). Bioresorbable stents may offer the next step in reducing disease recurrence while maintaining the natural arterial system.

The debulking of atherosclerotic lesions with atherectomy devices has also become somewhat commonplace depending on the characteristics of the lesion and ultimate treatment planned (Figure 11-20). Prior to any lesion treatment, however, is the need to cross the lesion if totally occluded. Various device designs are in existence with a variety of individual mechanical advantages. Thrombolytic therapies and new access techniques (Figure 11-21) continue to add to the feasibility of treating a lesion with endovascular methods. It remains to be seen if any of these individual techniques or devices will be superior in treating vascular disease in women. Studying the genders separately when evaluating new procedures will be extremely important for determining best treatment practices.

Open surgical procedures remain an important option for limb salvage in all patients, although as the complexity of the disease needing revascularization increases, so does the complexity of the procedures (Figure 11-22). Autogenous veins offer higher patency rates and lower infection rates than prosthetic bypass graft. Patency for open revascularization also remains higher in the short and long term than for endovascular approaches and no one has conclusively shown a difference in patency between the genders. Complications from open surgery exceed that from endovascular techniques, but costs have been found to be higher for the less-invasive procedures.[47]

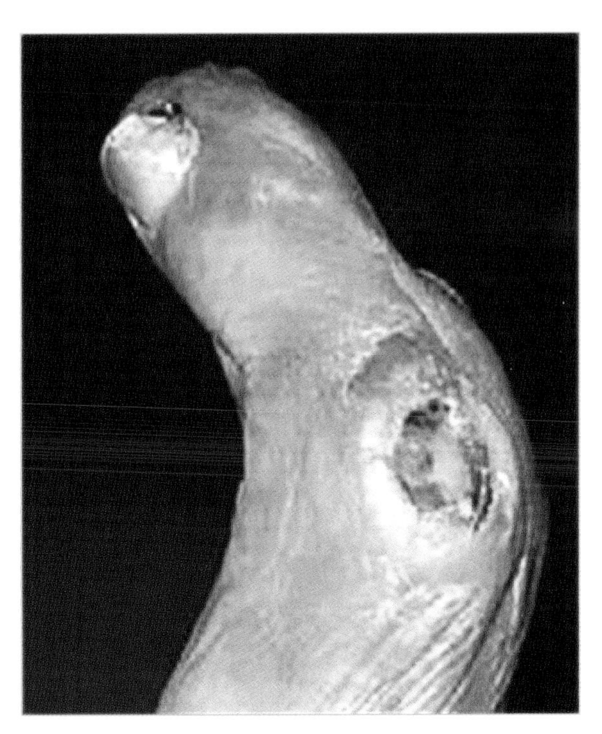

FIGURE 11-14 Ischemic foot ulcer caused by excess pressure on metatarsal head.

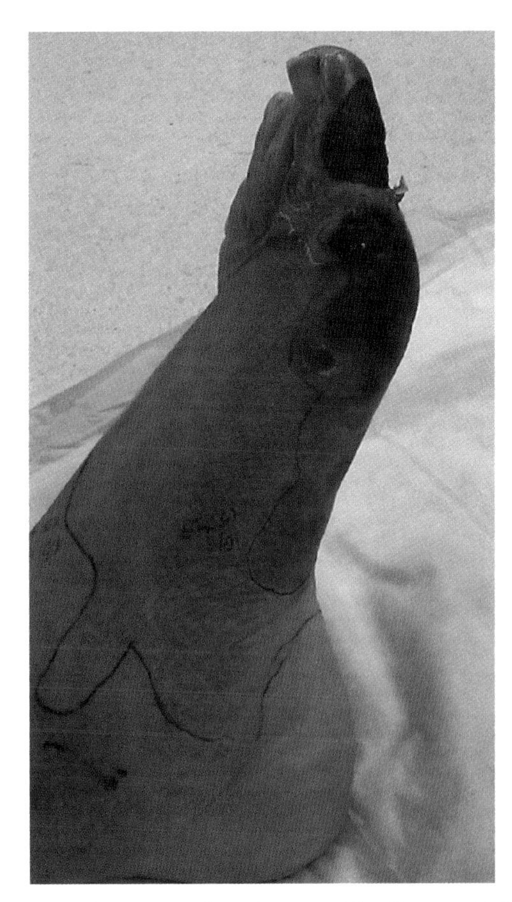

FIGURE 11-15 Gangrenous foot changes with adjacent cellulitis.

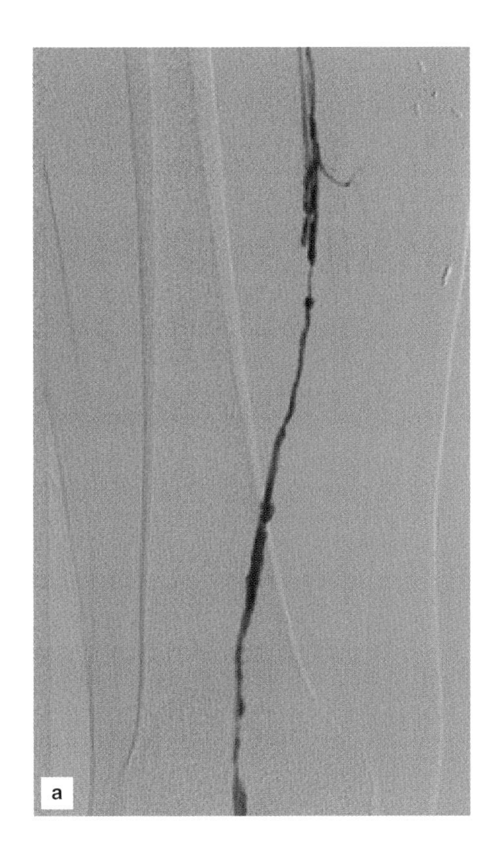

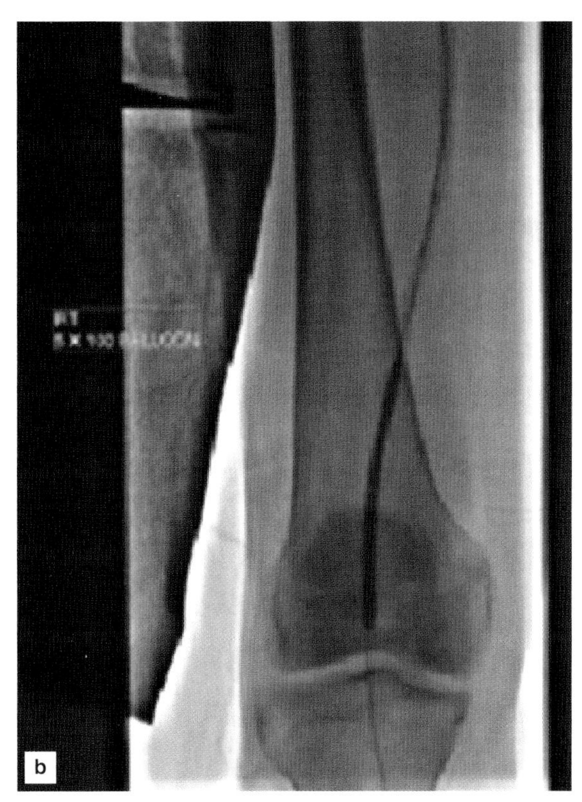

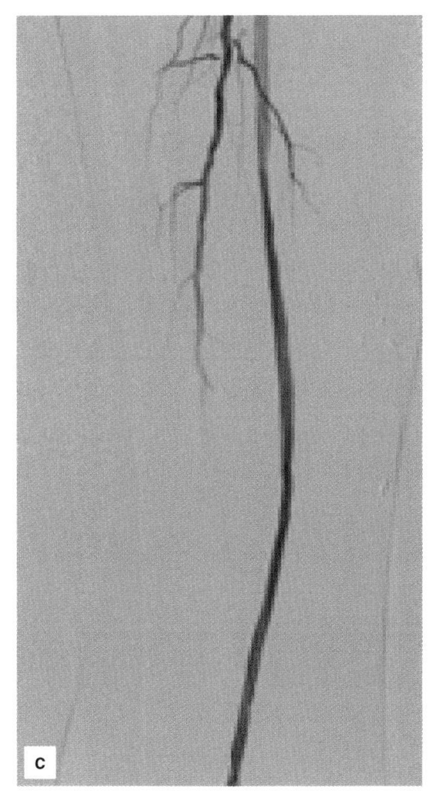

FIGURE 11-16 Angioplasty of right leg. (A) Preprocedural catheter-based angiogram showing severe superficial femoral (SFA) and popliteal arterial stenoses. (B) Angioplasty balloon inflation in popliteal artery. (C) Successful immediate angioplasty result.

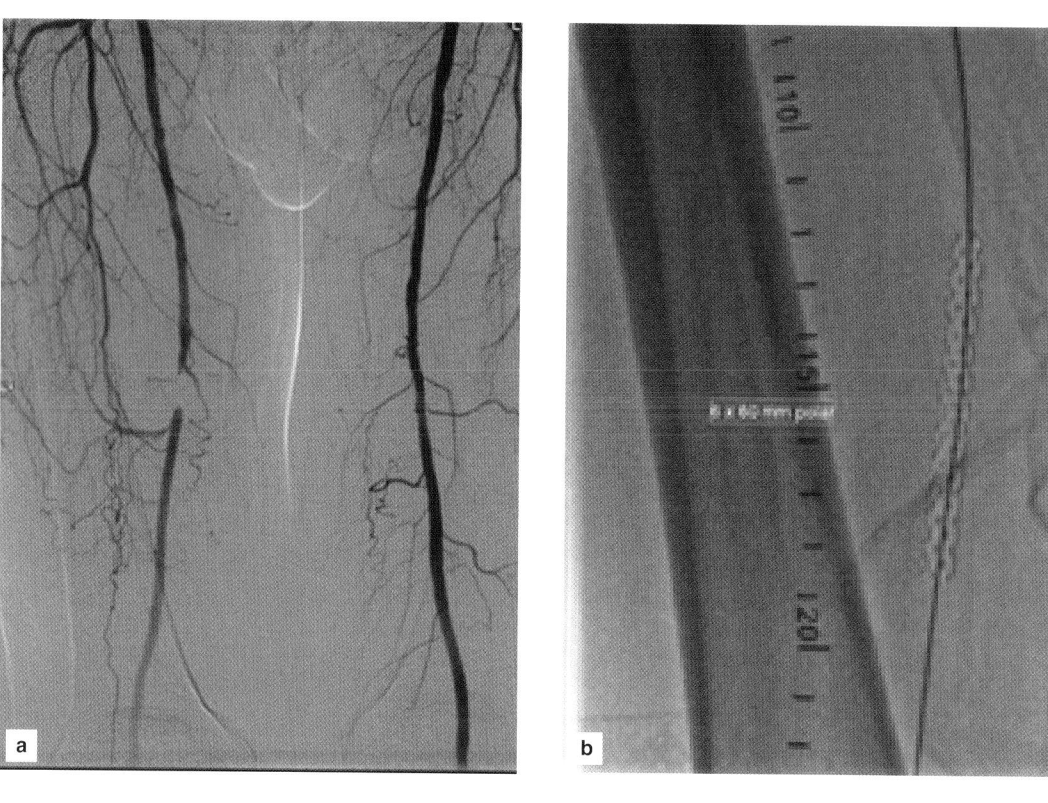

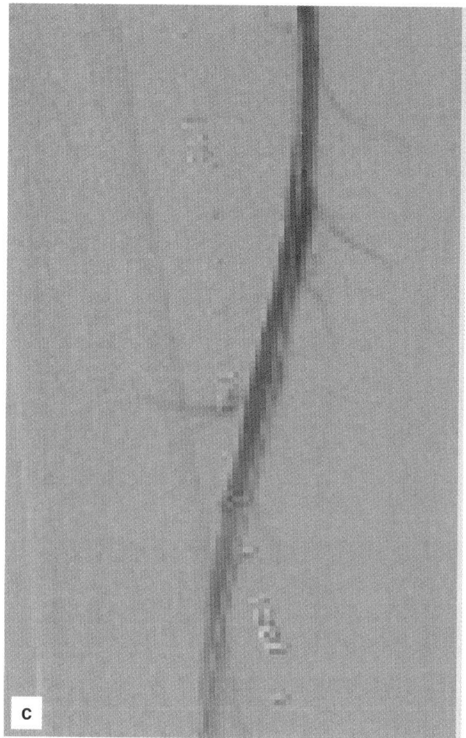

FIGURE 11-17 Cryoplasty of right leg. (A) Short-segment occlusion of right SFA. (B) Cryoplasty balloon inflated in mid-SFA. (C) Successful cryoplasty result.

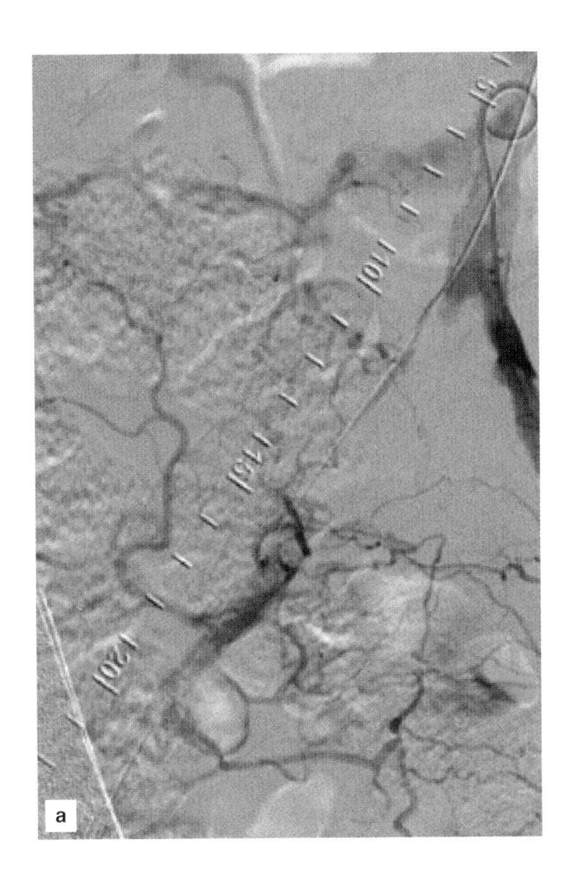

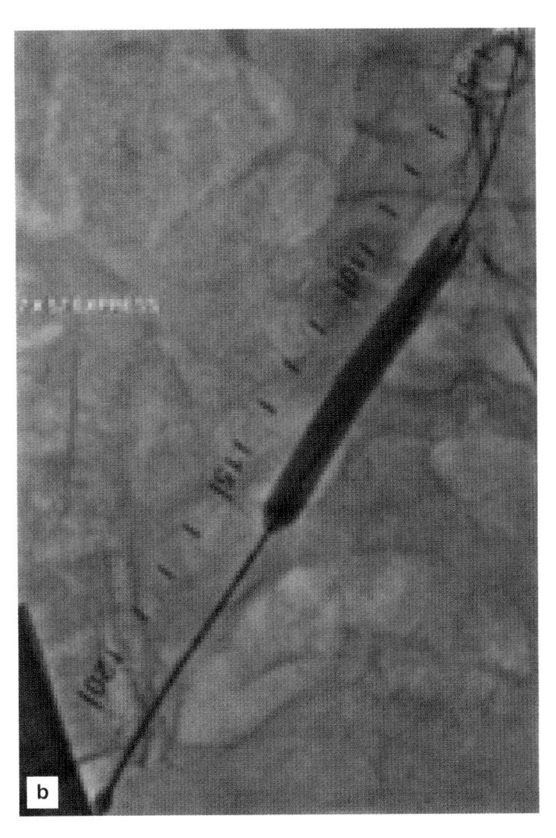

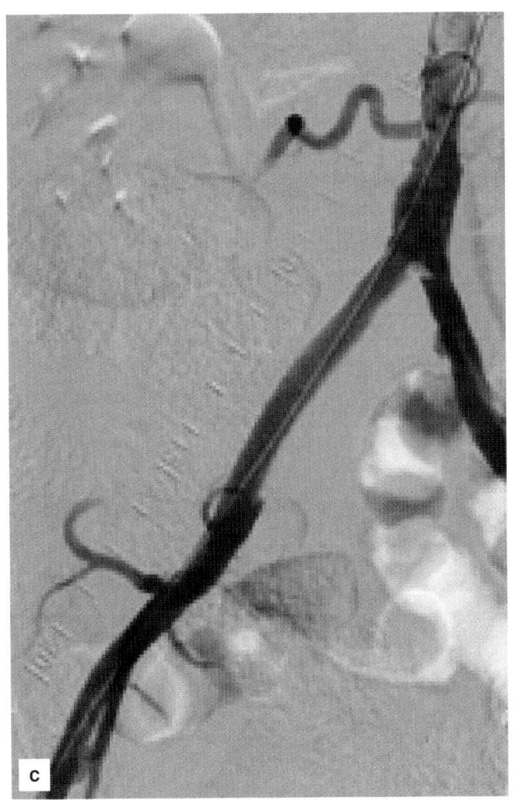

FIGURE 11-18 Stenting procedure of right common iliac artery (CI). (A) Right CI artery occlusion. (B) Balloon-expandable stent deployment. (C) Successful right iliac stent placement with widely patent lumen.

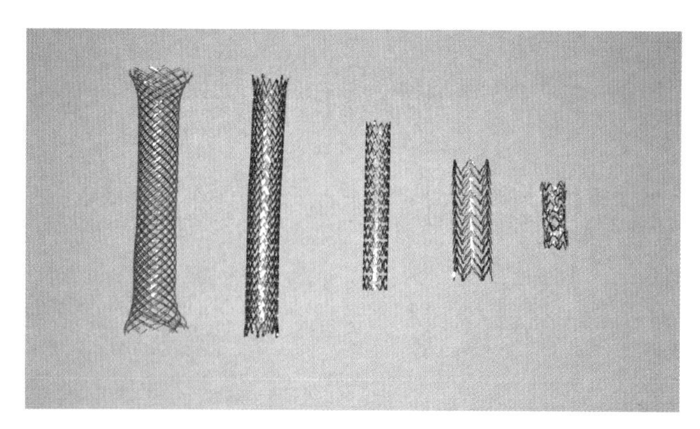

FIGURE 11-19 A variety of peripheral arterial stents.

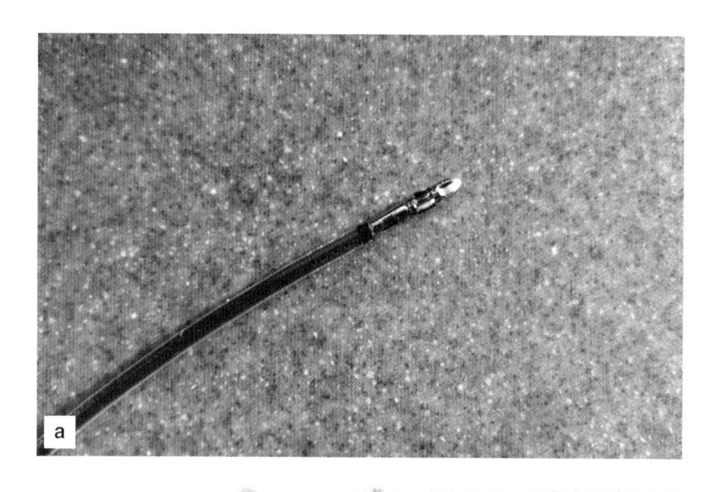

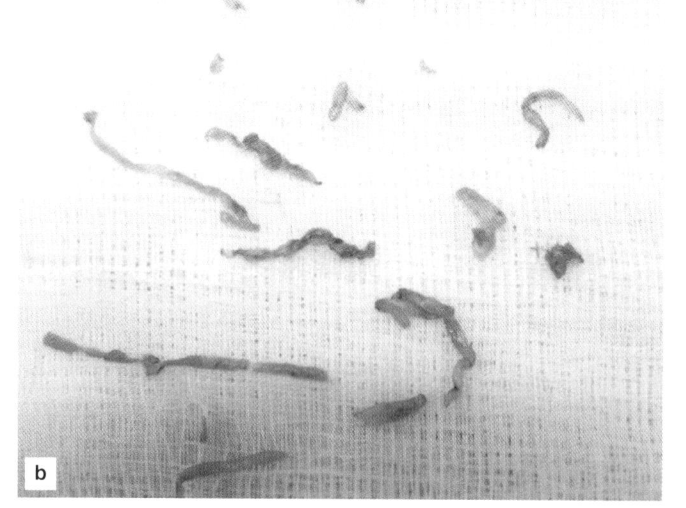

FIGURE 11-20 (A) Atherectomy device. (B) Atheroma removed with atherectomy device.

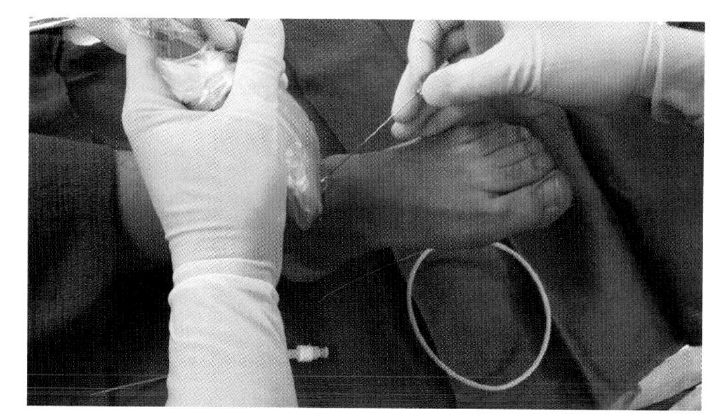

FIGURE 11-21 Percutaneous retrograde arterial access for treating a popliteal/tibial artery occlusion.

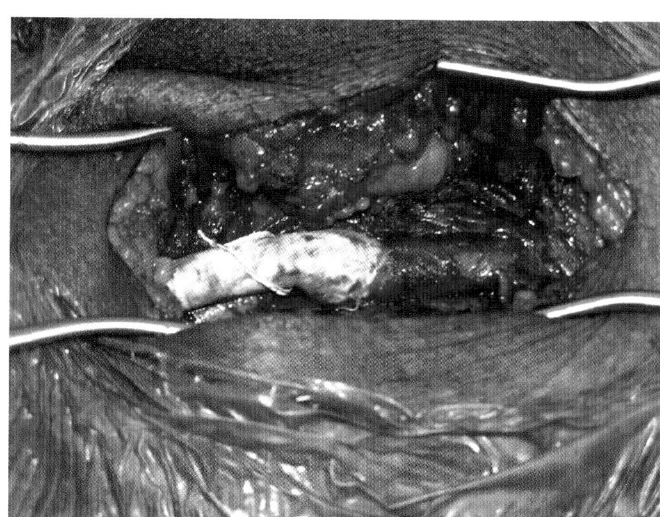

FIGURE 11-22 Proximal anastomosis of a femoral-popliteal PTFE prosthetic graft.

Women are older at presentation and require more complicated revascularization procedures. A greater percentage of women require an amputation on initial presentation than men. It is speculated that this late presentation may be due to a combination of factors: women tend to be caregivers for other family members and neglect their own needs, they may believe symptoms are from "old age," and there may be economic drawbacks to seeking medical care earlier.[1]

The PAD coalition of the Vascular Disease Foundation endorses the statements and recommendations of the American Heart Association in its 2012 document, in the areas of epidemiology, clinical presentation, diagnostic methods, treatment, awareness and knowledge of PAD, and national education and research programs.[48] This article focuses specifically on vascular disease in women and serves to educate the public and clinicians alike. When those who care for the patients with vascular disease recognize the gender differences and similarities, treatment can begin to be tailored for the individual through personalized medicine. This may in turn promote the development of devices and techniques to treat men and women more specifically in order to obtain better clinical outcomes. The future of these developments rests first on the study of vascular disease in women.

REFERENCES

1. Vouyouka AG, Kent KC. Arterial vascular disease in women. *J Vasc Surg*. 2007 December;46(6):1295-1302.
2. Kurrelmeyer K. Cardiovascular disease in women: the facts. *Methodist Debakey Cardiovasc J*. 2006;2(1):8-12.
3. Hansen F, Mangell P, Sonesson B, et al. Diameter and compliance in the human common carotid artery—variations with age and sex. *Ultrasound Med Biol*. 1995;21(1):1-9.
4. Rerkasem K, Gallagher PJ, Grimble RF, et al. Sex difference in composition of plaques of patients undergoing carotid endarterectomy. *Vascular*. 2010 March-April;18(2):77-81.
5. Ota H, Reeves MJ, Zhu DC, et al. Sex differences in patients with asymptomatic carotid atherosclerotic plaque: in vivo 3.0-T magnetic resonance study. *Stroke*. 2010 August;41(8):1630-1635.
6. Sangiorgi G, Roversi S, Biondi Zoccai G, et al. Sex-related differences in carotid plaque features and inflammation. *J Vasc Surg*. 2013 February;57(2):338-344.
7. Executive Committee for the Asymptomatic Carotid Atherosclerosis Study. Endarterectomy for asymptomatic carotid artery stenosis. *JAMA*. 1995;273:1421-1428.
8. Barnett HJ, Taylor DW, Eliasziw M, et al. Benefit of carotid endarterectomy in patients with symptomatic moderate or severe stenosis. North American Symptomatic Carotid Endarterectomy Trial Collaborators. *N Engl J Med*. 1998;339:1415-1425.
9. Randomised trial of endarterectomy for recently symptomatic carotid stenosis: final results of the MRC European Carotid Surgery Trial (ECST). *Lancet*. 1998;351:1379-1387.
10. Halliday A, Harrison M, Hayter E, et al. Asymptomatic Carotid Surgery Trial (ACST) Collaborative Group: 10-year stroke prevention after successful carotid endarterectomy for asymptomatic stenosis (ACST-1): a multicentre randomised trial. *Lancet*. 2010 September 25;376(9746):1074-1084.
11. Marquardt L, Fairhead JF, Rothwell PM. Lower rates of intervention for symptomatic carotid stenosis in women than in men reflect differences in disease incidence: a population-based study. *Stroke*. 2010 January;41(1):16-20.
12. Poisson SN, Johnston SC, Sidney S, et al. Gender differences in treatment of severe carotid stenosis after transient ischemic attack. *Stroke*. 2010 September;41(9):1891-1895.
13. Amaranto DJ, Abbas F, Krantz S, et al. An evaluation of gender and racial disparity in the decision to treat surgically arterial disease. *J Vasc Surg*. 2009 December;50(6):1340-1347.
14. Kapral MK, Degani N, Hall R, et al. Gender differences in stroke care and outcomes in Ontario. *Womens Health Issues*. 2011 March-April;21(2):171-176.
15. Mattos MA, Sumner DS, Bohannon WT, et al. Carotid endarterectomy in women: challenging the results from ACAS and NASCET. *Ann Surg*. 2001 October;234(4):438-445.
16. Baracchini C, Saladini M, Lorenzetti R, et al. Gender-based outcomes after eversion carotid endarterectomy from 1998 to 2009. *J Vasc Surg*. 2012 February;55(2):338-345.
17. Kapral MK, Wang H, Austin PC, et al. Sex differences in carotid endarterectomy outcomes: results from the Ontario Carotid Endarterectomy Registry. *Stroke*. 2003 May;34(5):1120-1125.
18. Ballotta E, Renon L, Da Giau G, et al. Carotid endarterectomy in women: early and long-term results. *Surgery*. 2000 March;127(3):264-271.
19. Grootenboer N, Hunink MG, Hoeks S, et al. The impact of gender on prognosis after non-cardiac vascular surgery. *Eur J Vasc Endovasc Surg*. 2011 October;42(4):510-516.
20. Yadav JS, Wholey MH, Kuntz RE, et al. Stenting and Angioplasty with Protection in Patients at High Risk for Endarterectomy Investigators. Protected carotid-artery stenting versus endarterectomy in high-risk patients. *N Engl J Med*. 2004 October 7;351(15):1493-1501.
21. Mas JL, Chatellier G, Beyssen B, et al. Endarterectomy versus stenting in patients with symptomatic severe carotid stenosis. *N Engl J Med*. 2006;355:1660-1671.
22. Brott TG, Hobson RW, 2nd, Howard G, et al; CREST Investigators. Stenting versus endarterectomy for treatment of carotid-artery stenosis. *N Engl J Med*. 2010 July 1;363(1):11-23.
23. De Rango P, Parlani G, Caso V, et al. A comparative analysis of the outcomes of carotid stenting and carotid endarterectomy in women. *J Vasc Surg*. 2010 February;51(2):337-344; discussion 344.
24. Goldstein LJ, Khan HU, Sambol EB, et al. Carotid artery stenting is safe and associated with comparable outcomes in men and women. *J Vasc Surg*. 2009 February;49(2):315-323; discussion 323-324.
25. Calonge N. Screening for abdominal aortic aneurysm recommendation. U.S. Preventive Services Task Force statement. *Ann Intern Med*. 2005 February 1;142(3):198-202.
26. Fleming C, Whitlock EP, Beil TL, et al. Screening for abdominal aortic aneurysm: a best-evidence systematic review for the U.S. Preventive Services Task Force. *Ann Intern Med*. 2005 February 1;142(3):203-211.

27. Lederle FA, Johnson GR, Wilson SE. Abdominal aortic aneurysm in women: Aneurysm Detection and Management Veterans Affairs Cooperative Study. *J Vasc Surg*. 2001 July; 34(1):122-126.

28. Derubertis BG, Trocciola SM, Ryer EJ, et al. Abdominal aortic aneurysm in women: prevalence, risk factors, and implications for screening. *J Vasc Surg*. 2007 October;46(4):630-635.

29. Brown LC, Powell JT. Risk factors for aneurysm rupture in patients kept under ultrasound surveillance. UK Small Aneurysm Trial Participants. *Ann Surg*. 1999 September;230(3):289-296; discussion 296-297.

30. McPhee JT, Hill JS, Eslami MH. The impact of gender on presentation, therapy, and mortality of abdominal aortic aneurysm in the United States, 2001-2004. *J Vasc Surg*. 2007 May;45(5): 891-899.

31. Mureebe L, Egorova N, McKinsey JF, et al. Gender trends in the repair of ruptured abdominal aortic aneurysms and outcomes. *J Vasc Surg*. 2010 April;51(4 suppl):9S-13S.

32. Brown PM, Sobolev B, Zelt DT. Selective management of abdominal aortic aneurysms smaller than 5.0 cm in a prospective sizing program with gender-specific analysis. *J Vasc Surg*. 2003 October;38(4):762-765.

33. Ouriel K, Greenberg RK, Clair DG, et al. Endovascular aneurysm repair: gender-specific results. *J Vasc Surg*. 2003 July;38(1):93-98.

34. Becker GJ, Kovacs M, Mathison MN, et al. Risk stratification and outcomes of transluminal endografting for abdominal aortic aneurysm: 7-year experience and long-term follow-up. *J Vasc Interv Radiol*. 2001 September; 12(9):1033-1046.

35. Mathison M, Becker GJ, Katzen BT, et al. The influence of female gender on the outcome of endovascular abdominal aortic aneurysm repair. *J Vasc Interv Radiol*. 2001 September; 12(9):1047-1051.

36. Wolf YG, Arko FR, Hill BB, et al. Gender differences in endovascular abdominal aortic aneurysm repair with the AneuRx stent graft. *J Vasc Surg*. 2002 May;35(5):882-886.

37. Katz DJ, Stanley JC, Zelenock GB. Gender differences in abdominal aortic aneurysm prevalence, treatment, and outcome. *J Vasc Surg*. 1997 March;25(3):561-568.

38. Norman PE, Powell JT. Abdominal aortic aneurysm: the prognosis in women is worse than in men. *Circulation*. 2007 June 5; 115(22):2865-2869.

39. Harthun NL, Cheanvechai V, Graham LM, et al. Prevalence of abdominal aortic aneurysm and repair outcomes on the basis of patient sex: should the timing of intervention be the same? *J Thorac Cardiovasc Surg*. 2004 February;127(2):325-328.

40. Allison MA, Ho E, Denenberg JO, et al. Ethnic-specific prevalence of peripheral arterial disease in the United States. *Am J Prev Med*. 2007 April;32(4):328-333.

41. Bhatt DL, Steg PG, Ohman EM, et al. REACH Registry Investigators. International prevalence, recognition, and treatment of cardiovascular risk factors in outpatients with atherothrombosis. *JAMA*. 2006 January 11;295(2):180-189.

42. Hirsch AT, Murphy TP, Lovell MB, et al. Peripheral Arterial Disease Coalition. Gaps in public knowledge of peripheral arterial disease: the first national PAD public awareness survey. *Circulation*. 2007 October 30; 116(18):2086-2094.

43. Ankle Brachial Index Collaboration, Fowkes FG, Murray GD, Butcher I, et al. Ankle brachial index combined with Framingham Risk Score to predict cardiovascular events and mortality: a meta-analysis. *JAMA*. 2008 July 9;300(2):197-208.

44. Norgren L, Hiatt WR, Dormandy JA, et al. TASC II Working Group. Inter-Society Consensus for the Management of Peripheral Arterial Disease (TASC II). *J Vasc Surg*. 2007 January;45(suppl S):S5-S67.

45. McDermott MM, Liu K, Greenland P, et al. Functional decline in peripheral arterial disease: associations with the ankle brachial index and leg symptoms. *JAMA*. 2004 July 28;292(4):453-461.

46. Egorova N, Vouyouka AG, Quin J, et al. Analysis of gender-related differences in lower extremity peripheral arterial disease. *J Vasc Surg*. 2010 February;51(2):372-378.

47. Sachs T, Pomposelli F, Hamdan A, et al. Trends in the national outcomes and costs for claudication and limb threatening ischemia: angioplasty vs bypass graft. *J Vasc Surg*. 2011 October;54(4):1021-1031.

48. Hirsch AT, Allison MA, Gomes AS, et al. American Heart Association Council on Peripheral Vascular Disease; Council on Cardiovascular Nursing; Council on Cardiovascular Radiology and Intervention; Council on Cardiovascular Surgery and Anesthesia; Council on Clinical Cardiology; Council on Epidemiology and Prevention. A call to action: women and peripheral artery disease: a scientific statement from the American Heart Association. *Circulation*. 2012 March 20;125(11):1449-1472.

12 PULMONARY HYPERTENSION IN WOMEN: GENDER MATTERS

Veronica Franco, MD, MSPH

INTRODUCTION

Pulmonary arterial hypertension (PAH) is rare and uniformly deadly disease characterized by extensive narrowing of the pulmonary vasculature, leading to progressive increases in pulmonary vascular resistance and ensuing right heart failure.[2] The underlying pathogenetic mechanisms of PAH are slowly being unraveled, but to a large degree remain poorly understood. Medial hypertrophy, intimal proliferative and fibrotic changes, perivascular inflammatory infiltrates, and thrombotic lesions are noted in the pulmonary arteries.

The nomenclature and classification of pulmonary hypertension was changed in 2009 by the World Health Organization (Table 12-1). Idiopathic PAH is now being used instead of primary pulmonary hypertension. The classification is easy to remember if we think of pulmonary hypertension as a "disease of triggers." In idiopathic or familial PAH, the trigger is a mutation or polymorphism. In PAH associated with connective tissue disease, congenital disease, HIV, anorexigens, or portal hypertension, the trigger is permissive phenotype. This will also help differentiate PAH from non-PAH etiologies. Non-PAH diseases could be triggered by high left atrial pressure (heart failure and valvular disease), hypoxia (lung disease), or emboli.

A right heart catheterization is mandatory to confirm the diagnosis of PAH (Figure 12-1). Important hemodynamic measurements that should be obtained are pulmonary wedge pressure, cardiac output, and pulmonary vascular resistance. Cardiac output in most cases is calculated by Fick method (using pulmonary artery saturation) because significant tricuspid regurgitation may alter the result of thermodilution method. Intracardiac shunting should be ruled out by saturation of the chambers. The diagnosis of PAH is defined as a mean pulmonary artery pressure ≥25 mm Hg at rest, in the setting of normal pulmonary capillary wedge pressure ≤15 mm Hg.[1,2] PAH remains a diagnosis of exclusion and other factors, like heart failure or emboli, should be evaluated and ruled out.

ESTROGEN AND PAH

Pulmonary arterial hypertension is more prevalent in women.[2] Given PAH worsens during the peripartium period, the association with oral contraceptives (possibly coincidental because of age and gender), and the known prothrombotic effects of estrogens, there is speculation that estrogens play a role in the initiation or progression of PAH. However, animal studies suggest that estrogen also has favorable effects in experimental PAH; there is better outcome in female animals, exacerbation of the disease after ovariectomy, and a strong protective effect of estrogen, a phenomenon known as the estrogen paradox[4] (Figure 12-2).

TABLE 12-1 Classification of pulmonary hypertension

1. Pulmonary arterial hypertension
   - Idiopathic
   - Heritable
   - Drug- and toxin induced
   - Associated with:
     - Collagen vascular disease
     - Congenital systemic-to-pulmonary shunts
     - HIV infection
     - Schistosomiasis
     - Chronic hemolytic anemia
   - Persistent pulmonary hypertension of the newborn
   - Associated with significant venous or capillary involvement
     - Pulmonary veno-occlusive disease
     - Pulmonary capillary hemangiomatosis
2. Pulmonary hypertension with left heart disease
   - Heart failure (systolic or diastolic)
   - Valvular heart disease
3. Pulmonary hypertension associated with lung disease and/or hypoxemia
   - Chronic obstructive pulmonary disease
   - Interstitial lung disease
   - Sleep-disordered breathing
   - Alveolar hypoventilation disorder
   - Chronic exposure to high altitude
   - Developmental abnormalities
4. Pulmonary hypertension due to chronic thromboembolic disease
5. Pulmonary hypertension with unclear multifactorial mechanisms
   - Hematologic disorders: myeloproliferative disorders, splenectomy
   - Systemic disorders: sarcoidosis, pulmonary Langerhans cell histiocytosis: lymphangioleiomyomatosis, neurofibromatosis, vasculitis
   - Metabolic disorders: glycogen storage disease, Gaucher disease, thyroid disorders
   - Others: tumoral obstruction, fibrosing mediastinitis, chronic renal failure on dialysis

The reason for the female predisposition is incompletely understood. PAH is associated with decreased bone morphogenetic protein receptor type 2 (BMPR2) expression.[1,2] Studies in multiple organ systems have shown cross-talk between signaling through the BMPR2 and estrogen pathways.[5] Increased exogenous estrogen decreases BMPR2 expression in cell culture. *BMPR2* gene expression is reduced in females compared to males in live humans and in mice, likely through direct estrogen receptor-α binding to the BMPR2 promoter. This reduced BMPR2 expression may contribute to the increased prevalence of PAH in females.

The effects of estrogens on pulmonary vasculature are well defined: (1) estradiol, via rapid, nongenomic mechanisms, increases prostacyclin release and production of nitric oxide and (2) through estrogen receptor-dependent mechanisms increases endothelial nitric oxide synthase mRNA levels and activity.[4] Furthermore, ovariectomy augments hypoxia-induced increase in endothelin-1 (ET-1). Low levels of prostacyclin and nitric oxide and increases in endothelin-1 lead to PAH.[1,2]

Right ventricular failure is a major cause of morbidity and mortality in patients with PAH. Female rats and swine compared with

- To measure wedge pressure or LVEDP
  - Scrutinize wedge tracings!!!!
  - Wedge saturation; end expiration
- To exclude or evaluate CHD
- To establish severity and prognosis
- To test vasodilator therapy

Catheterization is required for every patient with suspected pulmonary HTN.

LVEDP = left ventricular end diastolic pressure.

FIGURE 12-1 Cardiac catheterization to assess the diagnosis and severity of PAH.

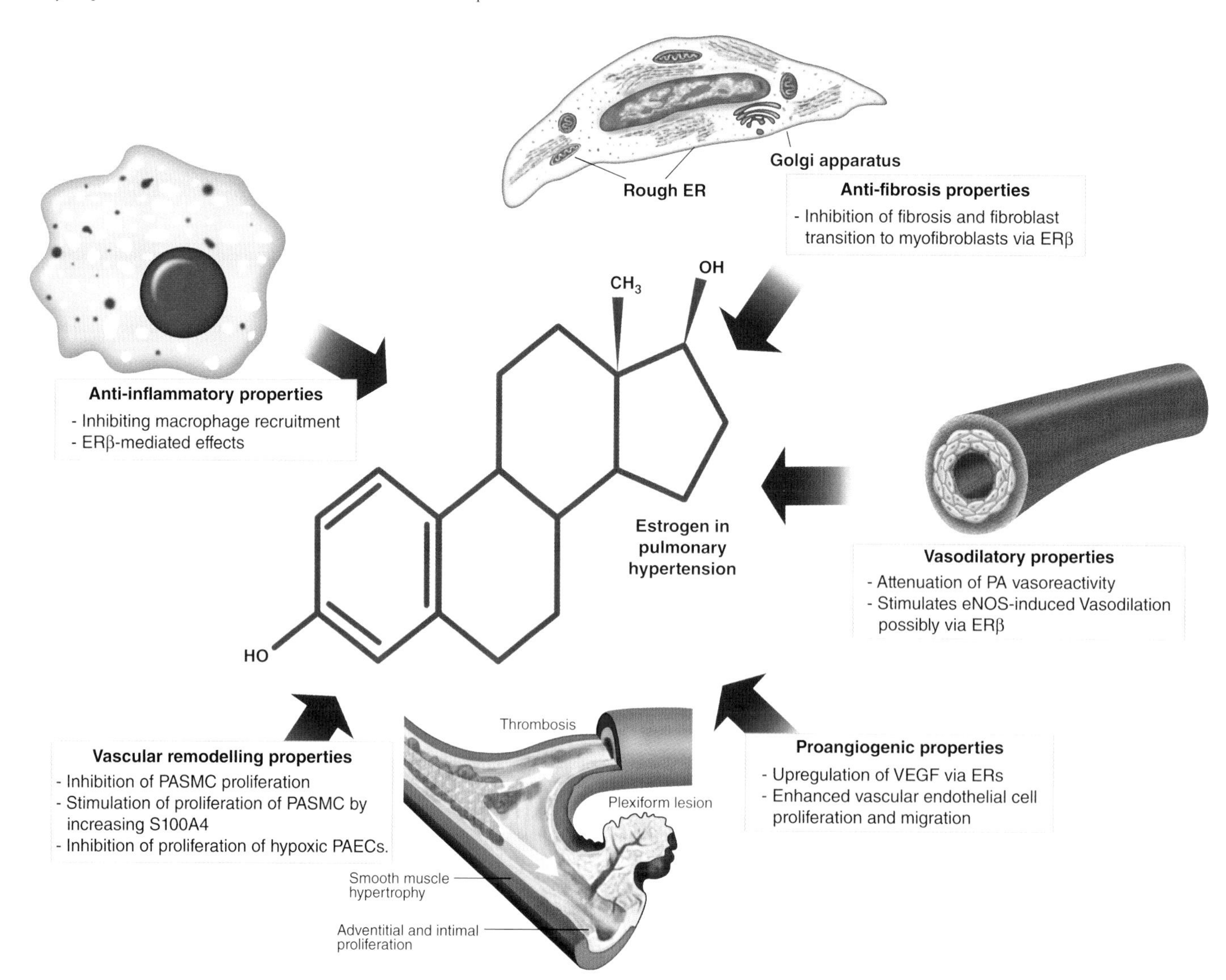

FIGURE 12-2 Summary of the likely protective effects of estrogen against PAH. Illustration of the possible beneficial effects of estrogen for the treatment of pulmonary hypertension.
Abbreviations: ER, estrogen receptor; eNOS, endothelial nitric oxide synthase; PA, pulmonary artery; PAEC, pulmonary artery endothelial cell; PASMC, pulmonary artery smooth muscle cell; VEGF, vascular endothelial growth factor.
Adapted from Umar et al. *Am J Respir Crit Care Med.* 2012;186:125-131.[4]

males, when exposed to chronic hypoxia develop less severe pulmonary hypertension, right ventricular hypertrophy, vascular remodeling, and polycythemia.[3] Estradiol may also cause myocardial vasodilatation and help the failing right ventricle. Furthermore, higher circulating estradiol levels are associated with better right-side heart function in postmenopausal women using hormone replacement therapy while higher levels of androgens are associated with greater right ventricular mass and volumes in both sexes.

Further studies are needed to resolve this paradox. To determine the estradiol metabolism, the vascular effects of its active metabolites and the potential benefit of estrogen-based therapies in PAH are required.

CHARACTERISTICS OF WOMEN WITH PAH

Pulmonary arterial hypertension afflicts predominantly women[2,6] and its prevalence among the female population is increasing. In the mid-1980s, the National Institute of Health registry of idiopathic PAH reported a 1.7:1 female-to-male ratio.[7] Similar US registries reported a 3.3:1 ratio in the period 1982 to 2006, 4.3:1 ratio for 1998 to 2001, and 4.1:1 ratio for 2006 to 2007.[6,8,9] National registries in France, Scotland, and China have reported ratios of 1.9:1, 2.3:1, and 2.4:1, respectively.[10-12] The Registry to Evaluate Early and Long-term Pulmonary Arterial Hypertension Disease Management (REVEAL Registry) has been the largest database to date.[6] It is a 55-US center, observational, prospective registry that includes approximately 3500 patients with new and previously diagnosed PAH. They were enrolled between March 2006 and September 2007 and followed for at least 5 years from time of enrollment. Characteristics of women with PAH are detailed in Table 12-2 and Figures 12-3 to 12-7.[6,13]

TABLE 12-2 Characteristics of those with pulmonary arterial hypertension by gender

	Females $n = 2318$	Males $n = 649$	*P* value
Age at diagnosis, years mean	48	46	0.01
Assisted care in home at enrollment (%)	65 (3)	39 (6)	0.001
Race, n (%)			0.001
Caucasian	1652 (71)	511 (79)	
African American	306 (13)	55 (9)	
Hispanic	218 (9)	46 (7)	
Other/unknown	142 (6)	37 (6)	
Hemodynamics at diagnosis			
mPAP (mm Hg)	51	53	0.013
Wedge (mm Hg)	9.9	10.3	0.027
mRAP (mm Hg)	9.2	9.8	0.037
PVR, Wood units	12	12	0.69
Svo_2 (%)	63	63	0.95
Fick or Thermodilution CI (L/min × m^2)	2.4	2.5	0.22

Women were older at diagnosis but time from onset of symptoms to diagnosis was similar to men. There were no differences in the time from symptom onset to treatment initiation. The delay in making the diagnosis and performing confirmatory RHCs was similar. With respect to hemodynamic parameters at diagnosis, men had a higher mPAP, mRAP, and PCWP than women.
Abbreviations: mPAP, mean pulmonary artery pressure; mRAP, mean right atrial pressure; PCWP, pulmonary capillary wedge pressure.
Adapted from Shapiro et al. *Chest.* 2012;141:363-373.

Females with PAH may respond better to certain specific vasodilators like endothelin receptor antagonists, as demonstrated in a pooled analysis of six randomized placebo-controlled trials where this medication was utilized.[14] The primary endpoint for this study was just 6-minute walk distance, which increased by 29.7 meters (95% CI, 3.7-55.7 m) greater in women than in men ($P = 0.03$). Importantly, the utility of walk distance as an endpoint is uncertain and has been extensively discussed in the PAH community as studies show that improvements in 6-minute walk distance does not reflect benefit in clinical outcomes.[15]

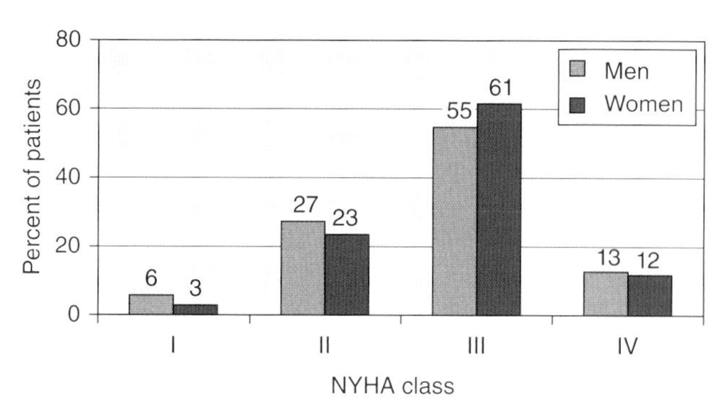

FIGURE 12-3 Dyspnea functional class by gender. More men had functional class dyspnea I to II, while more women had functional class dyspnea III, and similar proportions of men and women had functional class dyspnea IV at diagnosis ($P = 0.036$ overall).
Adapted from Shapiro et al. *Chest.* 2012;141:363-373.[6]

PREGNANCY AND PAH

Pregnancy poses a vast risk to women with PAH.[1,2] The first month after delivery represents the period of highest risk for patients with PAH (Figure 12-8).[16] Immediately postpartum, pulmonary vascular resistance increases and right ventricular contractility may decrease. These changes, in the face of a drop in preload, sets the stage for cardiovascular collapse in the PAH patient. Sudden death may also occur from numerous other mechanisms, including pulmonary embolism, arrhythmias, or stroke from intracardiac shunts.

Analysis of reported cases between 1978 and 1996 showed maternal mortality rates of 36% in Eisenmenger syndrome, 30% in primary pulmonary hypertension (now called idiopathic PAH), and 56% in pulmonary hypertension associated with other conditions (SVPH, secondary vascular pulmonary hypertension), $P < 0.08$ versus other 2 groups.[16] In this study, all fatalities occurred within 35 days after delivery, except for 3 prepartum deaths that occurred due to Eisenmenger syndrome.[4,16] Neonatal survival ranging from 87% to 89% was similar in the 3 groups. Late diagnosis ($P = 0.002$, odds ratio 5.4) and late hospital admission ($P = 0.01$, odds ratio 1.1 per week of pregnancy) were independent predictive risk factors of maternal mortality.

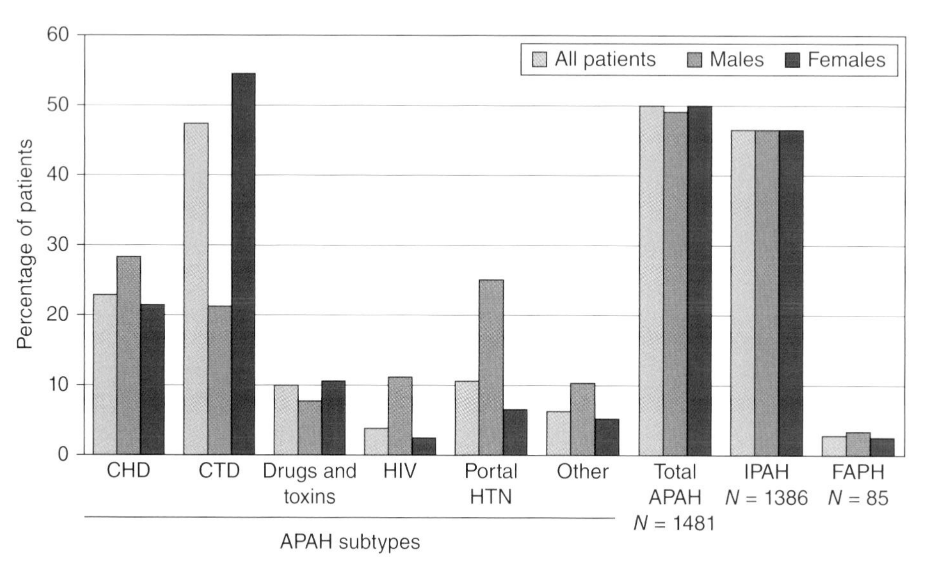

FIGURE 12-4 Etiologies of PAH by gender. There were no significant gender differences in cause at diagnosis among patients with idiopathic, familial, or associated PAH. However, among associated PAH subtypes, more women had connective tissue disease ($P < 0.001$) and congenital heart disease ($P = 0.017$) compared to men, and more men had HIV ($P < 0.001$) and portopulmonary hypertension ($P < 0.001$) compared to women.
Adapted from Shapiro et al. *Chest.* 2012;141:363-373.[6]

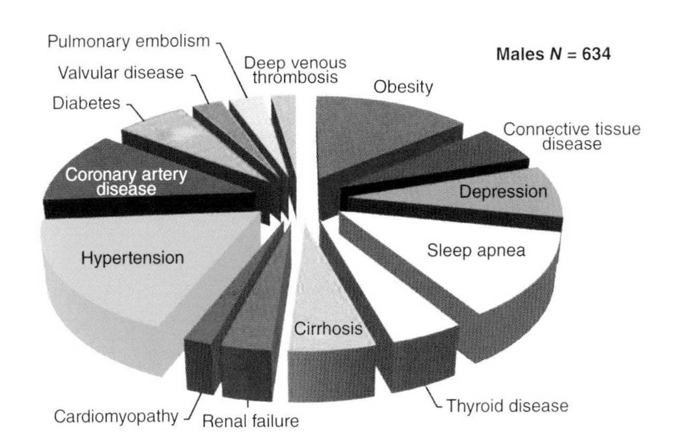

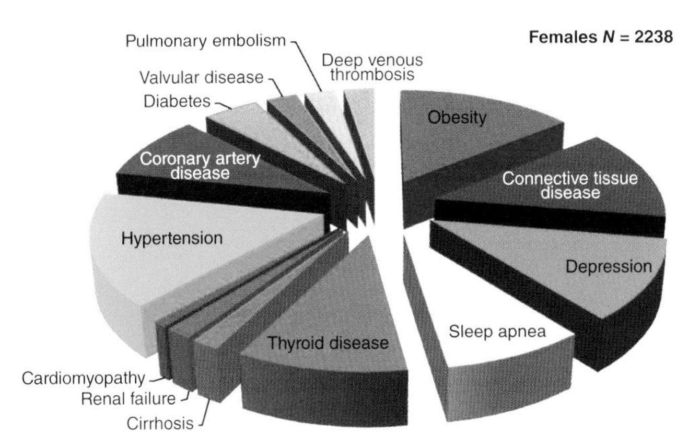

FIGURE 12-5 Comorbidities by gender. Women had more reported rates of depression, thyroid disease, obesity, and connective tissue disease ($P < 0.001$). Men had higher rates of history of sleep apnea ($P < 0.001$), cirrhosis ($P < 0.001$), renal insufficiency ($P = 0.003$), and cardiomyopathy ($P = 0.006$).
Adapted from Shapiro et al. *Chest.* 2012;141:363-373.[6]

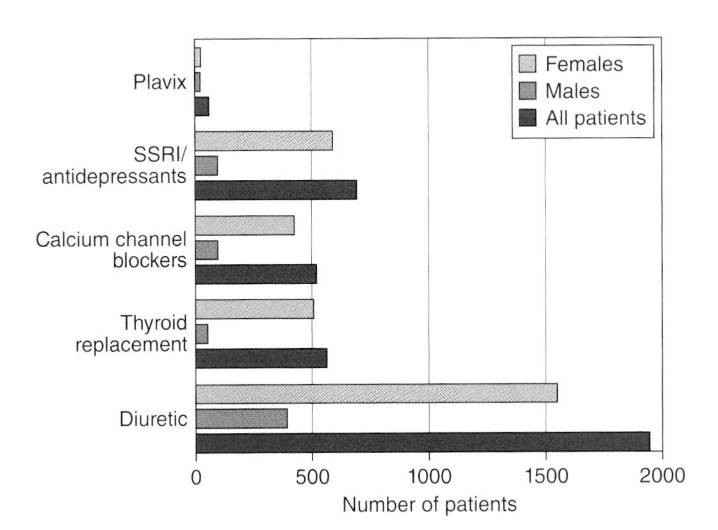

FIGURE 12-6 Medications used by women with PAH. There were no apparent differences in the use-specific vasodilators as phosphodiesterase type 5 inhibitors, endothelin receptor antagonists, or prostacyclin analogues. Both sexes used combination therapy with the same frequency. However, there were several differences in concomitant medications at enrollment. The use of diuretics, calcium channel blockers (as a concomitant medication not for the treatment of PAH), thyroid replacement, and selective serotonin reuptake inhibitors/antidepressants was greater among women than men.
Adapted from Shapiro et al. *Chest.* 2012;141:363-373.[6]

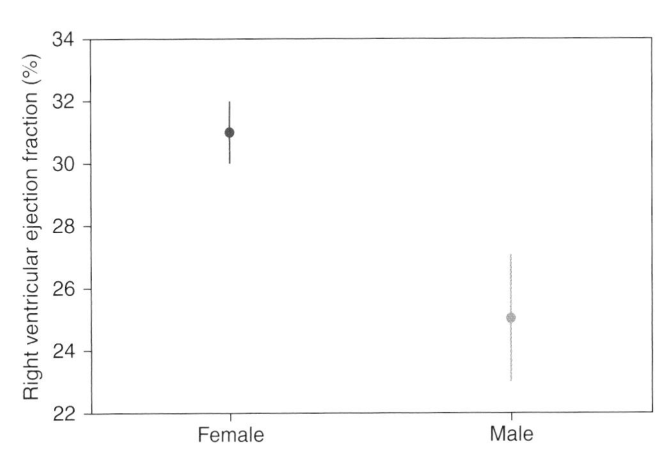

FIGURE 12-7 RVEF by gender. RVEF for males versus females (adjusted for age, pulmonary vascular resistance index, and LVEF) ($P = 0.02$).
Reproduced with permission from Kawut et al. *Chest.* 2009,135:752-759.[13]

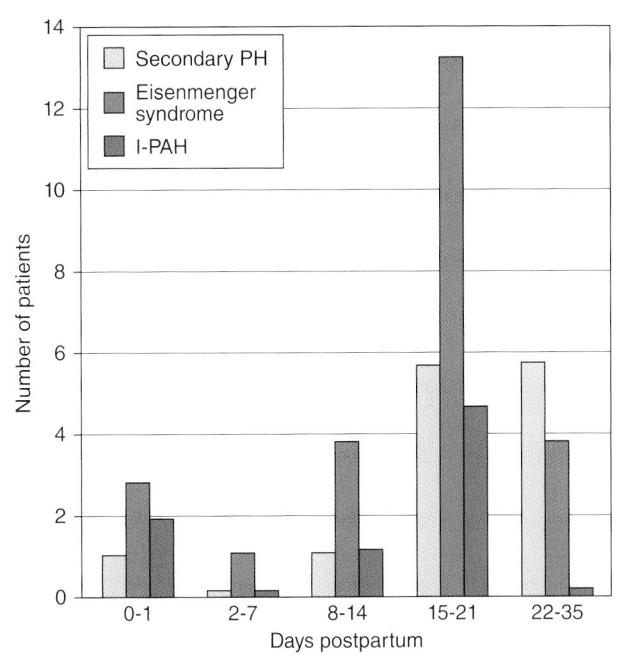

FIGURE 12-8 Time to maternal death. Time of maternal death in parturients with Eisenmenger syndrome ($N = 26$), PPH ($N = 8$), and SVPH ($N = 14$). The 0 to 1-day postpartum period includes 3 patients with Eisenmenger syndrome who died during pregnancy. The first month after delivery represents the period of highest risk for patients with PAH. The possible explanation is that even in healthy parturients, the lowest myocardial contractility is at delivery and immediately postpartum and there is slow cardiovascular recovery over the next 3 months. Other speculative explanations include an increased tendency toward thromboembolism, an exaggerated pulmonary vascular reactivity and/or a mismatch between declined myocardial contractility, and a too sudden decrease in blood volume after delivery. Maternal prognosis depends on the early diagnosis of PAH, early hospital admission, individually tailored treatment during pregnancy, and medical therapy and care focused on the postpartum period. The causes were Takayasu arteritis, pulmonary vasculitis of connective tissue (lupus erythematosus, scleroderma), sickle cell disease, illicit and appetite-suppressant drugs, chronic pulmonary thromboembolism, hepatitis, dwarfism with congenital hypothyroidism, and peripheral pulmonary artery stenoses.
Abbreviations: I-PAH, idiopathic pulmonary arterial hypertension; PAH, pulmonary arterial hypertension; SVPH, secondary vascular pulmonary hypertension.
Adapted from Weiss et al. *J Am Coll Cardiol.* 1998;31:1650-1657.[16]

Outcomes in PAH have improved since epoprostenol was approved by the FDA in 1995 (other PAH therapies were approved during the period 2001-2009).[17] Prospectively, data from pregnancies occurring between 2007 and 2010 in women with PAH was collected in 13 pulmonary hypertension centers in Europe, the United States, and Australia. There were a total of 26 pregnancies. Sixty-two percent (16 patients) had a healthy baby and no complications postdelivery; this group had a normal cardiac output prepregnancy. Interestingly, 50% of females who did well were considered "responders" to vasodilator testing and were on calcium channel blockers. All patients had a rigorous follow-up during pregnancy, with visits every 2 to 4 weeks, and some even had periodical catheterizations (French group). Thirty percent of patients who did well were on prostacyclins. None of the patients who died were on prostacyclins. Fifteen percent (4 patients) died or required lung transplantation. The other patients had a therapeutic abortion. Maternal mortality has been reported as 15% to 17% in the modern management era.[18-20] The lower maternal mortality may be related to an earlier diagnosis with prompt referral to an experienced pulmonary hypertension center and management that involved antepartum initiation of PAH therapy, particularly IV prostacyclins (Figure 12-9).

Case reports suggesting improved maternal survival are encouraging. Yet, the mortality rate of pregnant patients with severe PAH remains high and there is no consensus in the appropriate management of PAH in pregnancy. Therefore, current guidelines unanimously recommend pregnancy as being contraindicated in women with PAH and an effective method of contraception being

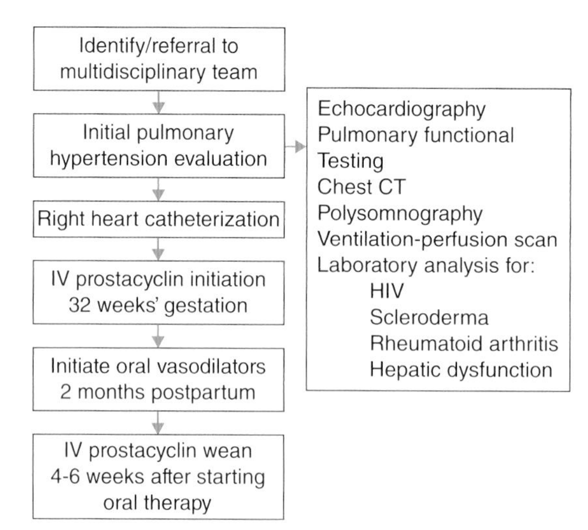

FIGURE 12-9 PAH evaluation and treatment algorithm in pregnancy. With the goal to improve maternal–fetal outcomes, pulmonary hypertension centers have established a standard treatment algorithm for PAH in the setting of pregnancy, tailored to each patient but with common components based on the known physiologic changes of pregnancy and delivery. Early recognition and referral to a center capable of extensive PAH evaluation and treatment is favorable. A multidisciplinary team, including a pulmonary hypertension specialist, maternal–fetal medicine specialist, cardiologist, and obstetric anesthesiologist, meets regularly to discuss each case. The team meets formally each month to discuss all pregnant patients, with additional time spent on those individuals at greatest risk. A detailed plan is formulated and documented, with updates occurring at the monthly meeting or earlier, depending on a patient's progress. On initial presentation a standard pulmonary hypertension evaluation is performed. Pregnancy alone induces the development of a hypercoagulable state though numerous mechanisms, including resistance to activated protein C, reduced levels of protein S, and increased levels of numerous other clotting factors. Therefore, patients are started on anticoagulation with subcutaneous enoxaparin. Other low-molecular-weight heparins or unfractionated heparins are also appropriate, with aggressive monitoring and dose adjustments based on partial thromboplastin time or anti-Xa levels, respectively. Anticoagulation is resumed 6 hours after vaginal birth and 12 hours following C-section if there is absence of excessive bleeding. Hypoxemia, if present, must be addressed with supplemental oxygen to maintain an oxygen saturation of >90% if possible. Notably, supplemental oxygen will not improve systemic oxygen saturation in the setting of a right-to-left shunt. It is important to remember that protocols are center specific and not based on current PAH treatment guidelines. Reproduced with permission from Smith et al. *Lung*. 2012;190:155-160.[19]

recommended in women of childbearing age. Therapeutic abortion should also be offered, particularly when early deterioration occurs. If this option is not accepted, IV prostacyclins should be considered promptly.[1,2,19]

SURVIVAL OF WOMEN WITH PAH

Although the prognosis of patients with PAH has markedly improved in the past decade with the development of new treatments, however it still remains poor. The median survival in the absence of treatment is 2.8 years.[1,2] Women had higher survival rates compared with men.[6,20,21] In the REVEAL Registry, there was a clear and significant difference in survival between men and women at 24 months from enrollment in the study (64% ± 3.6% vs 77.5% ± 1.6 %, respectively, $P < 0.001$). The estimated 5-year survival from diagnosis was 52% ± 3% for men and 62% ± 2% for women ($P = 0.005$) (Figure 12-10). Mortality was higher for males ≥60 years versus younger males or females at all ages (Figure 12-11).

It is not clear why men aged >60 years have worse survival than women and the role of gender and estrogen in the pathogenesis of PAH remains ambiguous. There have been concerns that estrogen may be a factor in causing PAH and that may be a reason for the disease being more prevalent in women; it would be interesting if it also had a protective role in prolonging women's lives with PAH. Studies have shown that females have better right ventricular ejection fraction compared to males at the time of diagnosis, which may contribute to a potential survival advantage.[13]

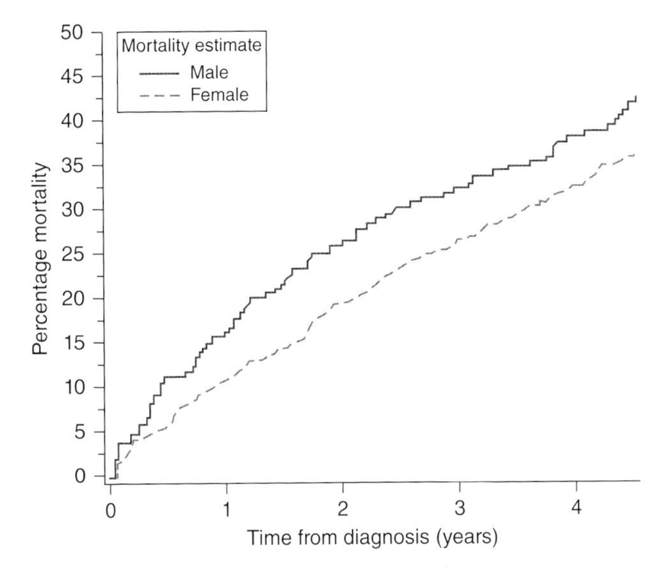

FIGURE 12-10 Mortality in PAH based in gender.
Adapted from Shapiro et al. *Chest*. 2012;141:363-373.[6]

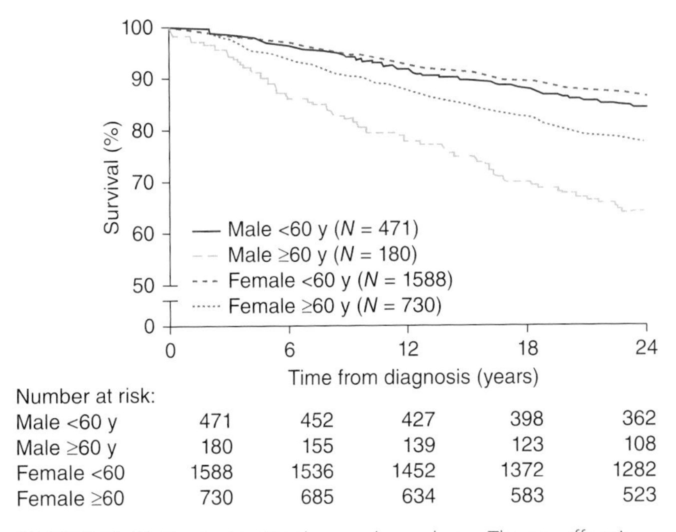

Number at risk:

Male <60 y	471	452	427	398	362
Male ≥60 y	180	155	139	123	108
Female <60	1588	1536	1452	1372	1282
Female ≥60	730	685	634	583	523

FIGURE 12-11 Survival in PAH by gender and age. The sex effect in mortality was absent in the subset of patients ≤60 years. The survival difference between sexes begins to appear in the ≥60 years of age, approximately 18 months after enrollment. Mortality is higher for males ≥60 years old versus younger males or females at all ages. Reproduced with permission from Shapiro et al. *Chest*. 2012;141:363-373.[6]

REFERENCES

1. Galie N, Hoeper MM, Humbert M, et al. Guidelines for the diagnosis and treatment of pulmonary hypertension. PAH guidelines. *Eur Heart J*. 2009;30:2493-2537.
2. McLaughlin VV, Archer SL, Badesch DB, et al. ACCF/AHA 2009 expert consensus document on pulmonary hypertension. *Circulation*. 2009;119:2250-2294.
3. Tofovic SP. Estrogens and development of pulmonary hypertension: interaction of estradiol metabolism and pulmonary vascular disease. *J Cardiovasc Pharmacol*. 2010;56:696-708.
4. Umar S, Rabinovitch M, Eghbali M. Estrogen paradox in pulmonary hypertension: current controversies and future perspectives. *Am J Respir Crit Care Med*. 2012;186:125-131.
5. Austin ED, Hamid R, Hemnes AR, et al. BMPR2 expression is suppressed by signaling through the estrogen receptor. *Biol Sex Differ*. 2012;3:6.
6. Shapiro S, Traiger GL, Turner M, et al. Sex differences in the diagnosis, treatment, and outcome of patients with pulmonary arterial hypertension enrolled in the registry to evaluate early and long-term pulmonary arterial hypertension disease management (REVEAL). *Chest*. 2012;141:363-373.
7. Rich S, Dantzker DR, Ayres SM, et al. Primary pulmonary hypertension. A national prospective study. *Ann Intern Med*. 1987;107:216-223.
8. Thenappan T, Shah SJ, Rich S, et al. A USA-based registry for pulmonary arterial hypertension: 1982-2006. *Eur Respir J*. 2007;30:1103-1110.
9. Walker AM, Langleben D, Korelitz JJ, et al. Temporal trends and drug exposures in pulmonary hypertension: an American experience. *Am Heart J*. 2006;152:521-526.
10. Humbert M, Sitbon O, Chaouat A, et al. Pulmonary arterial hypertension in France: results from a national registry. *Am J Respir Crit Care Med*. 2006;173:1023-1030.
11. Peacock AJ, Murphy NF, McMurray JJ, et al. An epidemiological study of pulmonary arterial hypertension. *Eur Respir J*. 2007;30:104-109.
12. Jing ZC, Xu XQ, Han ZY, et al. Registry and survival study in Chinese patients with idiopathic and familial pulmonary arterial hypertension. *Chest*. 2007;132:373-379.
13. Kawut SM, Al-Naamani N, Agerstrand C, et al. Determinants of right ventricular ejection fraction in pulmonary arterial hypertension. *Chest*. 2009;135:752-759.
14. Gabler NB, French B, Strom BL, et al. Race and sex differences in response to endothelin receptor antagonists for pulmonary arterial hypertension. *Chest*. 2012;141:20-26.
15. Savarese G, Paolillo S, Costanzo P, et al. Do changes of 6-minute walk distance predict clinical events in patients with pulmonary arterial hypertension?: a meta-analysis of 22 randomized trials. *J Am Coll Cardiol*. 2012;60:1192-1201.
16. Weiss BM, Zemp L, Seifert B, et al. Outcome of pulmonary vascular disease in pregnancy: a systematic overview from 1978 through 1996. *J Am Coll Cardiol*. 1998;31:1650-1657.
17. Jäis X, Olsson KM, Barbera JA, et al. Pregnancy outcomes in pulmonary arterial hypertension in the modern management era. *Eur Respir J*. 2012;40:881-885.
18. Duarte AG, Thomas S, Safdar Z, et al. Management of pulmonary arterial hypertension during pregnancy: a retrospective, multicenter experience. *Chest*. 2013;143:1330-1336.
19. Smith JS, Mueller J, Daniels CJ. Pulmonary arterial hypertension in the setting of pregnancy: a case series and standard treatment approach. *Lung*. 2012;190:155-160.
20. Humbert M, Sitbon O, Chaouat A, et al. Survival in patients with idiopathic, familial, and anorexigen-associated pulmonary arterial hypertension in the modern management era. *Circulation*. 2010;122:156-163.
21. Benza RL, Miller DP, Gomberg-Maitland M, et al. Predicting survival in pulmonary arterial hypertension: insights from the Registry to Evaluate Early and Long-Term Pulmonary Arterial Hypertension Disease Management (REVEAL). *Circulation*. 2010;122:164-172.

Page numbers followed by italic *f* or *t* denote figures or tables, respectively.

D